ANATOMY
TO COLOR AND STUDY

RAY PORITSKY, Ph.D.

Associate Professor
Department of Anatomy
Case Western University School of Medicine
Lecturer in Medical Illustration
Cleveland Institute of Art
Cleveland, Ohio

HANLEY & BELFUS, INC., Medical Publishers / Philadelphia
The C.V. Mosby Company / St. Louis • Toronto • London

Publisher: HANLEY & BELFUS, INC.
               210 S. 13th Street
               Philadelphia, PA 19107

North American and worldwide sales and distribution:
               THE C.V. MOSBY COMPANY
               11830 Westline Industrial Drive
               St. Louis, MO 63146

In Canada: THE C.V. MOSBY COMPANY
               5240 Finch Avenue East
               Unit 1
               Scarborough, Ontario M1S 4P2

Anatomy to Color and Study   ISBN   0-932883-18-4

Last digit is the print number: 9 8 7 6 5 4 3 2 1

Contents

Preface

This book is intended to present human anatomy about as simply and clearly as is possible and should be helpful to anyone studying gross anatomy. Its purpose is to augment and reinforce the student's anatomical knowledge by the coloring and labeling of key structures. It is expected that many students will also be engaged in dissections (*anatomy* is from Greek "to cut"), reading anatomy textbooks, and studying formal anatomical atlases, both artistic and photographic, all of which are essential to acquisition of a true working knowledge of the structures of a complex organism.

The book is arranged in regional order to follow the organization of most modern courses in anatomy. There are seven regions covered with 263 plates. An effort has been made to confine the labeling to structures that really need to be learned by anyone hoping to follow a career that requires some familiarity with human anatomy.

The use of the book should be fairly intuitive. The reader may choose any colors or art materials; however, the traditional color scheme or color code of anatomy textbooks and atlases is red for arteries, blue for veins, yellow for nerves, pink to reddish brown for muscles, and light tan for bones, roughly representing natural colors. Color pencils or color markers may be used. The reader will find that good quality, sharp, color pencils work quite well. One can employ many colors or just a few, depending on the time and effort one wishes to invest. Plate 13 illustrates how to shade muscles, bones, and blood vessels. According to students who have colored and labeled the author's drawings at his medical school, they are very useful for future reference and should be kept on file.

There is very little explanatory text. In a few places, short paragraphs have been added that impart important aspects of applied anatomy, but this book is not intended to serve as an anatomy textbook. Etymological cartoons are interspersed throughout for a brief change of pace and convey some information about Latin and Greek roots.

Pencils ready...go!

RAY PORITSKY, PH.D.
Cleveland, Ohio

Acknowledgments

The majority of the illustrations were drawn by the author, who has had formal training in anatomy and medical illustration. Additional drawings were done by Helen Williams, Susan Weil, Cheryl Owens, and James Bille. The author used the following texts as source materials: Spalteholz and Spanner: Atlas of Human Anatomy, 16th ed., Philadelphia, F.A. Davis, 1961; Wolf-Heidegger: Atlas of Systematic Human Anatomy, New York, Hafner, 1962; Hollingshead and Rosse: Textbook of Anatomy, 4th ed., Philadelphia, Harper and Row, 1985; Netter: The Ciba Collection of Medical Illustrations, Summit, NJ, Ciba Pharmaceutical Company, 1959, 1962; Clemente: Anatomy: A Regional Atlas of the Human Body, 3rd ed., Baltimore and Munich, Urban & Schwarzenberg, 1987; Rohen and Yokochi: Color Atlas of Anatomy: A Photographic Study of the Human Body, New York and Tokyo, Igaku-Shoin, 1984; Moore: Clinically Oriented Anatomy, Baltimore, Williams & Wilkins, 1982; Clemente: Anatomy of the Human Body, 13th ed., Philadelphia, Lea & Febiger, 1985; Williams and Warwick: Gray's Anatomy, 36th British ed., Edinburgh, Churchill Livingstone, 1980; Anson: Morris' Human Anatomy: A Complete Systematic Treatise, 12th ed., New York, McGraw-Hill, 1966; Pernkopf: Atlas of Topographical and Applied Human Anatomy, Munich, Urban & Schwarzenberg, 1980. I also found certain Somso anatomical models most helpful for several of the drawings.

I would like to thank Christine Haberecht and the pleasant people in the Department of Epidemiology and Biometry at Case Western Reserve Medical School for graciously affording me the opportunity to copy my Duoshade artwork on their wonderful Model 70 IBM copy machine, the best photocopier I could locate between Cleveland and Boston. The Duoshade 266 velum made by Ohio Graphics proved to be an amazingly facile method for producing shading dots for contours and gray tones.

I also thank Dr. Thomas Oelrich for his generous help relating to his work on pelvic anatomy, Dr. Marion Sherman for her comments and suggestions, and also the medical students at Case Western Reserve University School of Medicine for their suggestions, criticism, and encouragement.

Finally, I would like to thank and warmly dedicate this book to my wife Connie.

PART I: INTRODUCTION AND THORAX

PLATES 1-42

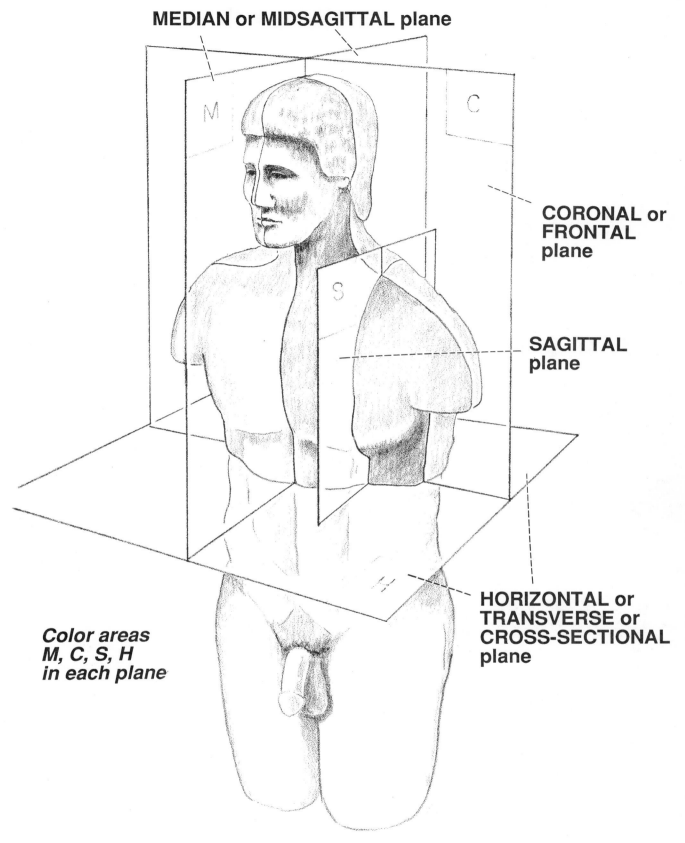

MEDIAN or MIDSAGITTAL plane

CORONAL or FRONTAL plane

SAGITTAL plane

HORIZONTAL or TRANSVERSE or CROSS-SECTIONAL plane

Color areas M, C, S, H in each plane

1 Planes of the body

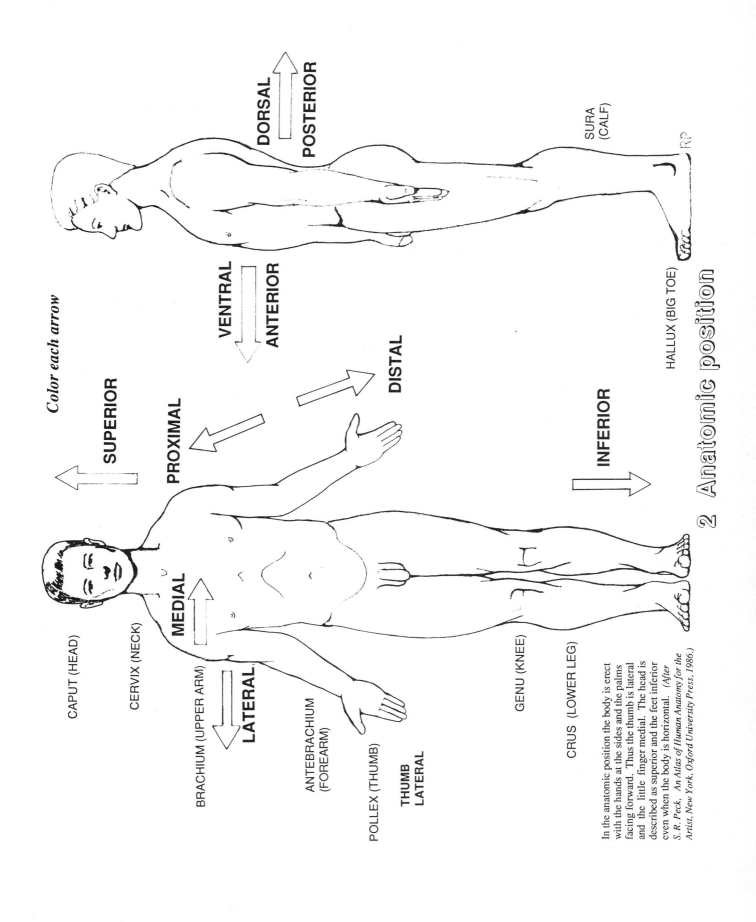

Color each arrow

DORSAL
POSTERIOR

SURA (CALF)

VENTRAL
ANTERIOR

SUPERIOR

PROXIMAL

DISTAL

INFERIOR

HALLUX (BIG TOE)

RP

MEDIAL

LATERAL

CAPUT (HEAD)

CERVIX (NECK)

BRACHIUM (UPPER ARM)

ANTEBRACHIUM (FOREARM)

POLLEX (THUMB)

THUMB LATERAL

GENU (KNEE)

CRUS (LOWER LEG)

In the anatomic position the body is erect with the hands at the sides and the palms facing forward. Thus the thumb is lateral and the little finger medial. The head is described as superior and the feet inferior even when the body is horizontal. (*After S. R. Peck, An Atlas of Human Anatomy for the Artist, New York, Oxford University Press, 1986.*)

2 Anatomic position

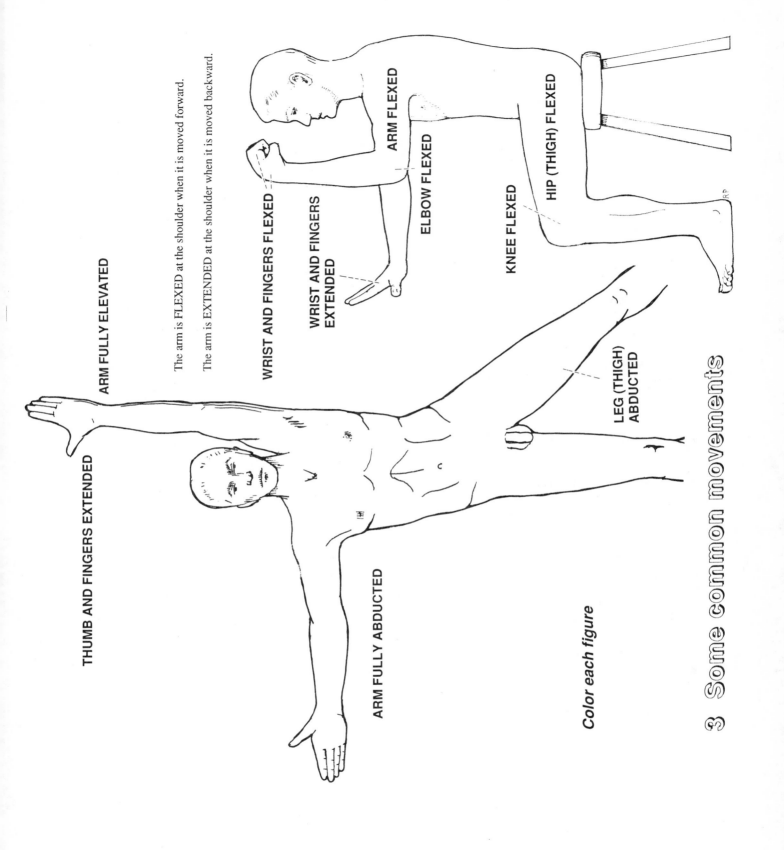

THUMB AND FINGERS EXTENDED

ARM FULLY ELEVATED

The arm is FLEXED at the shoulder when it is moved forward.

The arm is EXTENDED at the shoulder when it is moved backward.

WRIST AND FINGERS FLEXED

WRIST AND FINGERS EXTENDED

ARM FLEXED

ELBOW FLEXED

KNEE FLEXED

HIP (THIGH) FLEXED

LEG (THIGH) ABDUCTED

ARM FULLY ABDUCTED

Color each figure

3 Some common movements

4 An intestinal lining cell

(See opposite page)

Color and label

1 Nucleus
2 Nucleolus
3 Heterochromatin
4 Nuclear membrane or envelope (nucleolemma)
5 Outer nuclear membrane
6 Inner nuclear membrane
7 Nucleolemmal cistern
8 Cistern of endoplasmic reticulum continuous with nucleolemmal cistern
9 Nuclear pores
10 Centriole with 9 triplets of microtubules
11 One triplet of microtubules. *(Notice only inner microtubule is complete tube.)*
12 Golgi complex saccules
13 Convex proximal saccule (forming face)
14 Concave distal saccule (mature face)
15 Vesicles arising from mature face
16 Cistern rough (or granular) endoplasmic reticulum
17 Ribosomes
18 Mitochondrial outer membrane
19 Mitochondrial inner membrane
20 Mitochondrial cristae *(shelf-like)*
21 Outer chamber *(space between inner and outer membrane)* (intermembranous space)
22 Inner space *(space within inner membrane)*
23 Transverse tubular cristae
24 Longitudinal tubular cristae
25 Microvilli
26 Spot desmosome (macula adherens)
27 Tight junction (zonula occludens)
28 Belt desmosome (zonula adherens)
29 Gap junction (macula communicans) *(nexus)*
30 Tonofilaments
31 Adherens web
32 Core filament of microvilli

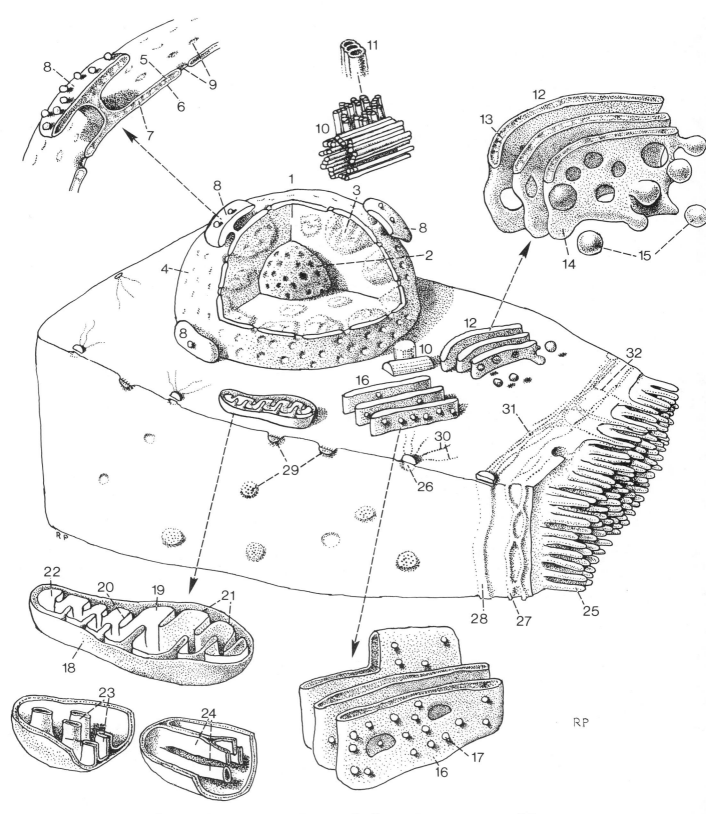

4 An intestinal lining cell

5 Sagitta (etymological cartoon)

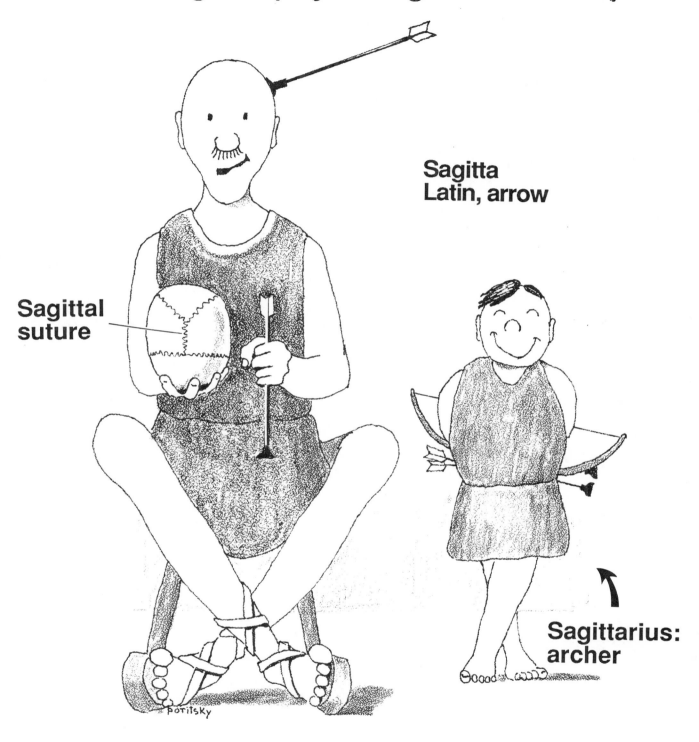

**Sagitta
Latin, arrow**

**Sagittal
suture**

**Sagittarius:
archer**

SAGITTA is *Latin* for arrow. The SAGITTAL plane of Anatomy takes its name from the
sagittal suture on the top of the skull, which runs between the two parietal bones in a
front-to-back direction. At the back of the skull the sagittal suture meets the inverted
V-shape of the lambdoid suture. With a bit of imagining one can visualize the sagittal
suture forming the shaft of an arrow and a portion of the lambdoid forming the feathers.

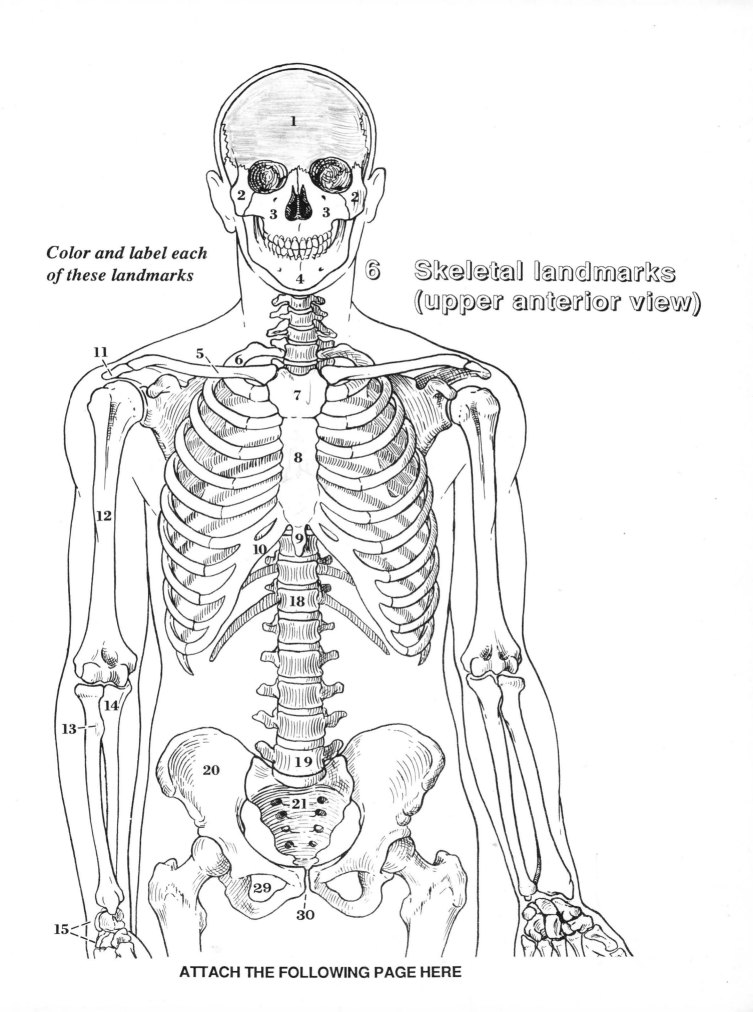

Color and label each of these landmarks

6 **Skeletal landmarks (upper anterior view)**

ATTACH THE FOLLOWING PAGE HERE

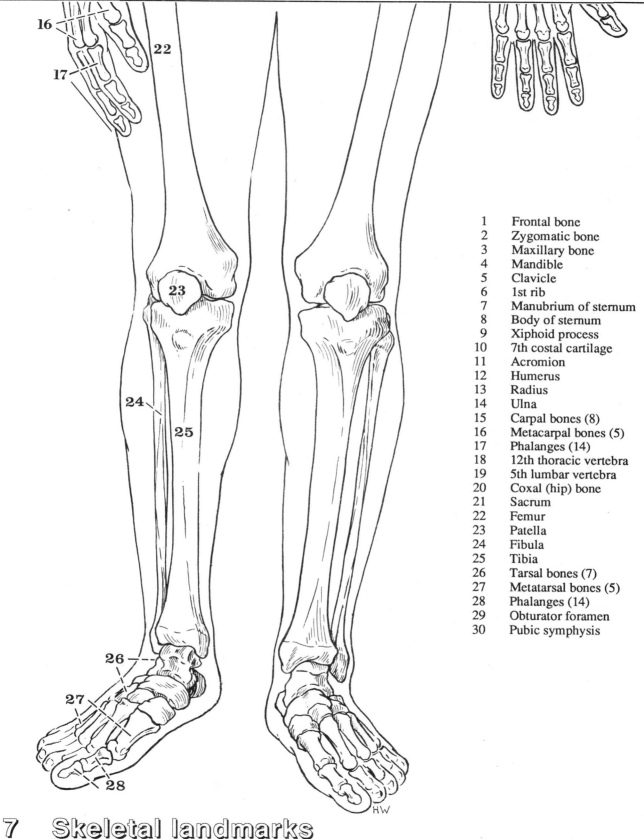

1   Frontal bone
2   Zygomatic bone
3   Maxillary bone
4   Mandible
5   Clavicle
6   1st rib
7   Manubrium of sternum
8   Body of sternum
9   Xiphoid process
10 7th costal cartilage
11 Acromion
12 Humerus
13 Radius
14 Ulna
15 Carpal bones (8)
16 Metacarpal bones (5)
17 Phalanges (14)
18 12th thoracic vertebra
19 5th lumbar vertebra
20 Coxal (hip) bone
21 Sacrum
22 Femur
23 Patella
24 Fibula
25 Tibia
26 Tarsal bones (7)
27 Metatarsal bones (5)
28 Phalanges (14)
29 Obturator foramen
30 Pubic symphysis

7 Skeletal landmarks (lower anterior view)

8 Skeletal landmarks (upper posterior view)

Color and label these bones

7 cervical vertebrae (numbers C1-C7)
12 thoracic vertebrae (numbers T1-T12)
5 lumbar vertebrae (numbers L1-L5)
12 pairs of ribs
Scapula
Clavicle
Humerus
Ulna
Radius
Carpal
Metacarpal
Phalanges
2 coxal bones
Sacrum
Femur
Fibula
Tibia
Tarsal
Metatarsal
Phalanges

Label these landmarks

1   Parietal bone
2   Occipital bone
3   Sagittal suture
4   Lambdoid suture
5   1st cervical vertebrae (atlas)
6   2nd cervical vertebrae (axis)
7   Acromion
8   Spine of scapula

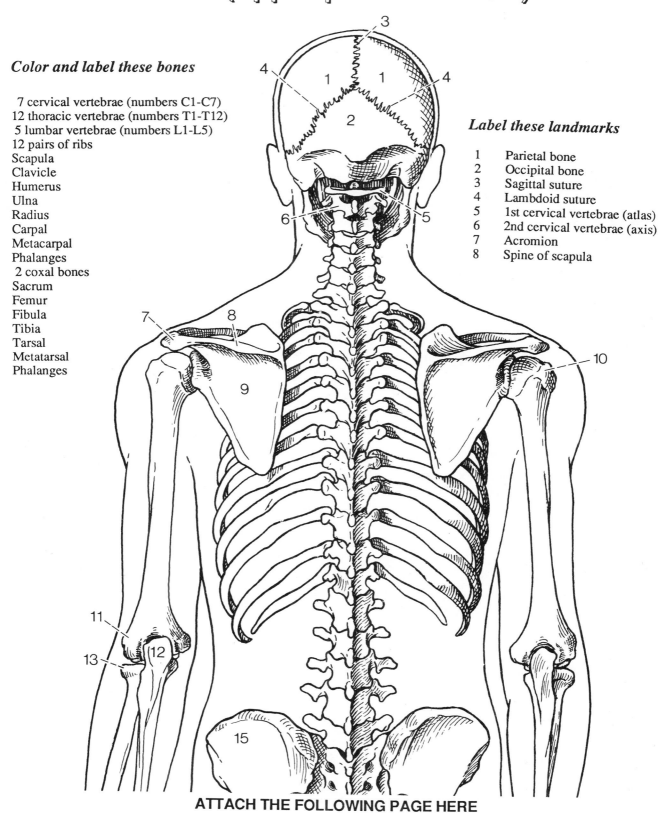

ATTACH THE FOLLOWING PAGE HERE

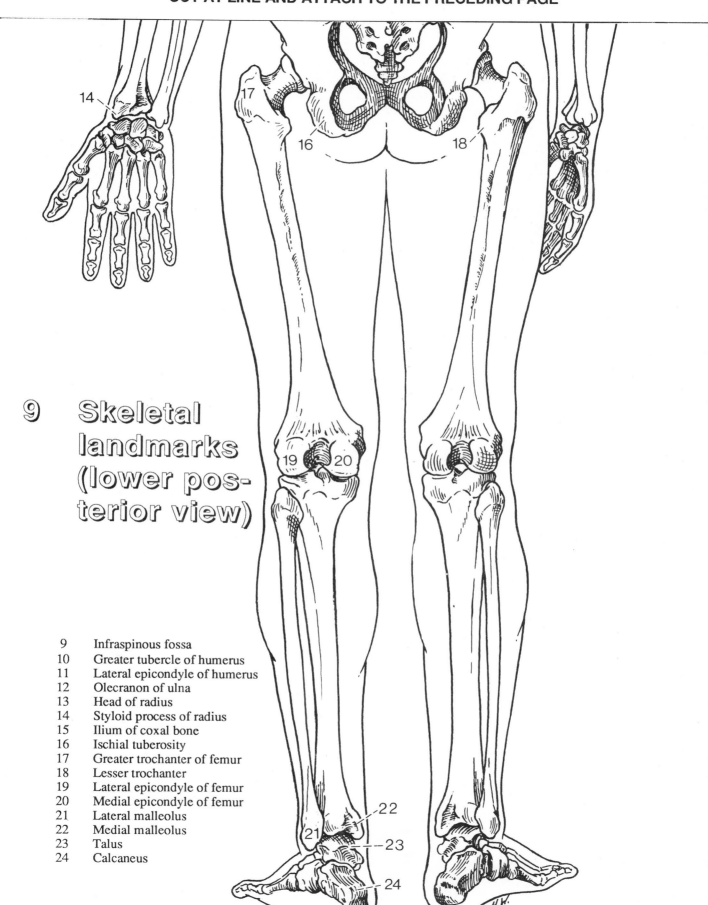

9   Skeletal landmarks (lower posterior view)

9	Infraspinous fossa
10	Greater tubercle of humerus
11	Lateral epicondyle of humerus
12	Olecranon of ulna
13	Head of radius
14	Styloid process of radius
15	Ilium of coxal bone
16	Ischial tuberosity
17	Greater trochanter of femur
18	Lesser trochanter
19	Lateral epicondyle of femur
20	Medial epicondyle of femur
21	Lateral malleolus
22	Medial malleolus
23	Talus
24	Calcaneus

10 Skeletal landmarks (thorax and upper arm)

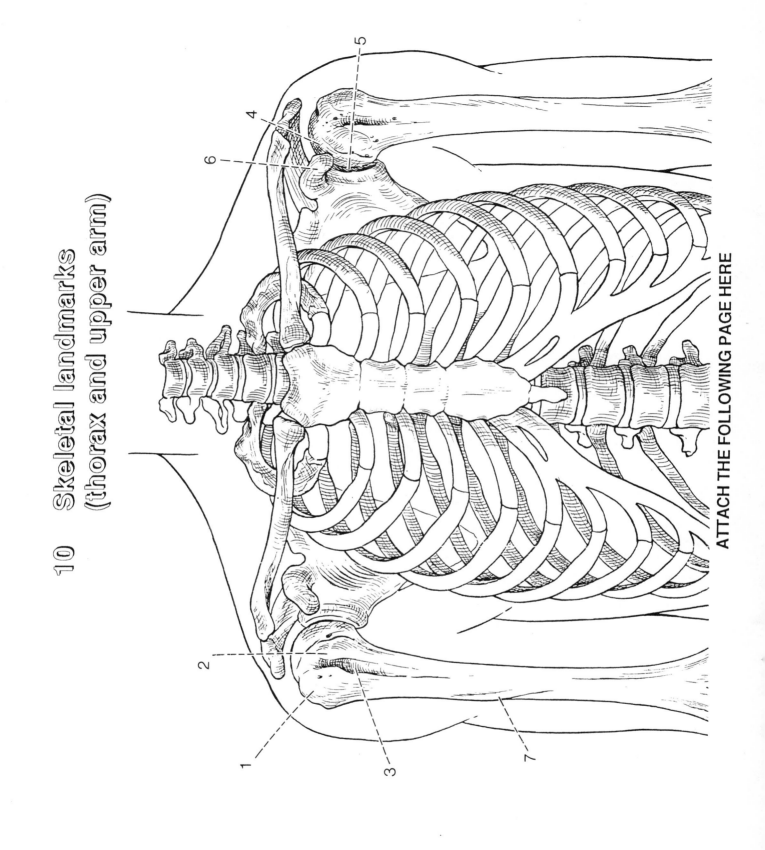

ATTACH THE FOLLOWING PAGE HERE

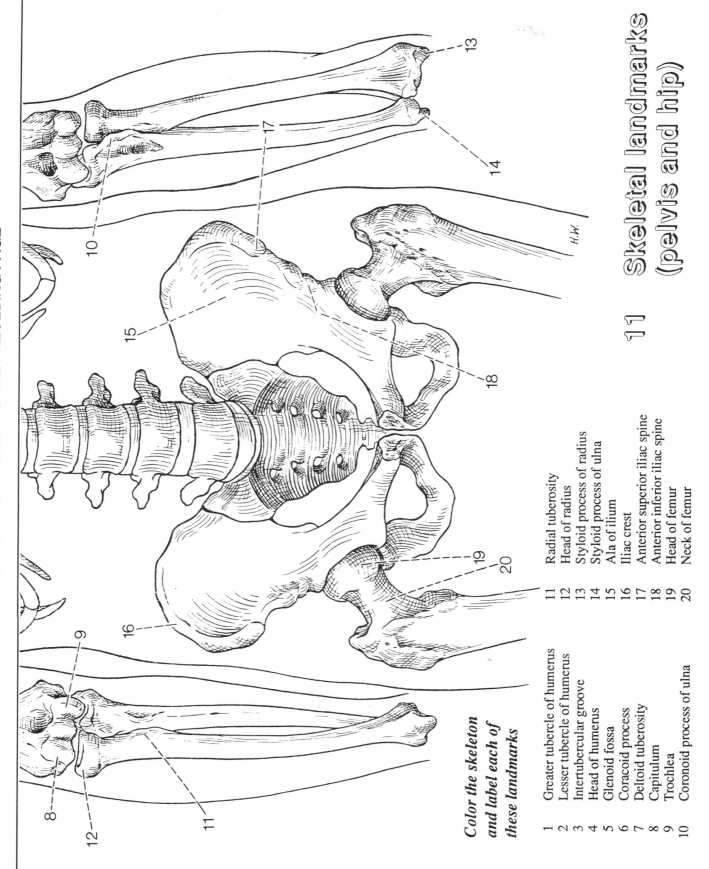

*Color the skeleton
and label each of
these landmarks*

1   Greater tubercle of humerus
2   Lesser tubercle of humerus
3   Intertubercular groove
4   Head of humerus
5   Glenoid fossa
6   Coracoid process
7   Deltoid tuberosity
8   Capitulum
9   Trochlea
10   Coronoid process of ulna

11   Radial tuberosity
12   Head of radius
13   Styloid process of radius
14   Styloid process of ulna
15   Ala of ilium
16   Iliac crest
17   Anterior superior iliac spine
18   Anterior inferior iliac spine
19   Head of femur
20   Neck of femur

11   **Skeletal landmarks
(pelvis and hip)**

12 Muscles of anterior thorax and abdomen

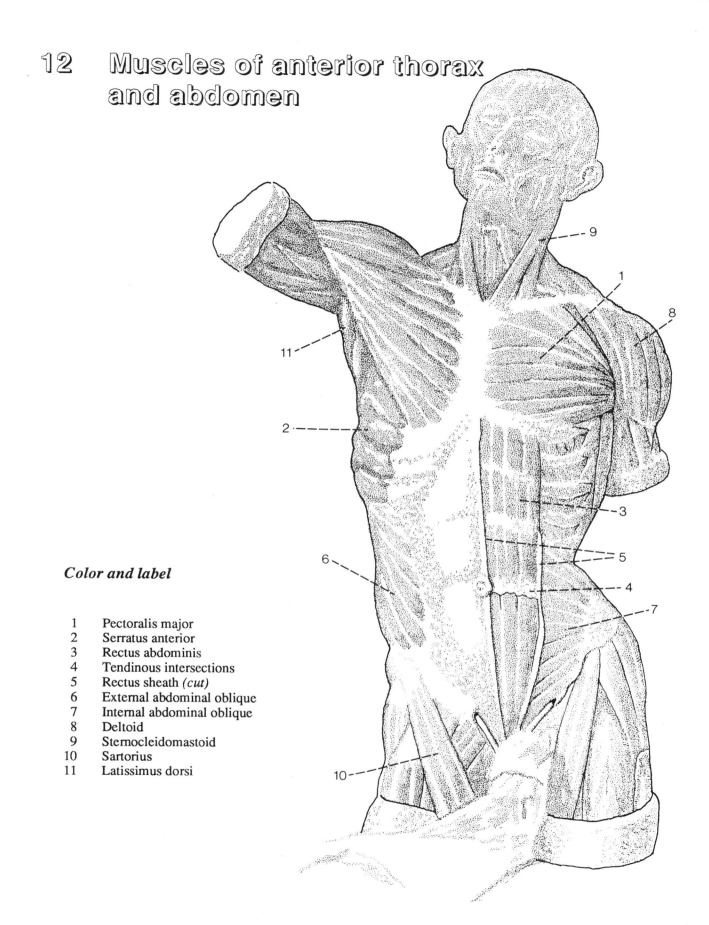

Color and label

1	Pectoralis major
2	Serratus anterior
3	Rectus abdominis
4	Tendinous intersections
5	Rectus sheath *(cut)*
6	External abdominal oblique
7	Internal abdominal oblique
8	Deltoid
9	Sternocleidomastoid
10	Sartorius
11	Latissimus dorsi

After E. A. Seeman, Fritz Schiders Plastisch-Anatomischer Handatlas (after Duval-Neelsen).
Leipzig, M. Averbach and Franz V. Stuck Verlag, 1929.

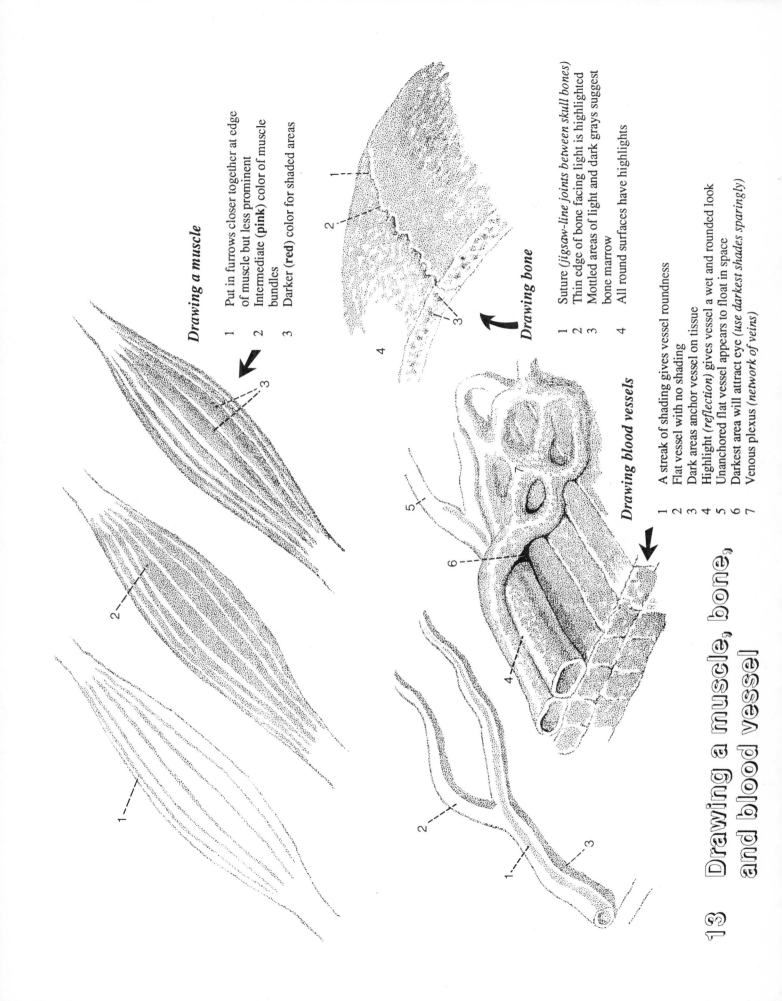

Drawing a muscle

1 Put in furrows closer together at edge of muscle but less prominent
2 Intermediate (**pink**) color of muscle bundles
3 Darker (**red**) color for shaded areas

Drawing bone

1 Suture (*jigsaw-line joints between skull bones*)
2 Thin edge of bone facing light is highlighted
3 Mottled areas of light and dark grays suggest bone marrow
4 All round surfaces have highlights

Drawing blood vessels

1 A streak of shading gives vessel roundness
2 Flat vessel with no shading
3 Dark areas anchor vessel on tissue
4 Highlight (*reflection*) gives vessel a wet and rounded look
5 Unanchored flat vessel appears to float in space
6 Darkest area will attract eye (*use darkest shades sparingly*)
7 Venous plexus (*network of veins*)

13 Drawing a muscle, bone, and blood vessel

14 Anterior thoracic muscles

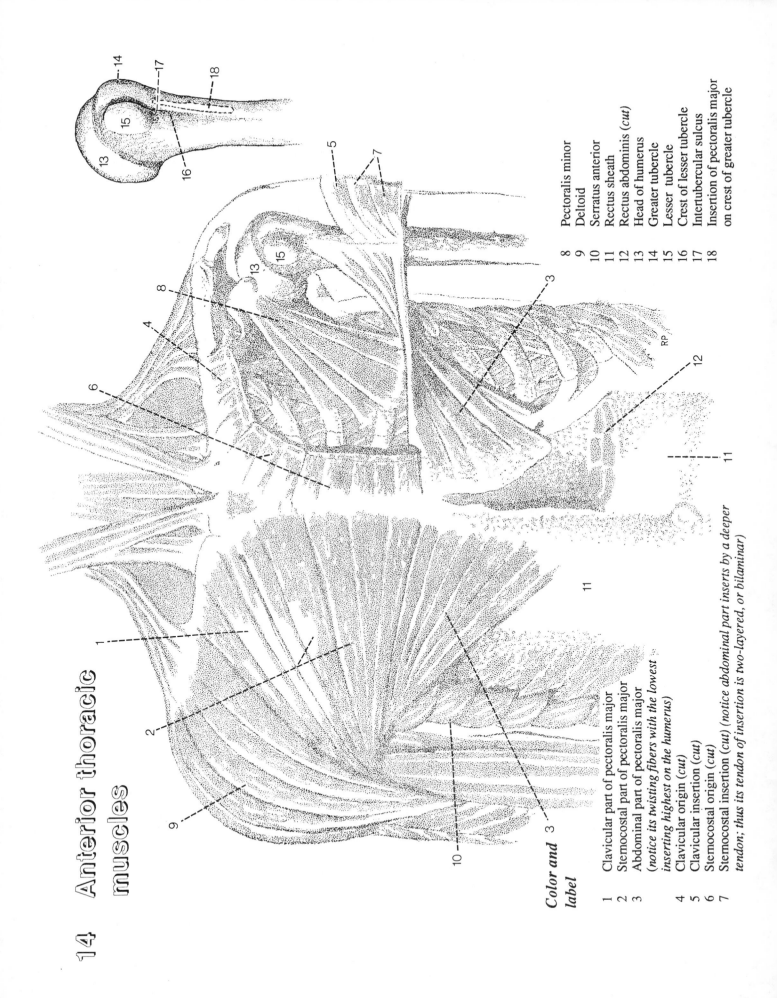

Color and label

1 Clavicular part of pectoralis major
2 Sternocostal part of pectoralis major
3 Abdominal part of pectoralis major
   (notice its twisting fibers with the lowest inserting highest on the humerus)
4 Clavicular origin (*cut*)
5 Clavicular insertion (*cut*)
6 Sternocostal origin (*cut*)
7 Sternocostal insertion (*cut*) *(notice abdominal part inserts by a deeper tendon; thus its tendon of insertion is two-layered, or bilaminar)*

8   Pectoralis minor
9   Deltoid
10 Serratus anterior
11 Rectus sheath
12 Rectus abdominis (*cut*)
13 Head of humerus
14 Greater tubercle
15 Lesser tubercle
16 Crest of lesser tubercle
17 Intertubercular sulcus
18 Insertion of pectoralis major on crest of greater tubercle

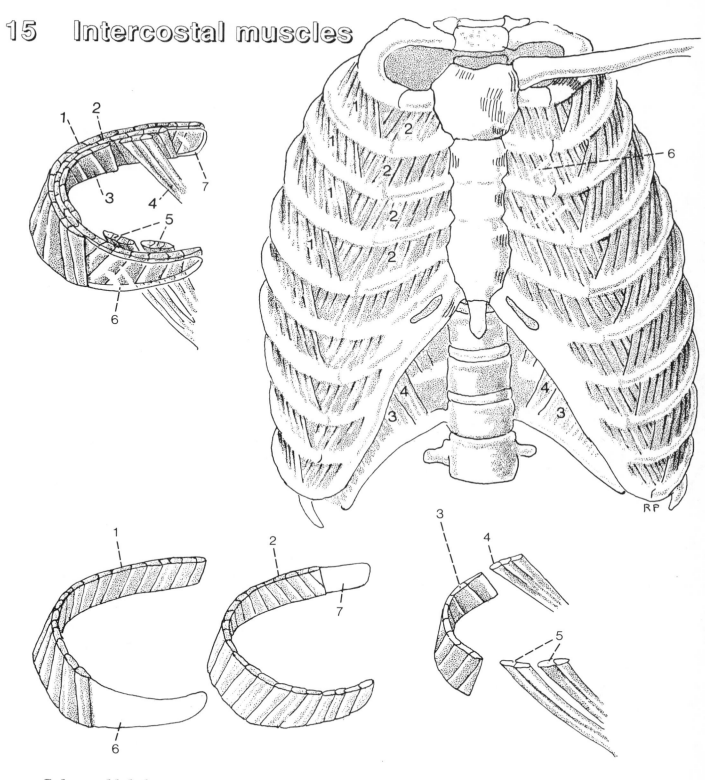

Color and label

1 External intercostal muscle
2 Internal intercostal muscle
3 Innermost intercostal muscle
4 Subcostal muscle
5 Transversus thoracis muscle
6 External intercostal membrane
7 Internal intercostal membrane

Notice direction of fibers in each layer. Also notice that neither the external intercostal nor the internal intercostal muscle fully extends from sternum to vertebral column; rather each has a membranous portion.

16 Anterior thoracic wall seen from inside

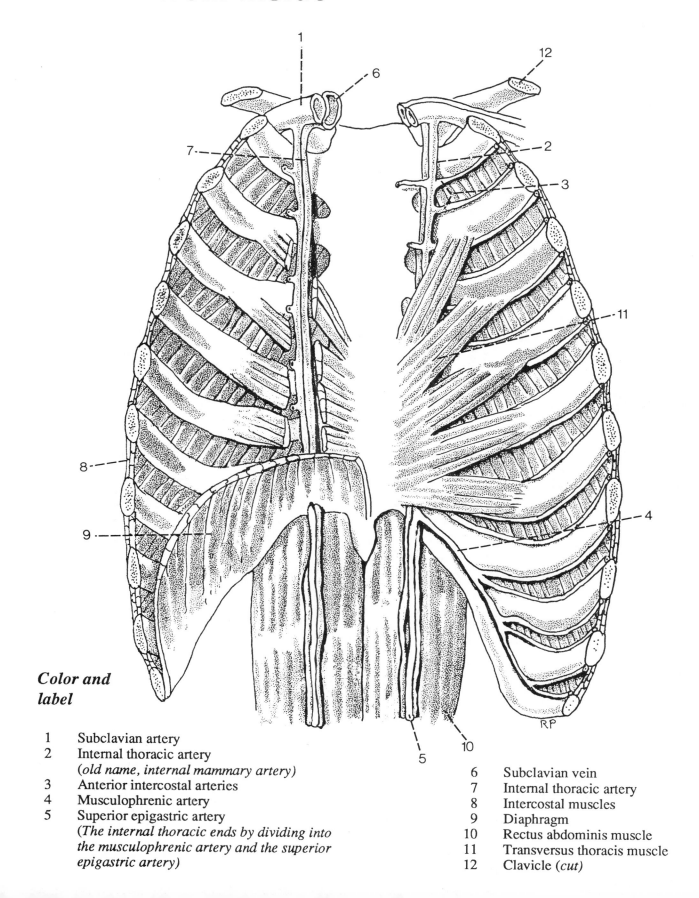

Color and label

1 Subclavian artery
2 Internal thoracic artery
 (*old name, internal mammary artery*)
3 Anterior intercostal arteries
4 Musculophrenic artery
5 Superior epigastric artery
 (*The internal thoracic ends by dividing into the musculophrenic artery and the superior epigastric artery*)

6 Subclavian vein
7 Internal thoracic artery
8 Intercostal muscles
9 Diaphragm
10 Rectus abdominis muscle
11 Transversus thoracis muscle
12 Clavicle (*cut*)

To the ancient Greeks and Romans contracted muscle looked like small mice running under the skin, so they named the fleshy red bundles of the body musculi, which means "little mice," musculus being the diminutive of mus, mouse.

A pedagogue or teacher orginally meant a leader of children and is derived from pais, a child, and agogos, to lead; hence, a leader of children.

Acropolis meant a "high city," from akron, peak, and polis, city. The acromion is the lateral peak or extremity of the shoulder blade or scapula (akron, peak, and omos, shoulder). Acrophobia is the fear of heights. Akron, Ohio, is built upon a hill.

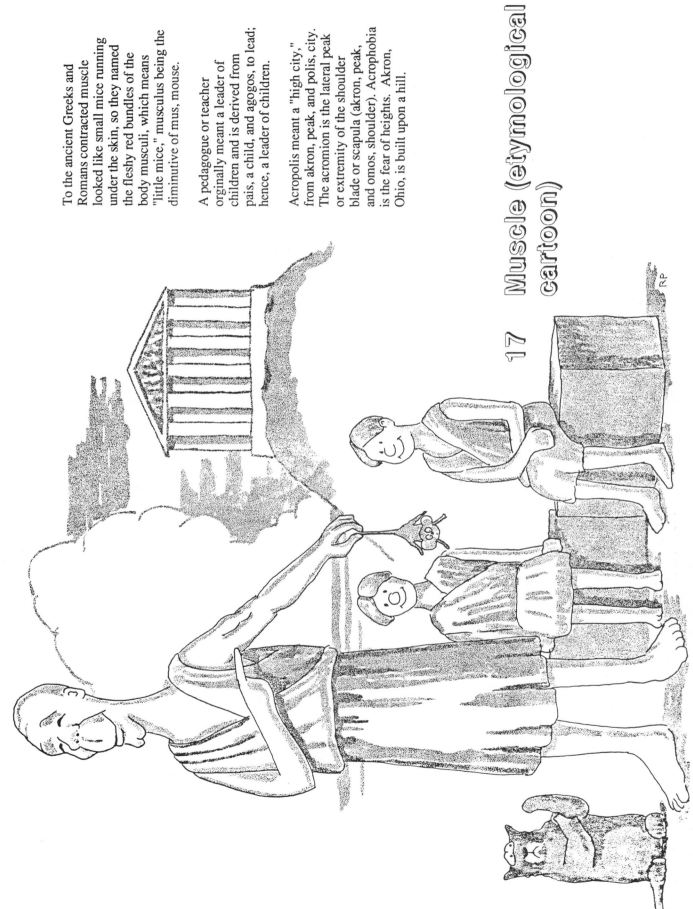

17 Muscle (etymological cartoon)

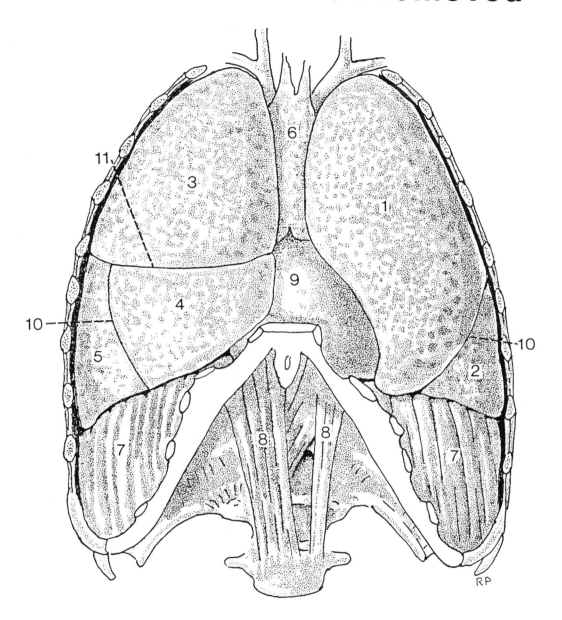

Color and label

1	Superior lobe of left lung	7	Diaphragm
2	Inferior lobe of left lung	8	Crura of diaphragm
3	Superior lobe of right lung	9	Pericardium
4	Middle lobe of right lung	10	Oblique fissures *(both lungs)*
5	Inferior lobe of right lung	11	Horizontal fissure *(right lung)*
6	Thymus *(remains)*		

1 Tibia meant a flute or pipe as well as the shinbone. The ancients probably made flutelike instruments from the shinbones of animals.

2 Fenestra was a window. Fenestrated means to contain little windows as in fenestrated capillaries.

3 Crista galli is Latin for cock's comb and is the name of the bony ridge at the top of the ethmoid bone.

4 Rostrum meant a beak or snout, or a ship's prow. The speaker's platform in the forum was decorated with the prows of ships captured in battle. Rostral means toward the nose.

5 Alveolus is Latin for a little hollow or bucket and is the diminutive of alveus, which could mean a trough, boat, hold of a ship, bathtub, bed of a stream, beehive, or gaming table.

6 Pecten is Latin for comb. Pectinate means comb-like. The pectinate muscles in the heart suggested a comb to earlier anatomists.

7 Putamen is Latin for "that which falls off with paring," such as a husk or a shell. The putamen is a mass of nerve cells in the brain in the shape of a shell.

8 Speculum is Latin for mirror. A speculum in medicine is an instrument with which a physician can examine passages and the interior of the body.

9 Acetabulum is the bony socket of the hip joint. It is derived from acetum, vinegar, and probably poculum, cup; hence, it means vinegar cup.

10 Galea meant helmet. The galea aponeurotica is a tough membrane that covers the top of the skull somewhat like the furry animal skins used as head coverings by ancient soldiers.

11 Cingulum meant a girdle or sword belt. The cinch is a girth or a saddle or pack. To an experienced hand it was an easy job; so easy, in fact, that "it was a cinch" to tie.

12 Fibula meant clasp, brooch, or buckle; in particular, the needle of the clasp or the tongue of the buckle. The long, thin fibula bone in the leg resembled the needle of a clasp to the Romans. Poorer Romans probably used the fibulas of animals as straight pins to hold clothes in place.

13 Capillus is Latin for hair of the head, being derived from caput, head, and pilus, hair. Capillaries are blood vessels so thin they were likened to the hair of the head.

14 Sella meant a chair or stool. The sella turcica, which houses the pituitary gland, suggested a Turkish saddle to the ancient anatomists.

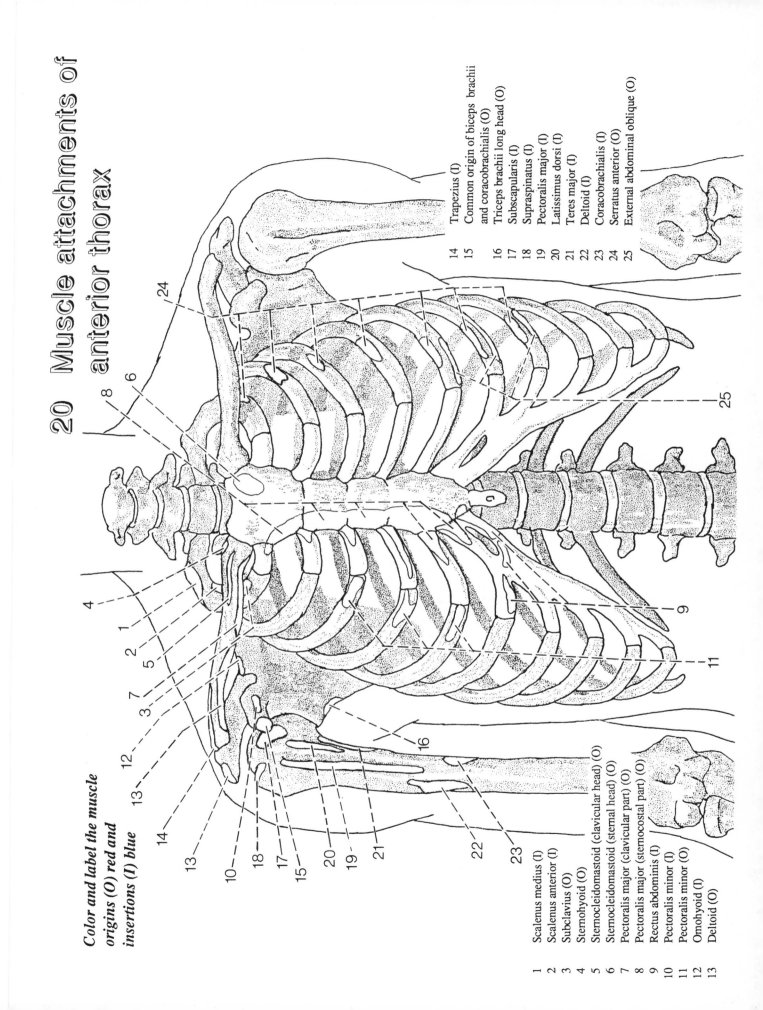

20 Muscle attachments of anterior thorax

Color and label the muscle origins (O) red and insertions (I) blue

1 Scalenus medius (I)
2 Scalenus anterior (I)
3 Subclavius (O)
4 Sternohyoid (O)
5 Sternocleidomastoid (clavicular head) (O)
6 Sternocleidomastoid (sternal head) (O)
7 Pectoralis major (clavicular part) (O)
8 Pectoralis major (sternocostal part) (O)
9 Rectus abdominis (I)
10 Pectoralis minor (I)
11 Pectoralis minor (O)
12 Omohyoid (I)
13 Deltoid (O)

14 Trapezius (I)
15 Common origin of biceps brachii and coracobrachialis (O)
16 Triceps brachii long head (O)
17 Subscapularis (I)
18 Supraspinatus (I)
19 Pectoralis major (I)
20 Latissimus dorsi (I)
21 Teres major (I)
22 Deltoid (I)
23 Coracobrachialis (I)
24 Serratus anterior (O)
25 External abdominal oblique (O)

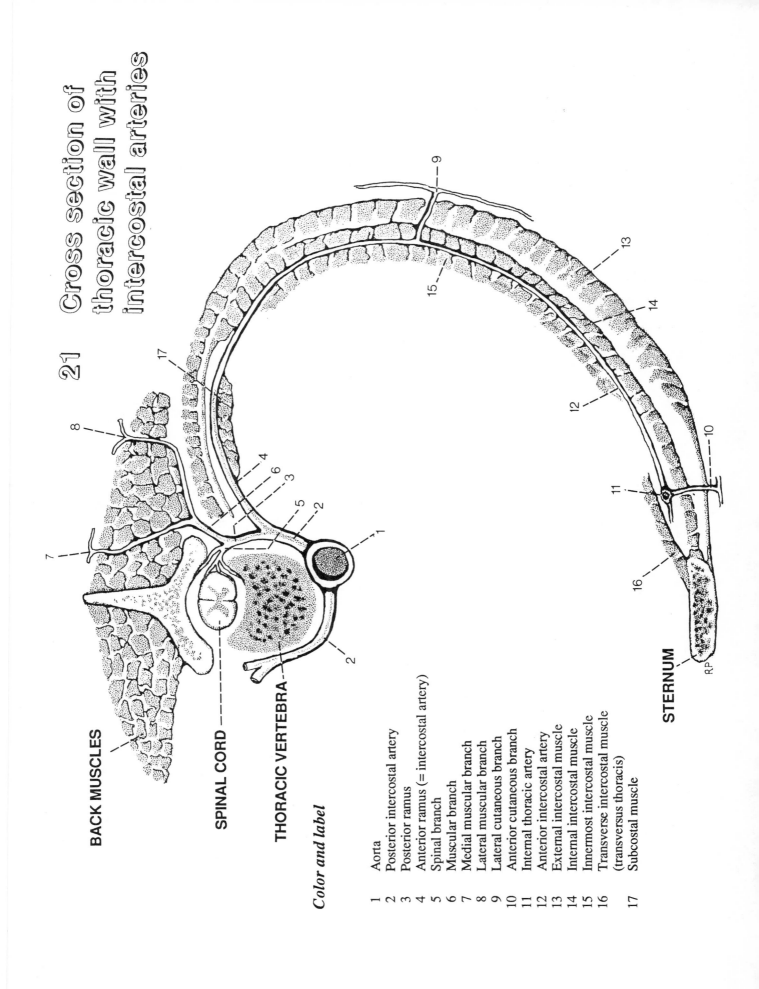

21 Cross section of thoracic wall with intercostal arteries

BACK MUSCLES

SPINAL CORD

THORACIC VERTEBRA

STERNUM

RP

Color and label

1   Aorta
2   Posterior intercostal artery
3   Posterior ramus
4   Anterior ramus (= intercostal artery)
5   Spinal branch
6   Muscular branch
7   Medial muscular branch
8   Lateral muscular branch
9   Lateral cutaneous branch
10 Anterior cutaneous branch
11 Internal thoracic artery
12 Anterior intercostal artery
13 External intercostal muscle
14 Internal intercostal muscle
15 Innermost intercostal muscle
16 Transverse intercostal muscle
    (transversus thoracis)
17 Subcostal muscle

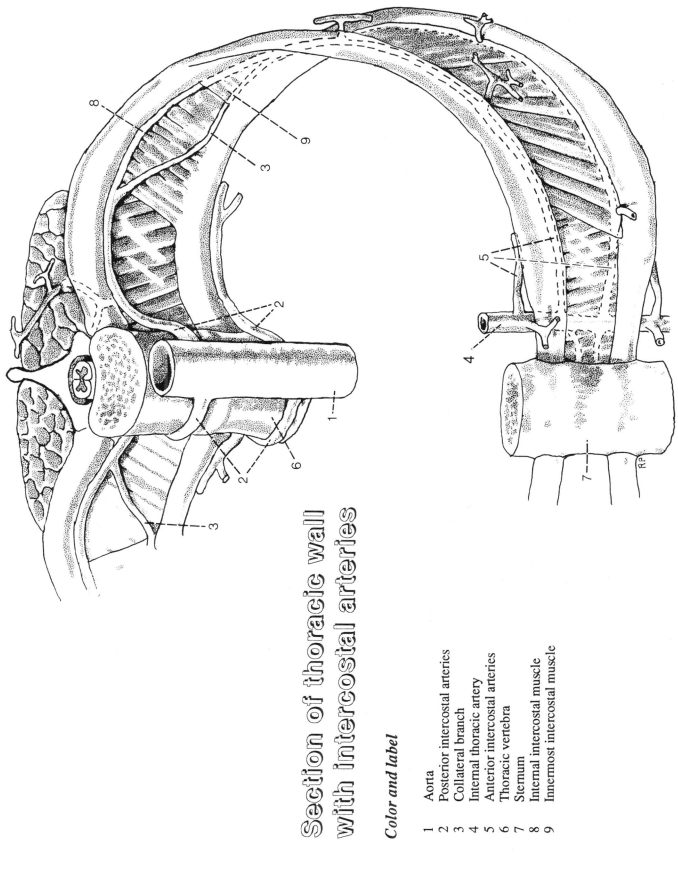

22   Section of thoracic wall
      with intercostal arteries

Color and label

1   Aorta
2   Posterior intercostal arteries
3   Collateral branch
4   Internal thoracic artery
5   Anterior intercostal arteries
6   Thoracic vertebra
7   Sternum
8   Internal intercostal muscle
9   Innermost intercostal muscle

Color and label

1   Ascending aorta
2   Brachiocephalic artery
3   Left common carotid artery
4   Right common carotid artery
5   Subclavian artery*
6   Vertebral artery
7   Thyrocervical artery
8   Inferior thyroid artery
9   Ascending cervical artery
10 Inferior laryngeal artery
11 Transverse cervical artery
12 Superficial branch of transverse cervical artery
13 Deep branch of transverse cervical artery
14 Ascending branch of superficial branch of transverse cervical artery
15 Descending branch of superficial branch of transverse cervical artery
16 Suprascapular artery
17 Internal thoracic (mammary) artery
18 Anterior intercostal arteries
19 Perforating branches
20 Musculophrenic artery
21 Superior epigastric artery
22 Deep cervical artery (branch of costocervical trunk)
23 Axillary artery*
24 Supreme thoracic artery
25 Thoracoacromial artery
26 Clavicular branch of thoracoacromial artery
27 Acromial branch
28 Deltoid branch
29 Pectoral branch(es)
30 Lateral thoracic artery (*usually it arises from thoracoacromial or subscapular artery and not from axillary artery as show here*)
31 Subscapular artery
32 Circumflex scapular artery
33 Thoracodorsal artery
34 Anterior humeral circumflex artery
35 Posterior humeral circumflex artery
36 Brachial artery*
37 Profunda brachii (deep brachial) artery
38 Radial collateral artery of deep brachial a.
39 Middle collateral artery of deep brachial a.
40 Superior ulnar collateral artery
41 Inferior ulnar collateral artery
42 Anterior ulnar recurrent artery
43 Posterior ulnar recurrent artery
44 Radial recurrent artery
45 Interosseous recurrent artery
46 Posterior interosseous artery
47 Anterior interosseous artery
48 Interosseous artery

*Notice that the subclavian artery becomes the axillary artery, which becomes the brachial artery.

23 Subclavian, axillary, and brachial arteries viewed from the front (anterior aspect)

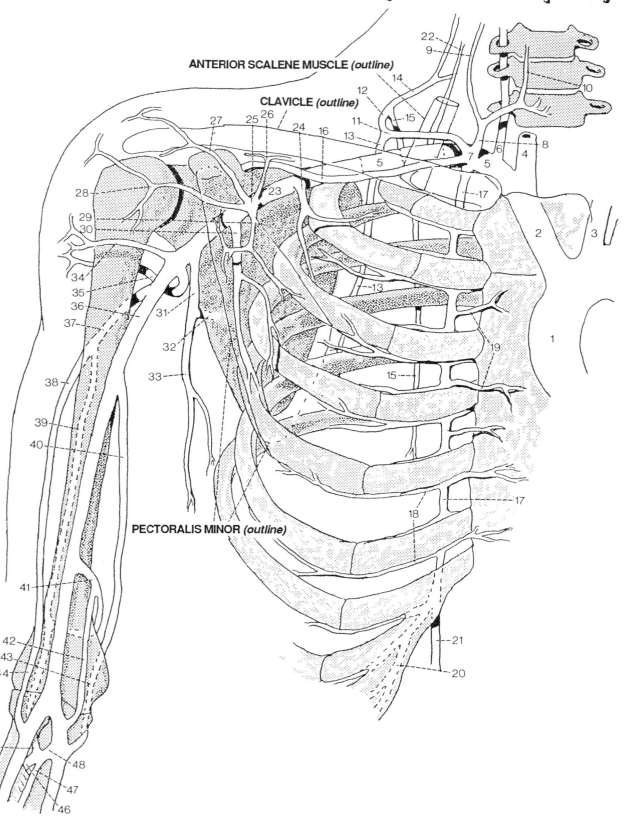

ANTERIOR SCALENE MUSCLE *(outline)*

CLAVICLE *(outline)*

PECTORALIS MINOR *(outline)*

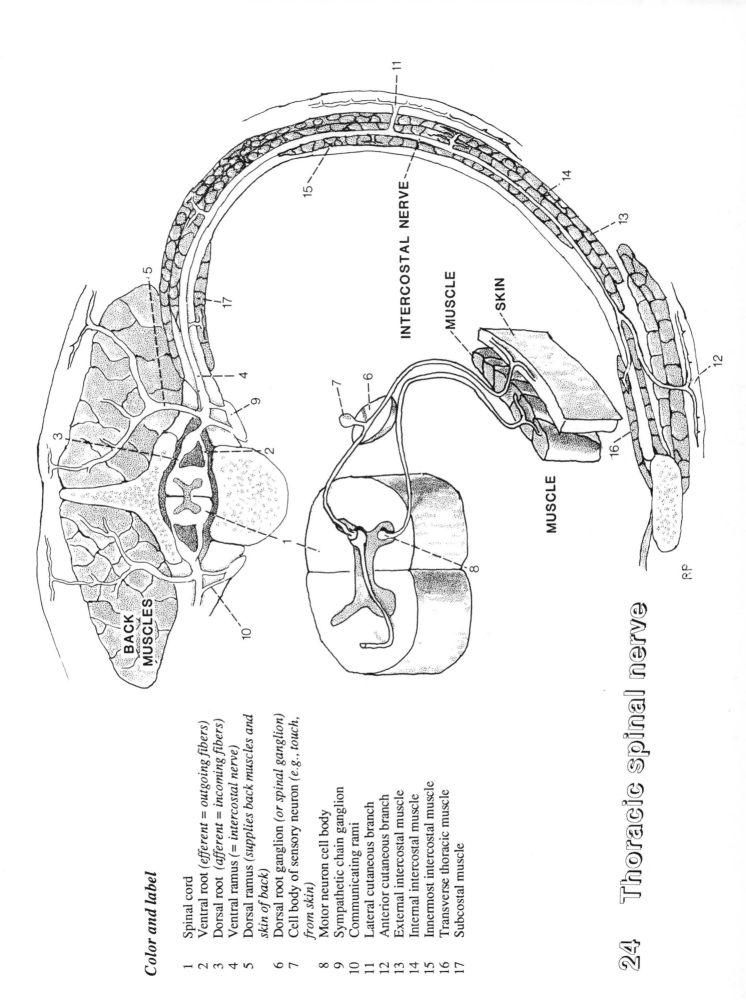

Color and label

1 Spinal cord
2 Ventral root (*efferent = outgoing fibers*)
3 Dorsal root (*afferent = incoming fibers*)
4 Ventral ramus (*= intercostal nerve*)
5 Dorsal ramus (*supplies back muscles and skin of back*)
6 Dorsal root ganglion (*or spinal ganglion*)
7 Cell body of sensory neuron (*e.g., touch, from skin*)
8 Motor neuron cell body
9 Sympathetic chain ganglion
10 Communicating rami
11 Lateral cutaneous branch
12 Anterior cutaneous branch
13 External intercostal muscle
14 Internal intercostal muscle
15 Innermost intercostal muscle
16 Transverse thoracic muscle
17 Subcostal muscle

24   Thoracic spinal nerve

The visceral and serous pericardium can be likened to pushing a fist into a soft balloon. The serous pericardium is thin and delicate. The outer fibrous pericardium is quite strong.

Color and label the edge of the balloon
1   "Parietal" layer *(paries, Latin, wall of a house)*
2   "Visceral" layer *(viscus, Latin, soft internal organ)*

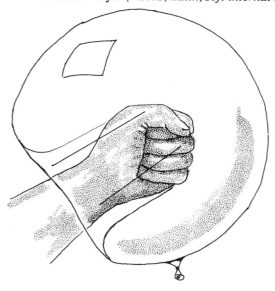

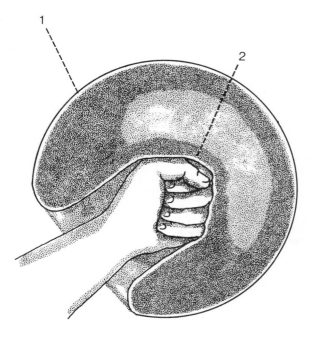

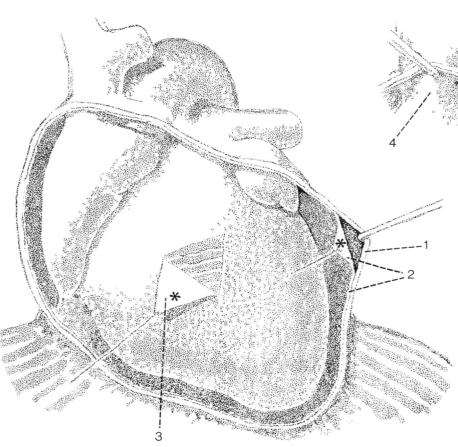

Color and label

1   Fibrous pericardium *(forms a strong sac that encloses heart)*
2   Parietal part of serous pericardium* *(lines inside of fibrous pericardium)*
3   Visceral part of serous pericardium* *(covers outside of heart; also called epicardium)*
4   Great vessels such as aorta penetrate pericardial sac and are covered by serous pericardium on their intra-pericardial parts.

Serous pericardium peeled off at asterisk

Color these veins violet (1-10)

1	Right brachiocephalic vein
2	Left brachiocephalic vein
3	Superior vena cava
4	Inferior vena cava
5	Right internal thoracic vein
6	Left internal thoracic vein
7	Right pericardiacophrenic vein
8	Left pericardiacophrenic vein
9	Anterior cardiac veins
10	Great cardiac vein
11	Pulmonary trunk (*also color violet*)

Color these arteries red (12-22)

12	Aorta
13	Brachiocephalic artery
14	Right internal artery
15	Right pericardiacophrenic artery
16	Left common carotid artery
17	Left subclavian artery
18	Left internal thoracic artery
19	Left pericardiacophrenic artery
20	Right coronary artery
21	Marginal branch
22	Anterior interventricular artery (*branch of left coronary artery*)
23	Cut edge of pericardium
24	Cut edge of pleura

Color these nerves yellow (25-28)

25	Right phrenic nerve
26	Left phrenic nerve
27	Left vagus nerve
28	Recurrent laryngeal nerve
29	Ligamentum arteriosum
30	Right auricle
31	Left auricle
32	Root of left lung

Coronary vessels lie under fat, which must be removed for vessels to be seen.

26 Exterior of heart

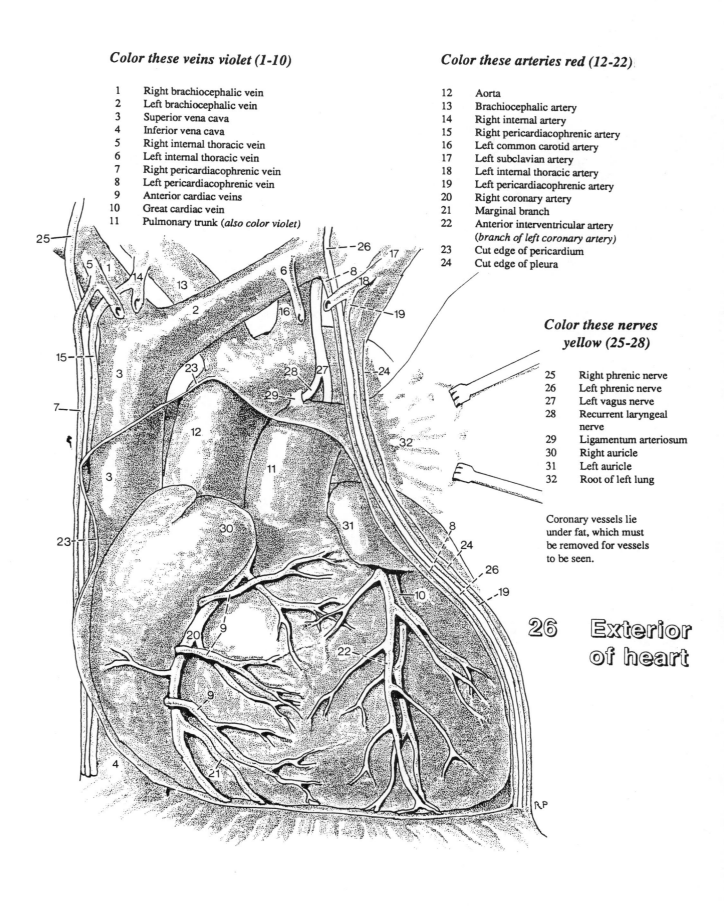

Trace the course of blood through the heart *(See opposite page)*

Blood returns from the head, arms and thorax via the superior vena cava (1), which empties into the right atrium. Blood returns from the legs and abdomen via the inferior vena cava (2). Blood returns from the heart itself via the coronary sinus (3). Blood leaves the right atrium through the tricuspid valve and enters the right ventricle (4). Ventricular contraction forces the blood through the pulmonary valve into the pulmonary trunk (5), which divides into the right pulmonary artery (6) and the left pulmonary artery (7). The right pulmonary artery is shown dividing into a superior branch (8) and an inferior branch (9). Blood returns from the lungs via four pulmonary veins (10-13), which empty into the left atrium. The blood then passes the tricuspid or mitral valve (14) into the left ventricle. Ventricular contraction will force the blood through the aortic valve into the aorta. Arrows 15 and 16 represent blood entering the right (15) and left (16) coronary arteries, which supply the heart and arise from the beginning of the aorta. Arrow 17 is within the ascending part of the aorta.

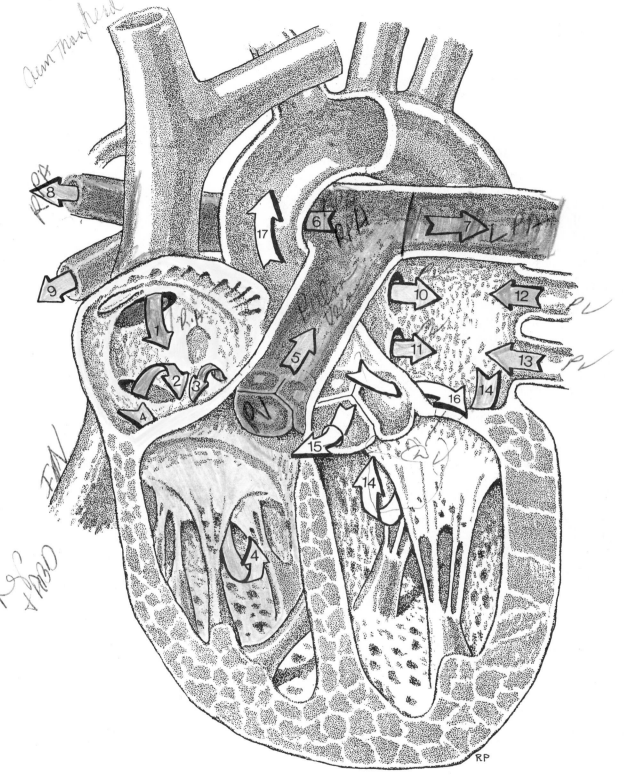

27   Trace the course of blood
      through the heart

Label and color these veins blue or violet

1 Right brachiocephalic vein
2 Left brachiocephalic vein
3 Superior vena cava
4 Azygos vein
5 Inferior vena cava

Label and color the interior of the right atrium

6 Ostium (opening) of superior vena cava
7 Ostium of inferior vena cava
8 Ostium of coronary sinus
9 Fossa ovalis
10 Musculi pectinati
11 Crista terminalis
12 Sinoatrial node *(pacemaker)*
13 Right auricle

Label and color the interior of the right ventricle

14 Anterior cusp of tricuspid valve
15 Chordae tendineae
16 Anterior papillary muscle
17 Trabeculae carneae
18 Septomarginal trabecula (moderator band)
19 Conus arteriosus
20 Anterior valvule of pulmonary valve
21 Myocardium *(color pink)*
22 Endocardium *(leave white)*
23 Epicardium *(leave white)*
24 Interventricular septum
25 Pulmonary trunk
26 Right pulmonary artery
27 Left pulmonary artery
28 Superior branch of right pulmonary artery
29 Inferior branch of right pulmonary artery

Label and color the left atrium

30 Ostia (openings) of right pulmonary veins
31 Left pulmonary veins

Label and color the left ventricle

32 Anterior cusp of mitral valve
33 Posterior cusp of mitral valve
34 Chordae tendineae
35 Anterior papillary muscle
36 Left valvule of aortic valve
37 Ostium (opening) of left coronary artery
38 Aortic arch
39 Brachiocephalic artery
40 Left common carotid artery
41 Left subclavian artery

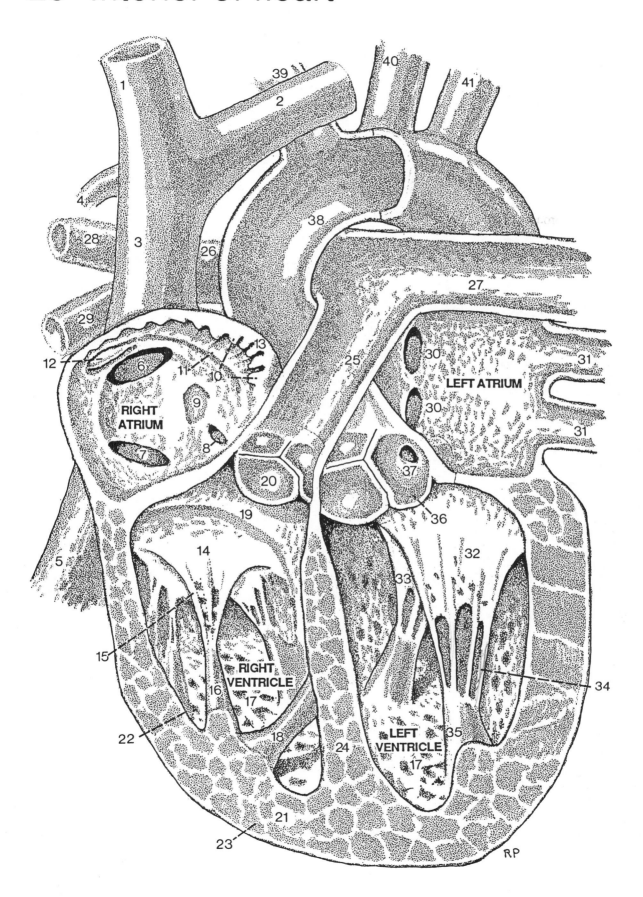

RP

Color and label

1 Right coronary artery
2 Left coronary artery
3 Anterior interventricular branch of the left coronary artery (left anterior descending branch)
4 Circumflex branch of left coronary artery
5 Anterior cusp of tricuspid valve

6 Septal cusp of tricuspid valve
7 Posterior cusp of tricuspid valve
8 Anterior cusp of mitral valve
9 Posterior cusp of mitral valve
10 Anterior cusp (valvule) of pulmonary valve
11 Right cusp (valvule) of pulmonary valve
12 Left cusp (valvule) of pulmonary valve
13 Right cusp (valvule) of aortic valve
14 Left cusp (valvule) of aortic valve
15 Posterior cusp (valvule) of aortic valve

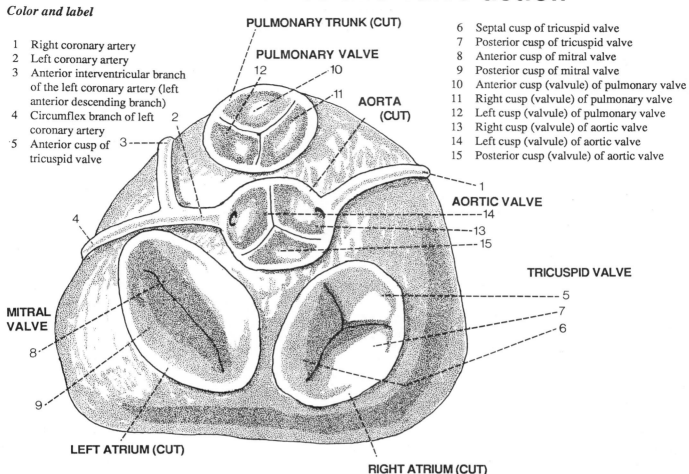

PULMONARY TRUNK (CUT)

PULMONARY VALVE

AORTA (CUT)

AORTIC VALVE

TRICUSPID VALVE

MITRAL VALVE

LEFT ATRIUM (CUT)

RIGHT ATRIUM (CUT)

The mitral valve is also called the bicuspid valve. The tricuspid valve and the mitral valve are also referred to as the atrioventricular valves (AV valves), whereas the pulmonary valve and the aortic valve are called the semilunar valves.

SEMILUNAR VALVES CLOSED

SEMILUNAR VALVES OPEN

DIASTOLE
AV VALVES OPEN

SYSTOLE
AV VALVES CLOSED

RP

Color and label

Coronary arteries (most common pattern):

1 Right coronary artery and its branches
2 Main atrial branch (usually called artery of sinoatrial node)
3 Sinoatrial nodal artery *(arises from right coronary artery in 55% of hearts examined; from circumflex branch of left coronary artery in 45%)*
4 Right conus artery
5 Right anterior ventricular rami
6 Right marginal artery *(reaches apex of heart in 93% of hearts examined)*
7 Right posterior ventricular rami
8 Posterior interventricular artery
9 Atrioventricular nodal artery *(supplies AV node)*
10 Anterior atrial rami
11 Left coronary artery and its branches
12 Circumflex artery
13 Anterior interventricular artery (also called left anterior descending artery)
14 Left conus artery
15 Left diagonal artery *(present in 33-50% of hearts)*
16 Left anterior ventricular arteries
17 Anterior septal rami *(supplies anterior interventricular septum)*
18 Posterior septal rami
19 Left marginal artery *(present in 90% of hearts)*

ANTERIOR VIEW OF HEART
Shaded vessels are on posterior surface

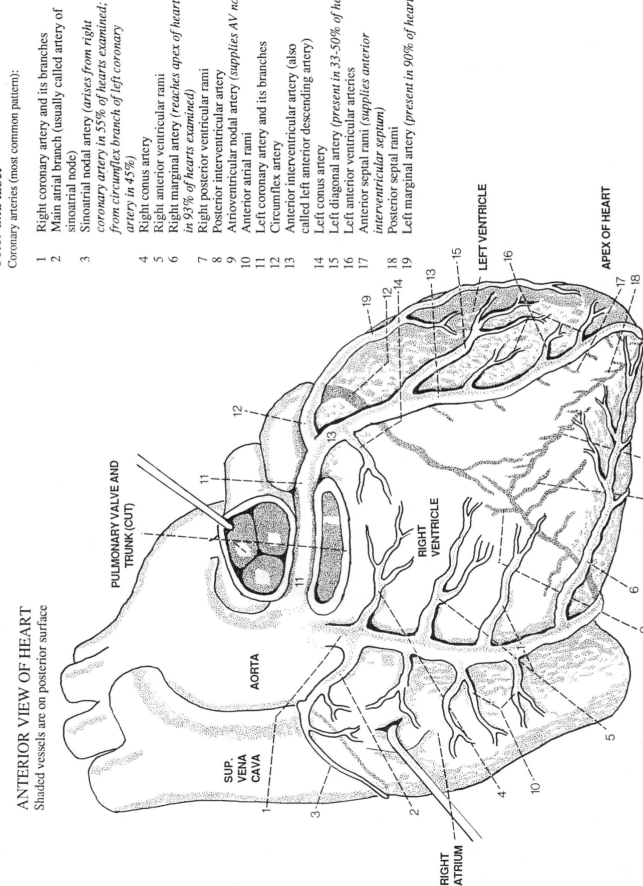

LEFT VENTRICLE

APEX OF HEART

PULMONARY VALVE AND TRUNK (CUT)

AORTA

SUP. VENA CAVA

RIGHT VENTRICLE

RIGHT ATRIUM

30 Coronary arteries

Based on Williams and Warwick: Gray's Anatomy, 36th Brit. ed. Edinburgh, Churchill Livingstone, 1980, pp 669-673.

Color and label

VENOUS DRAINAGE OF THE HEART

Principal veins of the heart:

1 Coronary sinus (*on posterior surface of heart*)*
2 Orifice (*opening*) of coronary sinus into right atrium
3 Great cardiac vein
4 Left marginal vein
5 Small cardiac vein
6 Right marginal vein (*usually ends in right atrium as shown here; less frequently it drains into small cardiac vein, which drains into coronary sinus*)
7 Middle cardiac vein
8 Posterior vein of left ventricle
9 Anterior cardiac veins (*notice these usually drain directly into right atrium*)

*The coronary sinus is the main vein that drains blood from the heart itself.

ANTERIOR VIEW OF HEART

Shaded vessels are on posterior surface

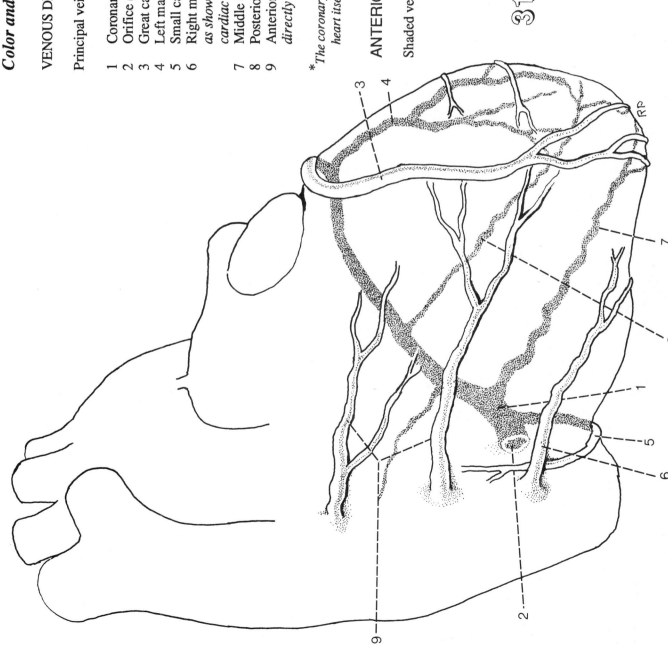

31 Coronary veins

32　Cardiac conducting system

Color and label

1　Sinoatrial node *(pacemaker)*
2　Atrioventricular node
3　Atrioventricular bundle (of His; common bundle)
4　Right bundle branch
5　Left bundle branch(es)
6　Anterior internodal tract
7　Middle internodal tract
8　Posterior internodal tract
9　Septomarginal trabecula (moderator band)
10　Interventricular septum *(cut)*
11　Right atrium
12　Right ventricle
13　Left ventricle
14　Pulmonary valve and artery *(cut)*
15　Superior vena cava
16　Subendocardial plexus

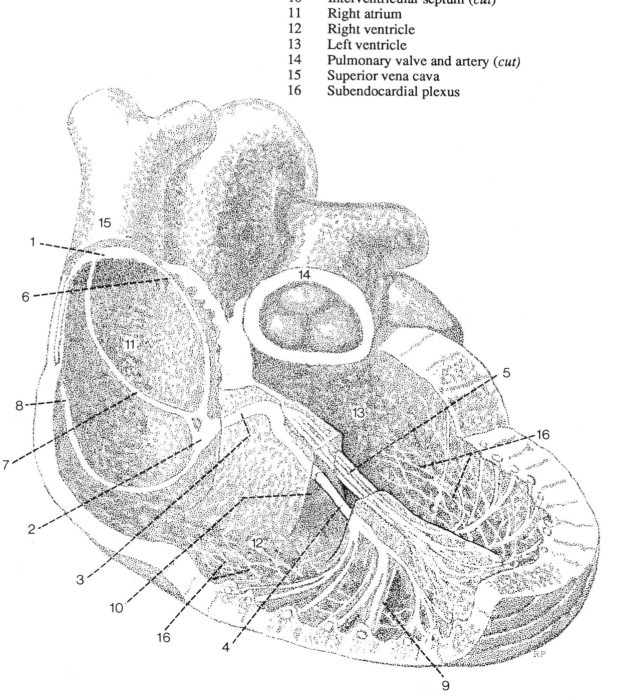

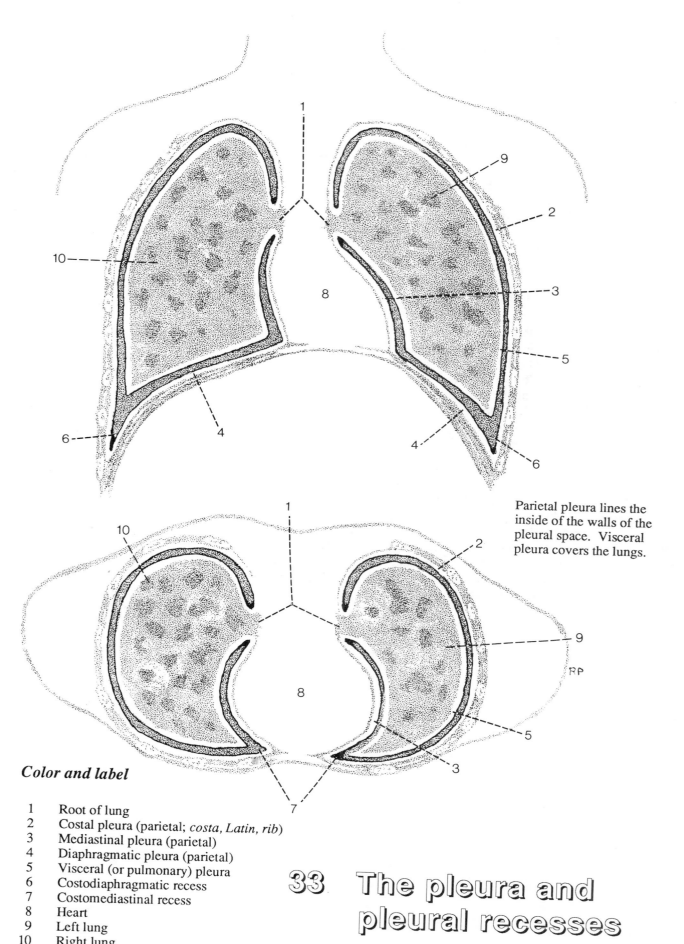

Parietal pleura lines the
inside of the walls of the
pleural space. Visceral
pleura covers the lungs.

RP

Color and label

1	Root of lung
2	Costal pleura (parietal; *costa, Latin, rib*)
3	Mediastinal pleura (parietal)
4	Diaphragmatic pleura (parietal)
5	Visceral (or pulmonary) pleura
6	Costodiaphragmatic recess
7	Costomediastinal recess
8	Heart
9	Left lung
10	Right lung

33 The pleura and pleural recesses

(See opposite page)

Color and label

1 Principal bronchus
2 Pulmonary artery *(blue)*
3 Pulmonary veins *(red)*
4 Cut edge of pleura
5 Pulmonary ligament

Label

6 Oblique fissure
7 Horizontal fissure *(right lung only)*
8 Diaphragmatic surface *(base)*
9 Groove of aorta
10 Anterior surface and margin
    (sharp border)
11 Posterior surface and margin
    (round border)

The trachea divides into a right and a left principal bronchus. The right principal bronchus divides into three lobar bronchi, superior, middle, and inferior. The left principal bronchus divides into two, superior and inferior. The lobar bronchi divide into segmental bronchi (1-10), each of which supplies a bronchopulmonary segment numbered identical to its segmental bronchus.

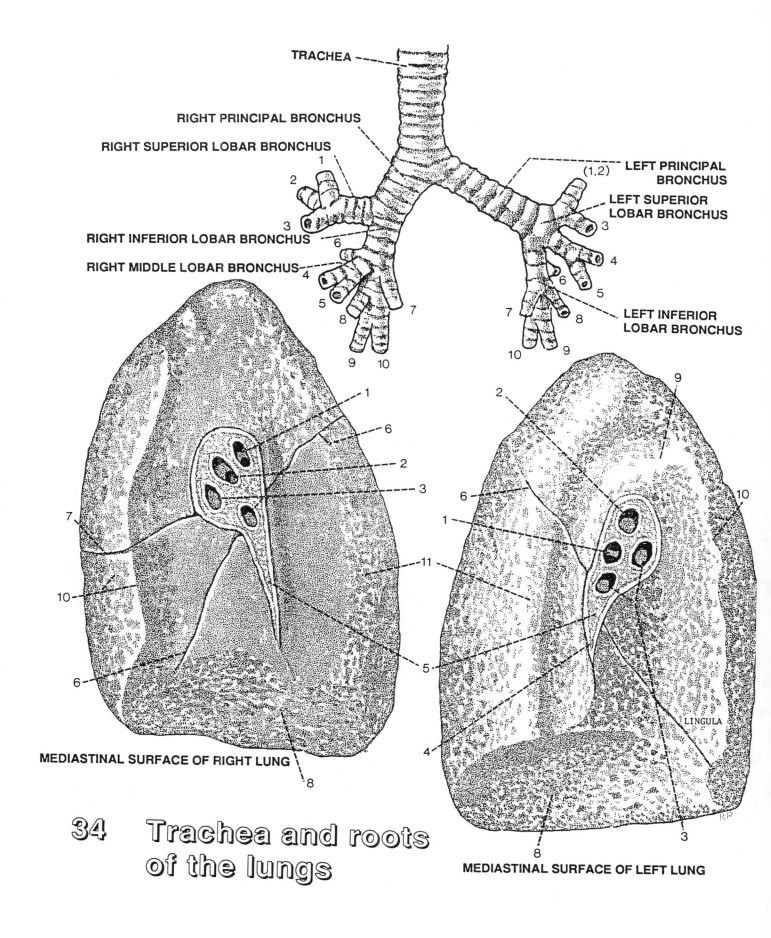

TRACHEA

RIGHT PRINCIPAL BRONCHUS

RIGHT SUPERIOR LOBAR BRONCHUS

LEFT PRINCIPAL BRONCHUS

LEFT SUPERIOR LOBAR BRONCHUS

RIGHT INFERIOR LOBAR BRONCHUS

RIGHT MIDDLE LOBAR BRONCHUS

LEFT INFERIOR LOBAR BRONCHUS

(1,2)

MEDIASTINAL SURFACE OF RIGHT LUNG

LINGULA

MEDIASTINAL SURFACE OF LEFT LUNG

34 Trachea and roots
of the lungs

Each segmental bronchus and its branches remain entirely within a single bronchopulmonary segment. Color the segmental bronchus and its branches tan.

The accompanying segmental artery may send branches* into adjacent bronchopulmonary segments. Color the artery and its branches blue (for deoxygenated blood).

Veins tend to lie both within the bronchopulmonary segments (as segmental or intrasegmental veins) and between the bronchopulmonary segments (as intersegmental or infrasegmental veins). Color the veins red (for oxygenated blood).

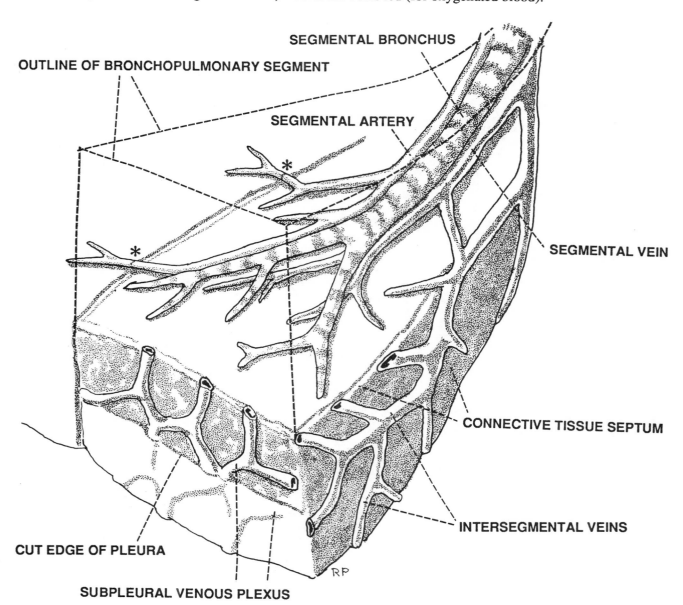

SEGMENTAL BRONCHUS

OUTLINE OF BRONCHOPULMONARY SEGMENT

SEGMENTAL ARTERY

SEGMENTAL VEIN

CONNECTIVE TISSUE SEPTUM

INTERSEGMENTAL VEINS

CUT EDGE OF PLEURA

SUBPLEURAL VENOUS PLEXUS

Thus, resection (surgical removal) of one bronchopulmonary segment along its connective tissue borders (septa) should not cut any air passageways. However, some arteries* will probably be cut and the intersegmental veins that lie in the septa between the bronchopulmonary segments will necessarily be cut.

35   Bronchopulmonary segments

Color each segmental bronchus (1-10) the same color as the bronchopulmonary segment (1-10) that it supplies

Notice that the right lung has three lobes and the left lung has two lobes. The boundaries of the bronchopulmonary segments are not visible on the lung surface as pictured here. Notice also that in the right lung the upper lobe has three bronchopulmonary segments (1, 2, 3), the middle lobe has two segments (4, 5), and the lower lobe has five segments (6-10).

After E. Pernkopf.

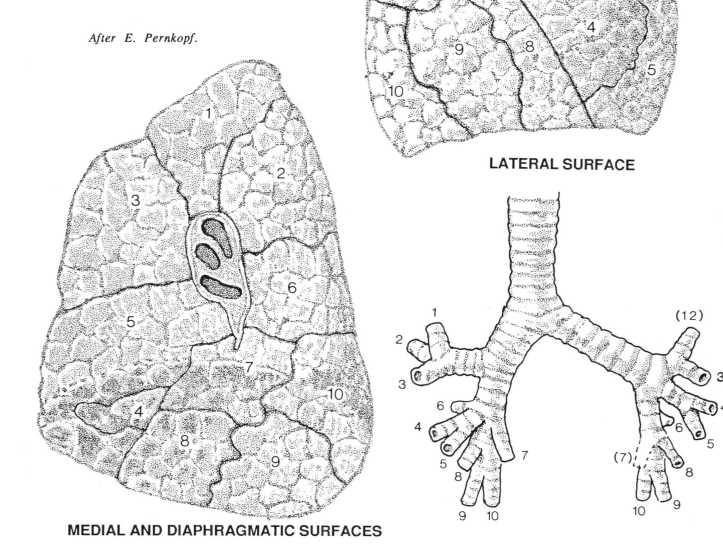

LATERAL SURFACE

MEDIAL AND DIAPHRAGMATIC SURFACES

36   Bronchopulmonary segments (right lung)

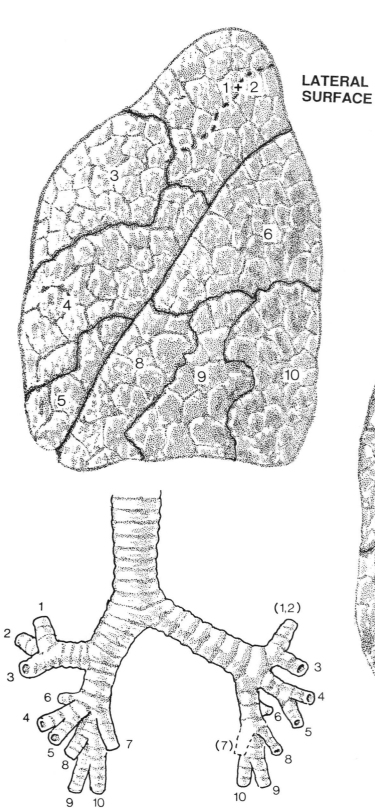

LATERAL SURFACE

Notice that the left lung contains only two lobes separated by the oblique fissure. Usually the upper lobe of the left lung contains four bronchopulmonary segments; segments 1 and 2 are supplied by a single segmental bronchus and, hence, function as a single segment. The lower lobe usually contains five segments, although bronchopulmonary segment 7 is missing in the lung pictured here.

After E. Pernkopf.

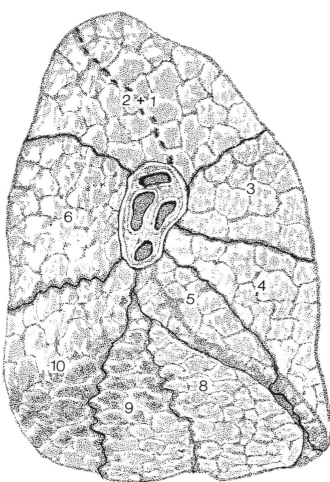

MEDIAL AND DIAPHRAGMATIC SURFACES

Color each segmental bronchus (1-10) the same color as the bronchopulmonary segment (1-10) that it supplies

37 Bronchopulmonary segments (left lung)

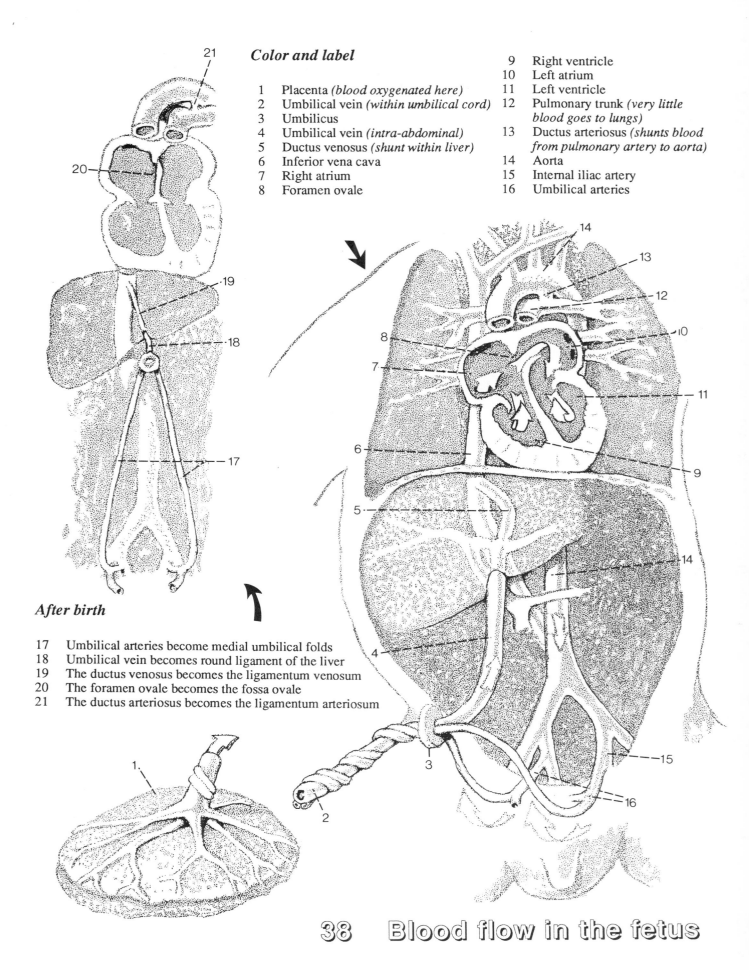

Color and label

1 Placenta *(blood oxygenated here)*
2 Umbilical vein *(within umbilical cord)*
3 Umbilicus
4 Umbilical vein *(intra-abdominal)*
5 Ductus venosus *(shunt within liver)*
6 Inferior vena cava
7 Right atrium
8 Foramen ovale

9 Right ventricle
10 Left atrium
11 Left ventricle
12 Pulmonary trunk *(very little blood goes to lungs)*
13 Ductus arteriosus *(shunts blood from pulmonary artery to aorta)*
14 Aorta
15 Internal iliac artery
16 Umbilical arteries

After birth

17 Umbilical arteries become medial umbilical folds
18 Umbilical vein becomes round ligament of the liver
19 The ductus venosus becomes the ligamentum venosum
20 The foramen ovale becomes the fossa ovale
21 The ductus arteriosus becomes the ligamentum arteriosum

38   Blood flow in the fetus

Notice that the greater splanchnic nerve ends in the celiac ganglion. The lesser splanchnic nerve ends in the aorticorenal ganglion, and the lowest splanchnic nerve ends in the renal plexus.

Color yellow and label

1   Greater splanchnic nerve
2   Lesser splanchnic nerve
3   Lowest splanchnic nerve
4   Celiac ganglion
5   Aorticorenal ganglion
6   Renal plexus
7   Sympathetic ganglia
8   Rami communicantes

Label

9   Aorta
10   Celiac trunk
11   Suprarenal gland
12   Crus of diaphragm
13   Renal artery
14   Kidney

39 Thoracic splanchnic nerves

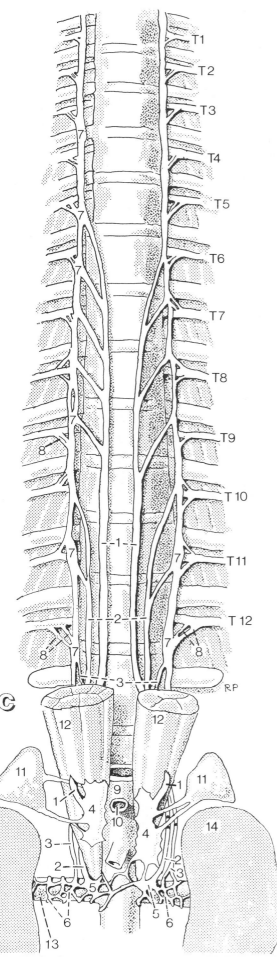

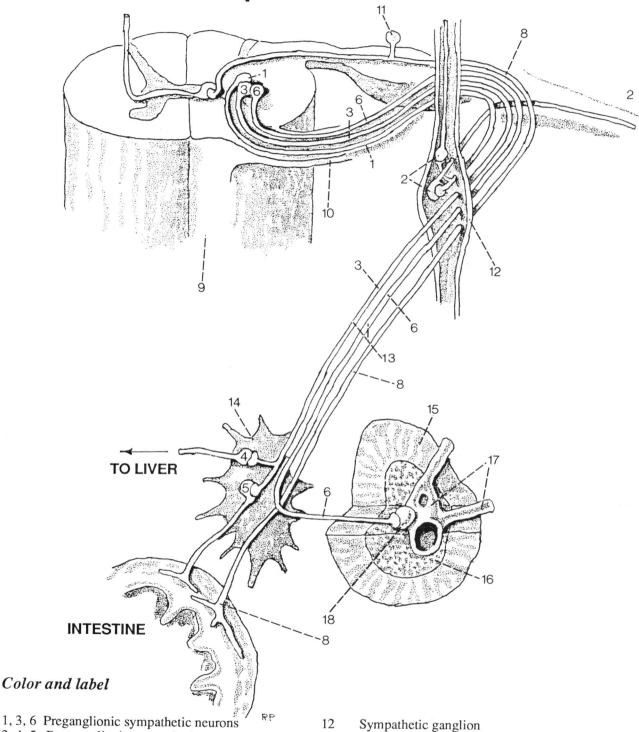

TO LIVER

INTESTINE

Color and label

RP

1, 3, 6 Preganglionic sympathetic neurons
2, 4, 5 Postganglionic sympathetic neurons
    8 Afferent (incoming) fiber
    9 Spinal cord
   10 Ventral root of spinal nerve
       containing efferent (outgoing)
       fibers
   11 Afferent neuron cell body in dorsal
       root ganglion

   12 Sympathetic ganglion
   13 Preganglionic sympathetic fibers in
       splanchnic nerve
   14 Celiac ganglion
   15 Cortex of suprarenal gland
   16 Medulla of suprarenal gland
   17 Blood vessels in suprarenal medulla
   18 Epinephrine-secreting cell in
       suprarenal medulla

(See opposite page)

Color and label

1 Lymph nodes
2 Cisterna chyli
3 Thoracic duct
4 Ostium of thoracic duct into subclavian vein at its junction with internal jugular vein
5 Azygos vein
6 Hemiazygos vein
7 Accessory hemiazygos vein
8 Posterior intercostal veins
9 Posterior intercostal arteries (aorta has been removed)
10 Intercostal nerves
11 Sympathetic ganglia
12 Greater splanchnic nerve
13 Ascending lumbar vein
14 Lumbar veins
15 Subcostal vein
16 Left renal vein
17 Connection between left renal and hemiazygos veins
18 Inferior vena cava
19 Connection between azygos vein and inferior vena cava
20 Superior vena cava
21 Opening of azygos vein into superior vena cava
22 Brachiocephalic vein
23 Internal jugular vein
24 Subclavian vein
25 Left superior intercostal vein
26 Right superior intercostal vein
27 Innermost intercostal muscle
28 Subcostal muscle
29 Diaphragm *(partially resected)*
30 Crus of diaphragm
31 Outline of aortic hiatus in diaphragm
32 Variable connection

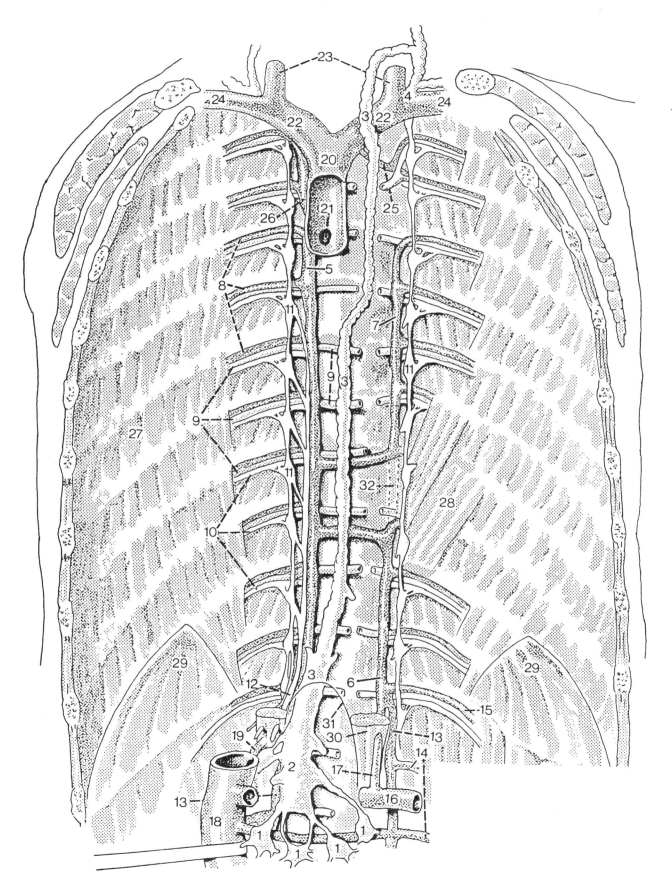

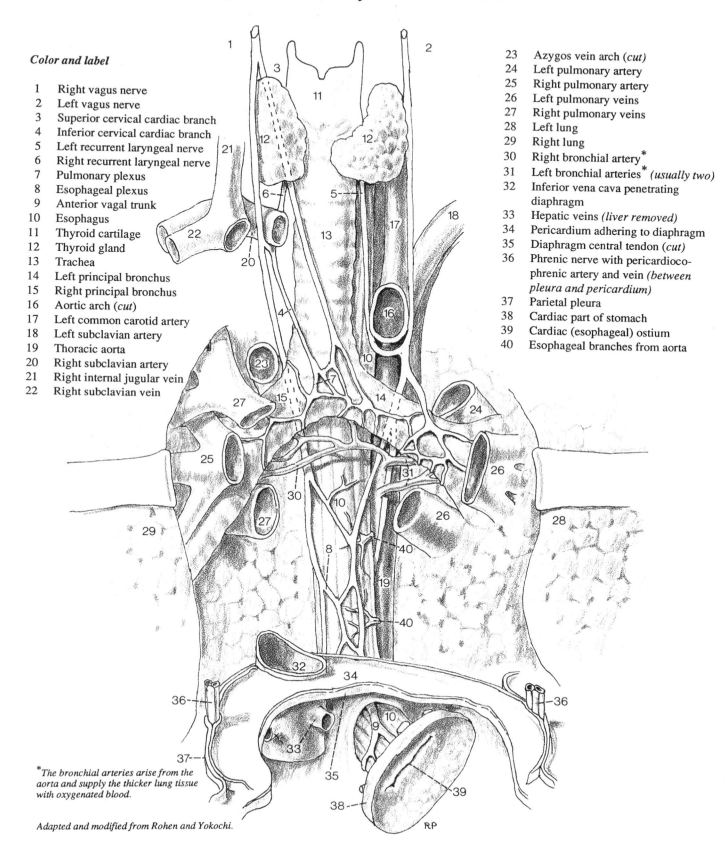

Color and label

1 Right vagus nerve
2 Left vagus nerve
3 Superior cervical cardiac branch
4 Inferior cervical cardiac branch
5 Left recurrent laryngeal nerve
6 Right recurrent laryngeal nerve
7 Pulmonary plexus
8 Esophageal plexus
9 Anterior vagal trunk
10 Esophagus
11 Thyroid cartilage
12 Thyroid gland
13 Trachea
14 Left principal bronchus
15 Right principal bronchus
16 Aortic arch (cut)
17 Left common carotid artery
18 Left subclavian artery
19 Thoracic aorta
20 Right subclavian artery
21 Right internal jugular vein
22 Right subclavian vein

23 Azygos vein arch (cut)
24 Left pulmonary artery
25 Right pulmonary artery
26 Left pulmonary veins
27 Right pulmonary veins
28 Left lung
29 Right lung
30 Right bronchial artery*
31 Left bronchial arteries* (usually two)
32 Inferior vena cava penetrating diaphragm
33 Hepatic veins (liver removed)
34 Pericardium adhering to diaphragm
35 Diaphragm central tendon (cut)
36 Phrenic nerve with pericardiaco-phrenic artery and vein (between pleura and pericardium)
37 Parietal pleura
38 Cardiac part of stomach
39 Cardiac (esophageal) ostium
40 Esophageal branches from aorta

*The bronchial arteries arise from the aorta and supply the thicker lung tissue with oxygenated blood.

Adapted and modified from Rohen and Yokochi.

PART II: ABDOMEN

PLATES 43-69

Color and label

1 Rectus abdominis muscle
2 Tendinous intersections
(*there are usually three of these*)
3 Origin of rectus abdominis on pubic crest and symphysis
4 Insertion of rectus abdominis on costal cartilages of ribs 5, 6, and 7
5 Linea alba
6 External abdominal oblique muscle
7 Internal abdominal oblique muscle
8 Transverse abdominal muscle (transversus abdominis)
9 Aponeurosis* of external oblique
10 Aponeurosis of internal oblique (*notice that it splits into two layers, with one passing in front of and one behind the rectus abdominis*)
11 Slips of origin of external oblique
12 Digitations of serratus anterior
13 Superficial inguinal ring and opening
14 Inguinal ligament
15 Rectus sheath (anterior layer, formed by aponeurosis of external oblique and anterior division of aponeurosis of internal oblique)

*An aponeurosis is a flat tendon.

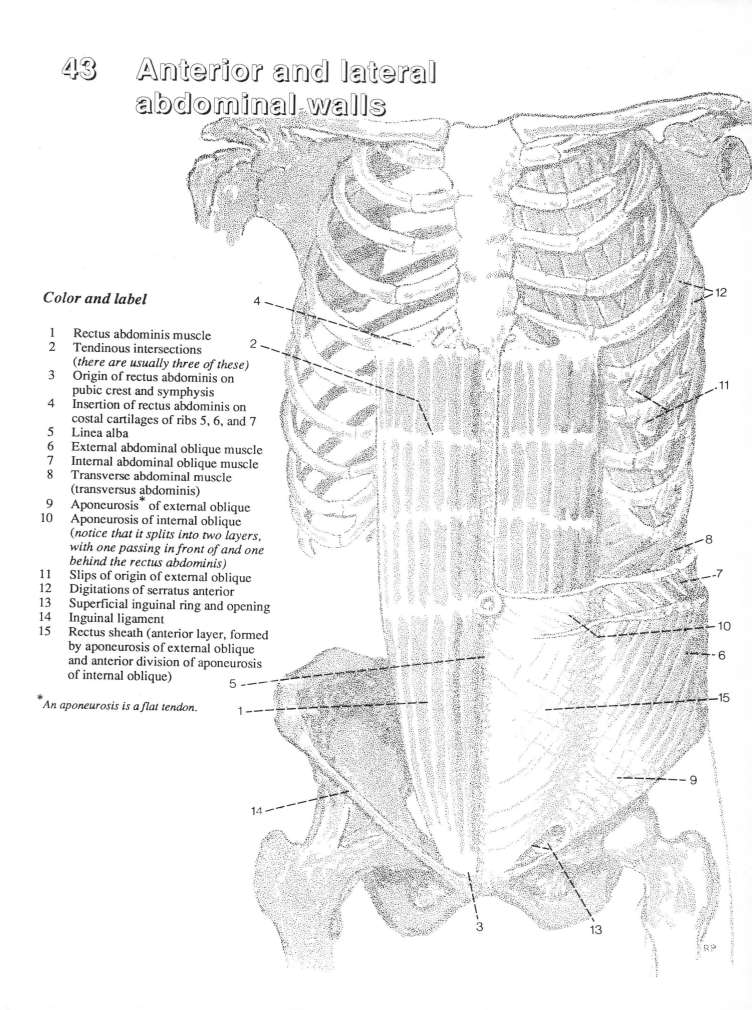

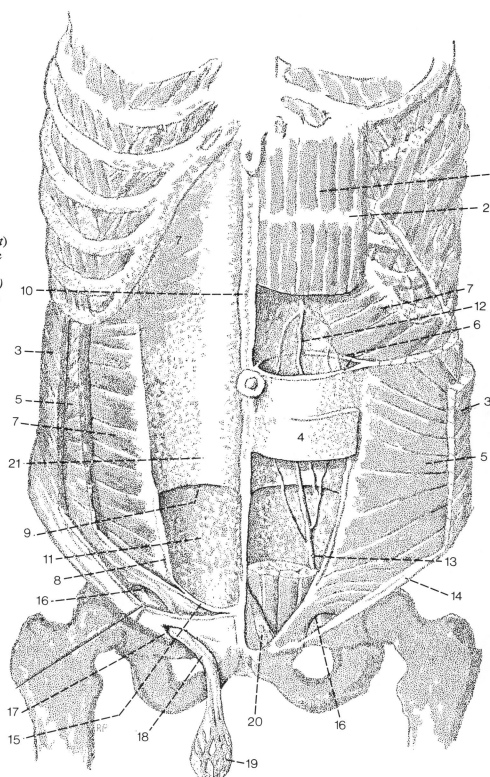

Color and label

1   Rectus abdominis *(cut)*
2   Tendinous intersections
3   External abdominal oblique *(cut)*
4   Aponeurosis of external oblique *(cut)*
5   Internal abdominal oblique *(cut)*
6   Aponeurosis of internal oblique *(cut)*
7   Transversus abdominis
8   Aponeurosis of transversus abdominis
9   Arcuate line
10 Linea alba
11 Transversalis fascia
12 Superior epigastric artery
13 Inferior epigastric artery
14 Inguinal ligament
15 Conjoint tendon
16 Opening of internal oblique and transversus
17 Superficial inguinal ring
18 Spermatic cord
19 Testis
20 Pyramidalis muscle
21 Posterior layer of rectus sheath, consisting of posterior layer of internal oblique aponeurosis, transversus aponeurosis, and transversus muscle

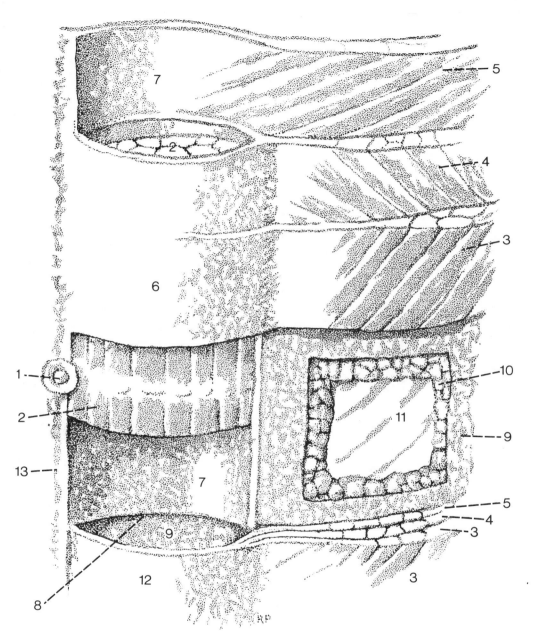

Color and label

1 Umbilicus
2 Rectus abdominis muscle (*cut*)
3 External abdominal oblique muscle
4 Internal abdominal oblique muscle
5 Transverse abdominal muscle
6 Anterior layer of rectus sheath (*made up of aponeurosis of external oblique and internal oblique anterior layer*)
7 Posterior layer of rectus sheath (*made up of posterior layer of internal oblique aponeurosis and transverse aponeurosis*)

8 Arcuate line (*lower border of posterior layer of rectus sheath*)
9 Transversalis fascia
10 Preperitoneal fat
11 Peritoneum
12 Below the arcuate line all three aponeuroses go in front of the rectus abdominis and form the anterior layer of the rectus sheath
13 Linea alba

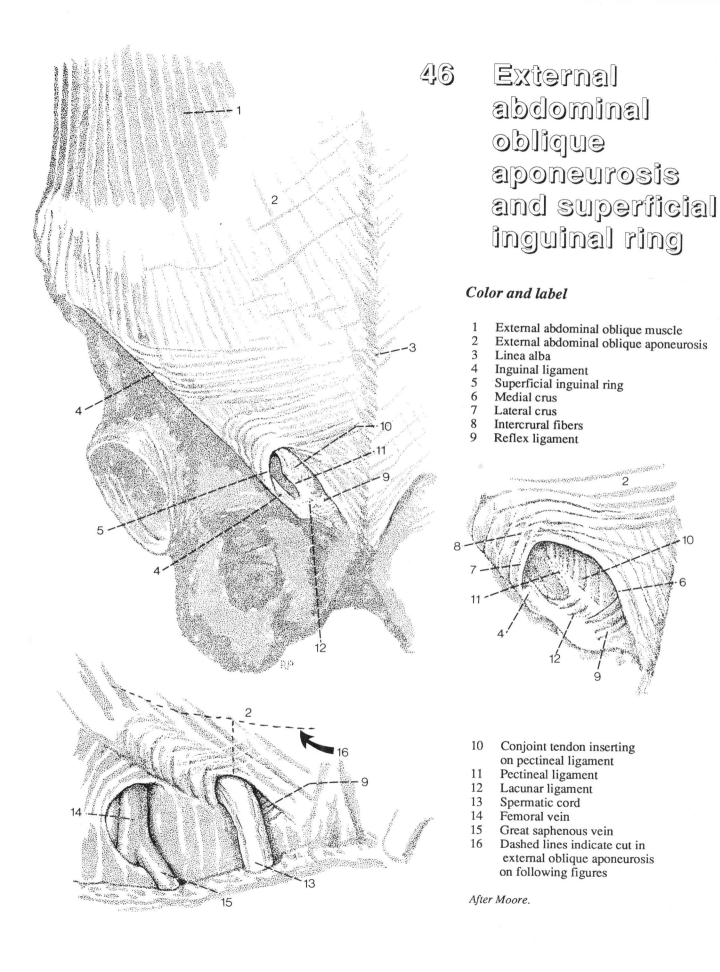

46 External abdominal oblique aponeurosis and superficial inguinal ring

Color and label

1 External abdominal oblique muscle
2 External abdominal oblique aponeurosis
3 Linea alba
4 Inguinal ligament
5 Superficial inguinal ring
6 Medial crus
7 Lateral crus
8 Intercrural fibers
9 Reflex ligament

10 Conjoint tendon inserting
    on pectineal ligament
11 Pectineal ligament
12 Lacunar ligament
13 Spermatic cord
14 Femoral vein
15 Great saphenous vein
16 Dashed lines indicate cut in
    external oblique aponeurosis
    on following figures

After Moore.

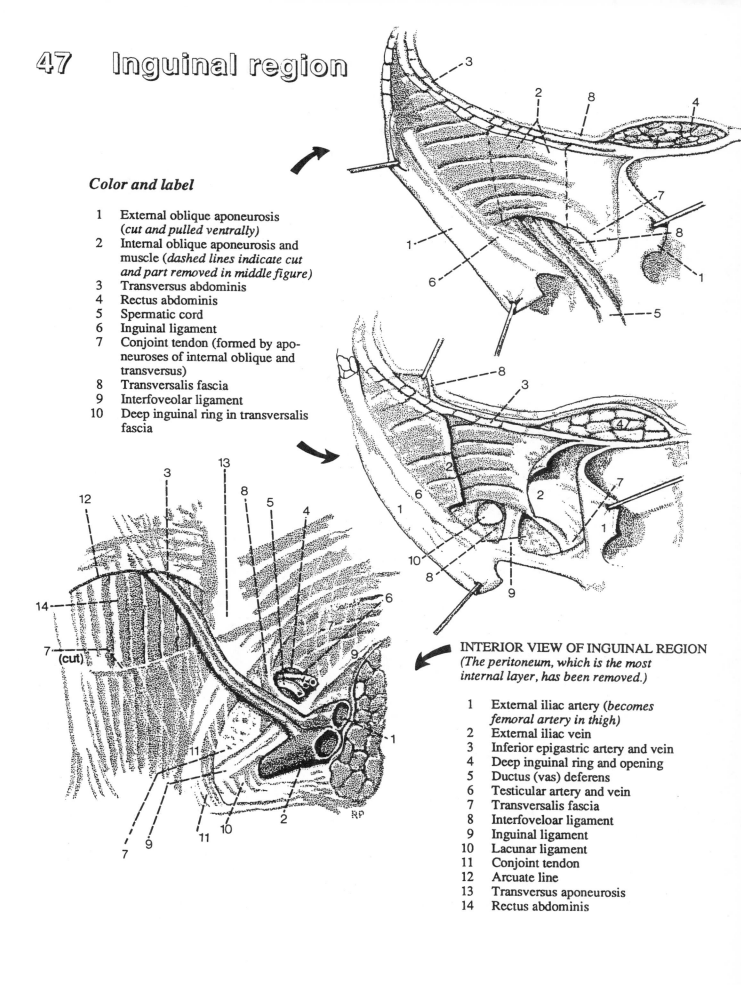

Color and label

1 External oblique aponeurosis (*cut and pulled ventrally*)
2 Internal oblique aponeurosis and muscle (*dashed lines indicate cut and part removed in middle figure*)
3 Transversus abdominis
4 Rectus abdominis
5 Spermatic cord
6 Inguinal ligament
7 Conjoint tendon (formed by aponeuroses of internal oblique and transversus)
8 Transversalis fascia
9 Interfoveolar ligament
10 Deep inguinal ring in transversalis fascia

INTERIOR VIEW OF INGUINAL REGION
(*The peritoneum, which is the most internal layer, has been removed.*)

1 External iliac artery (*becomes femoral artery in thigh*)
2 External iliac vein
3 Inferior epigastric artery and vein
4 Deep inguinal ring and opening
5 Ductus (vas) deferens
6 Testicular artery and vein
7 Transversalis fascia
8 Interfoveolar ligament
9 Inguinal ligament
10 Lacunar ligament
11 Conjoint tendon
12 Arcuate line
13 Transversus aponeurosis
14 Rectus abdominis

Inguinal ligament and related structures *(See opposite page)*

Color and label

1 Inguinal ligament (= thickened) inferior margin of external oblique aponeurosis)
2 Aponeurosis of external abdominal oblique muscle *(cut)*
3 Lacunar ligament
4 Reflected (inguinal) ligament
5 Pectineal ligament (superior pubic ligament)
6 Superficial inguinal ring
7 Lateral crus
8 Medial crus
9 Conjoined tendon (falx inguinalis)
10 Aponeurosis of internal abdominal oblique muscle
11 Aponeurosis of transverse abdominal muscle
12 Sacrospinous ligament
13 Sacrotuberous ligament
14 Base of sacrum (body)
15 Lateral part of sacrum (ala)
16 Iliac crest
17 Iliac fossa
18 Ischial spine
19 Ischial tuberosity
20 Coccyx
21 Greater sciatic foramen
22 Lesser sciatic foramen

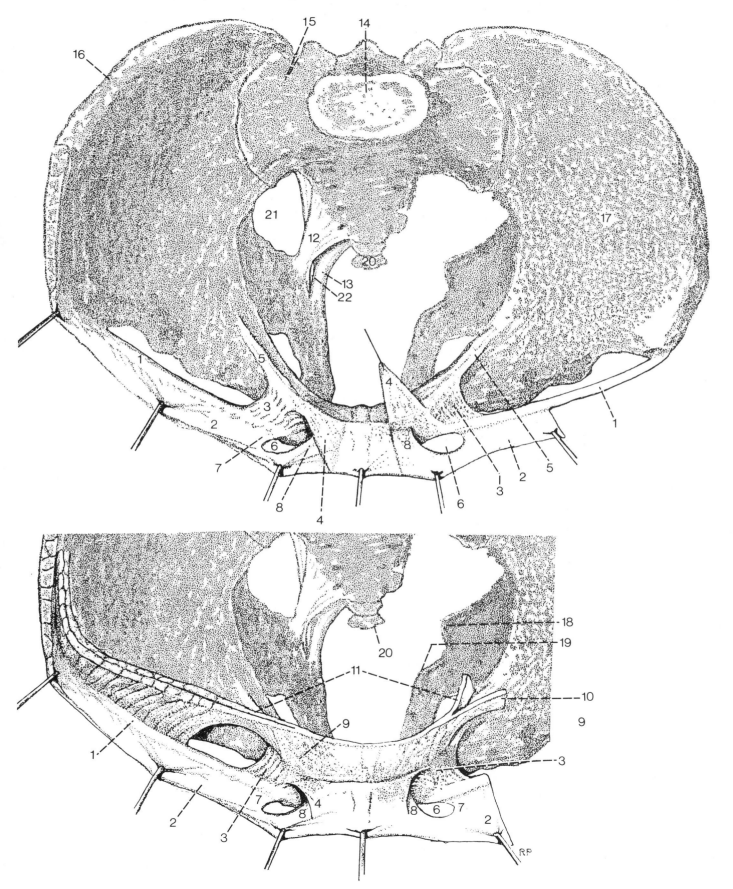

Color and label

1 Aponeurosis of external oblique (*cut*)
2 Inguinal ligament (*actually it is a thickening of the lower border of the aponeurosis of the external oblque*)
3 Aponeurosis of internal oblique (*cut*)
4 Aponeurosis of transversus abdominis (*notice that all three aponeuroses pass in front of the rectus abdominis at this point*)
5 Rectus sheath anterior layer (*formed by all three aponeuroses at this level*)
6 Conjoint tendon (falx inguinalis; *formed by aponeuroses of internal oblique and transversus*)
7 Spermatic cord
8 Deep inguinal ring in transversalis fascia
9 Transversalis fascia
10 Interfoveolar ligament
11 Internal abdominal oblique muscle
12 Transverse abdominal muscle (transversus abdominis)
13 Rectus abdominis
14 Preperitoneal fat

15 Peritoneum
16 External spermatic fascia (*continous with and derived from deep fascia of external oblique*)
17 Cremasteric fascia and cremasteric muscle (*derived from internal oblique and transversus*)
18 Internal spermatic fascia (*derived from transversalis fascia*)
19 Ductus (vas) deferens
20 Testicular artery and pampiniform plexus
21 Inferior epigastric artery and vein
22 Femoral vein
23 Femoral artery
24 Great saphenous vein
25 Saphenous hiatus (opening)
26 Fascia lata (deep fascia of thigh)
27 Subcutaneous fat (superficial fascia)
28 Skin of thigh
29 Medial crus of superficial inguinal ring
30 Lateral crus
31 Reflex ligament
32 Superficial inguinal ring

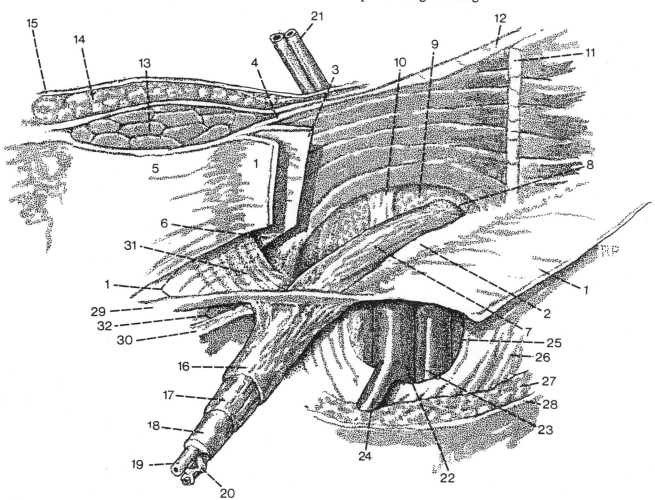

49 Inguinal canal dissection

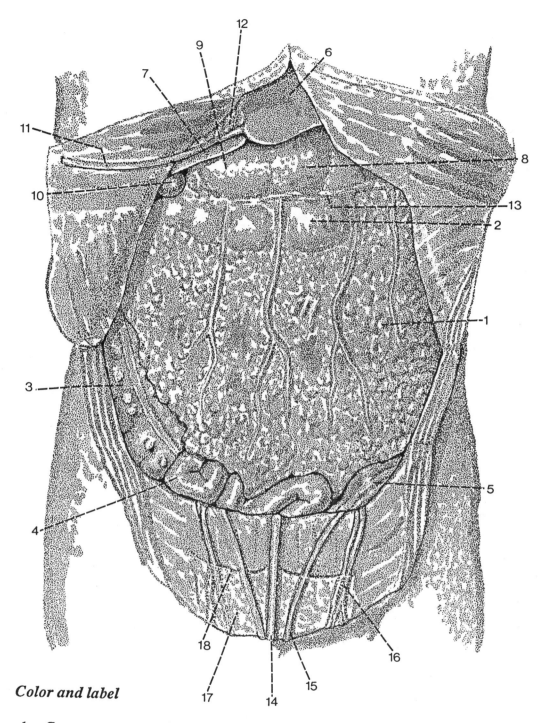

After Clemente.

Color and label

1 Greater omentum (*contains varying amounts of fat*)
2 Transverse colon (large intestine)
3 Ascending colon (large intestine)
4 Ileum (third part of small intestine)
5 Sigmoid colon (large intestine)
6 Liver (left lobe)
7 Liver (right lobe)
8 Stomach
9 Pyloric antrum of stomach
10 Gallbladder
11 Round ligament of the liver (ligamentum teres hepatis; umbilical vein in fetus)

12 Falciform ligament
13 Gastroepiploic vessels
14 Median umbilical fold (urachus; *derived from fetal allantois*)
15 Medial umbilical folds (*derived from fetal umbilical arteries*)
16 Inferior epigastric artery and vein (*form lateral umbilical folds*)
17 Rectus sheath (posterior layer)
18 Arcuate line (lower border of posterior layer of rectus sheath)

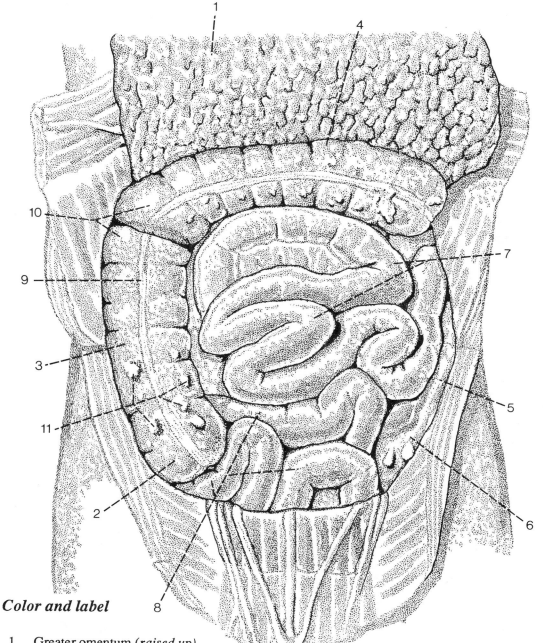
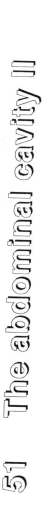

Color and label

1   Greater omentum (*raised up*)
2   Cecum (beginning of large intestine)
3   Ascending colon
4   Transverse colon
5   Descending colon
6   Sigmoid colon
7   Jejunum (second part of small intestine)
8   Ileum (third part of small intestine)
9   Taenia coli (longitudinal strip of smooth muscle; *there are three of these on the large intestine*)*
10 Haustra coli (outpouchings or sacculations)*
11 Appendices epiploicae (epiploic appendices; fatty appendices)*

*Found only on the large intestine (which is also called the colon or large bowel).

After Clemente.

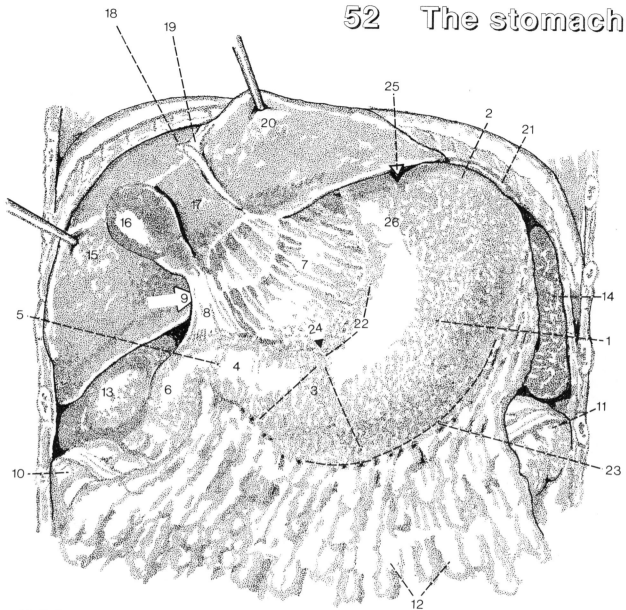

Color and label

1	Stomach (body, corpus)
2	Stomach (fundus)
3	Pyloric antrum
4	Pyloric canal
5	Pylorus (pyloric sphincter)
6	Duodenum
7	Lesser omentum (peritoneum extending from liver to stomach lesser curvature; *this part of lesser omentum is also called hepatogastric ligament*)
8	Hepatoduodenal ligament (*part of lesser omentum; consists of peritoneum surrounding common bile duct, proper hepatic artery, and portal vein*)
9	Arrow in omental foramen (old names: epiploic foramen, foramen of Winslow)
10	Hepatic (or right) flexure of colon
11	Splenic (or left) flexure of colon

12	Greater omentum
13	Right kidney
14	Spleen
15	Liver, right lobe
16	Gallbladder
17	Quadrate lobe
18	Round ligament of liver
19	Falciform ligament
20	Left lobe of liver
21	Diaphragm
22	Lesser curvature
23	Greater curvature
24	Angular incisure
25	Cardiac incisure
26	Cardiac part

After Netter.

Color and label

1. Round ligament of the liver *(obliterated umbilical vein)*
2. Falciform *(Latin, sickle-shaped)* ligament*
3. Right coronary ligament, anterior layer*
4. Left coronary ligament, anterior layer* *(the coronary ligament has been cut near its attachment to the diaphragm)*
5. Right triangular ligament*
6. Left triangular ligament*
7. Fibrous appendix
8. Right lobe of liver
9. Left lobe of liver
10. Gallbladder
11. Bare area *(not covered with peritoneum)*

*These ligaments are peritoneal reflections which attach the liver to the diaphragm and body wall.

LIVER,
SUPERIOR
VIEW

Color and label

1. Falciform ligament
2. Coronary ligament
3. Right triangular ligament
4. Left triangular ligament
5. Fibrous appendix
6. Bare area
7. Inferior vena cava
8. Left lobe
9. Right lobe
10. Caudate lobe
11. Hepatic vein
12. Esophageal impression
13. Ligament of vena cava

Color and label

1   Right lobe
2   Left lobe
3   Caudate lobe (*so named because of its tail-like process*)
4   Quadrate lobe
5   Caudate process of caudate lobe
6   Gallbladder
7   Inferior vena cava
8   Hepatic veins
9   Ligament of the inferior vena cava
10 Round ligament of the liver
11 Ligamentum venosum (*obliterated ductus venosus which shunted the blood from the umbilical vein to the inferior vena cava*)
12 Portal vein
13 Left branch of portal vein
14 Common bile duct
15 Cystic duct
16 Aorta
17 Celiac trunk (*viewed through a transparent aorta*)
18 Common hepatic artery
19 Proper hepatic artery
20 Right posterior layer of coronary ligament
21 Left posterior layer of coronary ligament
22 Right triangular ligament
23 Left triangular ligament
24 Lesser omentum (*cut, vertical part*)
25 Lesser omentum (*horizontal part*)
26 Bare area

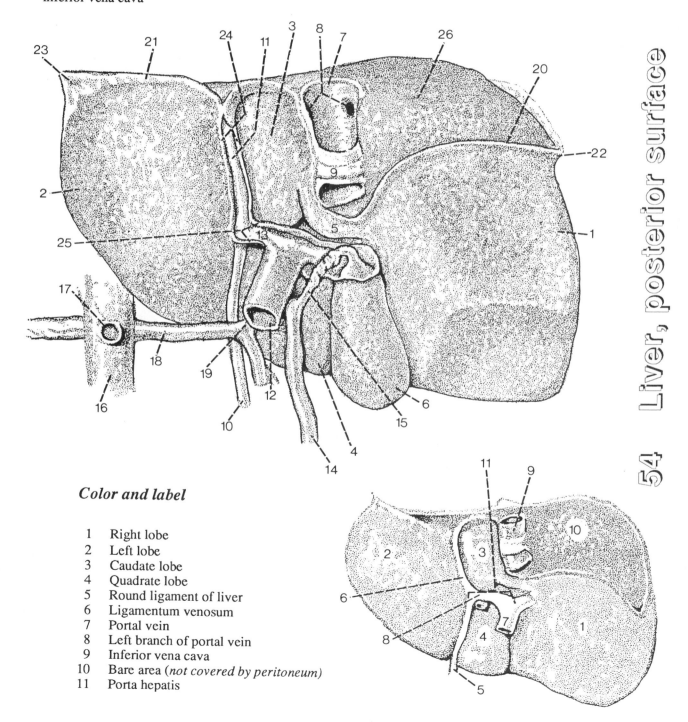

Color and label

1   Right lobe
2   Left lobe
3   Caudate lobe
4   Quadrate lobe
5   Round ligament of liver
6   Ligamentum venosum
7   Portal vein
8   Left branch of portal vein
9   Inferior vena cava
10 Bare area (*not covered by peritoneum*)
11 Porta hepatis

54 Liver, posterior surface

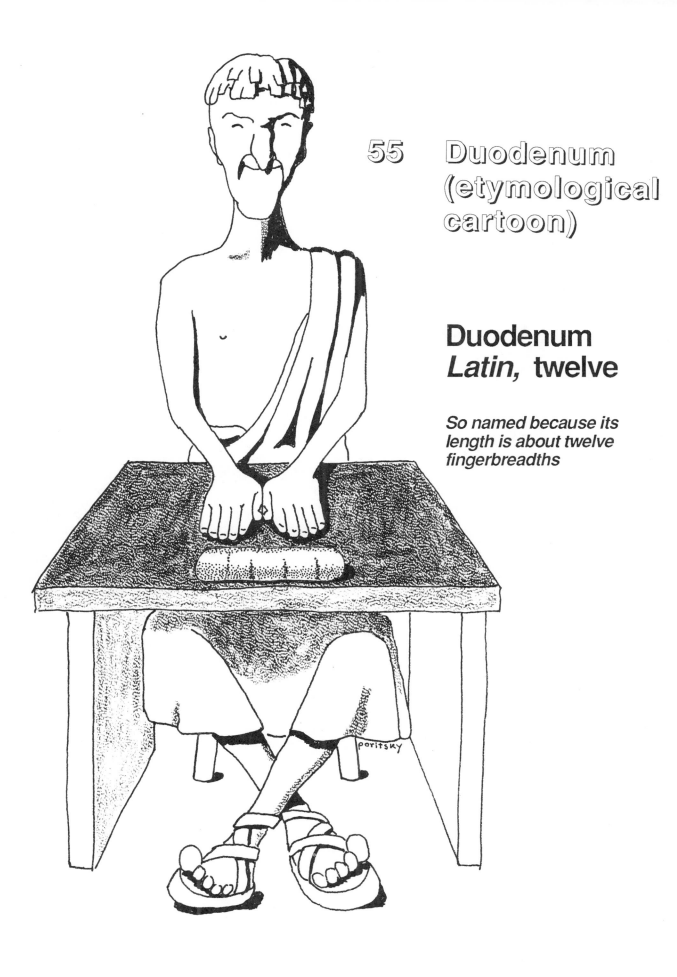

55 Duodenum (etymological cartoon)

Duodenum
Latin, twelve

So named because its length is about twelve fingerbreadths

Color and label

1 Abdominal aorta
2 Celiac trunk
3 Common heptic artery
4 Proper hepatic artery
5 Right gastric artery
6 Gastroduodenal artery
7 Superior pacreaticoduodenal arteries (anterior and posterior)
8 Left gastric artery
9 Esophageal branch of left gastric artery
10 Splenic artery (*seen through stomach*)
11 Short gastric arteries
12 Left gastroepiploic artery
13 Spleen
14 Esophagus
15 Right gastroepiploic artery

After Hollinshead and Rosse.

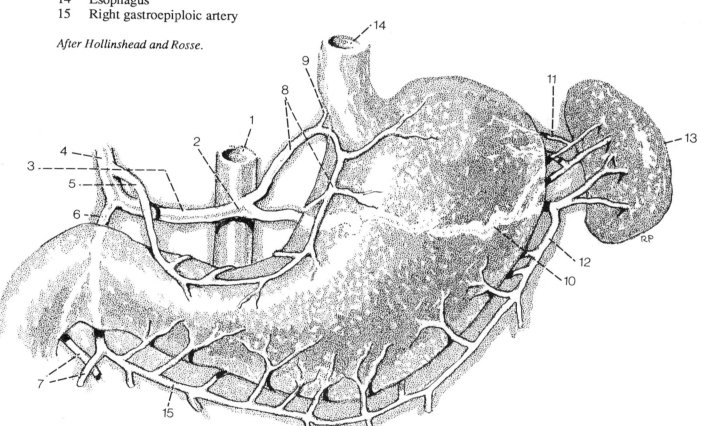

56   Blood supply of the
stomach

(See opposite page)

Color and label

1   Esophagus
2   Cardiac orifice and cardiac region of stomach
3   Fundus of stomach
4   Body of stomach
5   Pyloric antrum
6   Pyloric canal
7   Pyloric opening
8   Pyloric sphincter muscle (*pylorus*, Greek for gatekeeper)
9   Duodenum (first part, superior part, "duodenal bulb")
10 Duodenum (second part, descending part)
11 Duodenum (third part, horizontal part)
12 Duodenum (fourth part, ascending part)
13 Probe in greater duodenal papilla (common opening of common bile duct and pancreatic duct)
14 Lesser duodenal papilla (opening of accessory pancreatic duct)
15 Pancreatic duct (head of pancreas partially removed)
16 Accessory of pancreatic duct
17 Head of pancreas (*cut*)
18 Circular folds in duodenum (plicae circulares)
19 Common bile duct
20 Cystic duct
21 Common hepatic duct
22 Right hepatic duct
23 Left hepatic duct
24 Gallbladder
25 Gastric ridges (rugae; *gaster* is Greek for stomach or belly)
26 Aorta (abdominal)
27 Celiac trunk
28 Left gastric artery
29 Splenic artery
30 Common hepatic artery
31 Proper hepatic artery
32 Left hepatic artery
33 Right hepatic artrey
34 Middle hepatic artery
35 Right gastric artery
36 Gastroduodenal artery
37 Superior mesenteric vein
38 Superior mesenteric artery

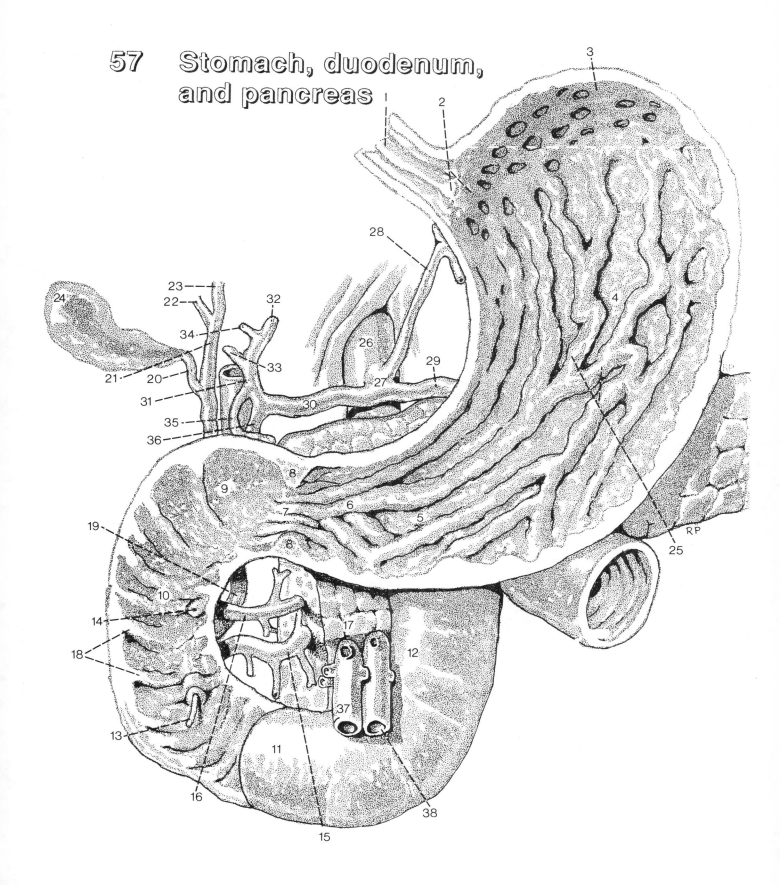

(See opposite page)

Color and label

1 Gallbladder
2 Stomach *(cut)*
3 Spleen
4 Duodenum
5 Jejunum
6 Pancreas
7 Celiac trunk
8 Left gastric artery
9 Splenic artery
10 Common hepatic artery
11 Proper hepatic artery
12 Right gastric artery *(cut)*
13 Right hepatic ramus
14 Middle hepatic ramus
15 Left hepatic ramus
16 Supraduodenal artery
17 Gastroduodenal artery
18 Anterior superior pancreaticoduodenal artery
19 Posterior superior pancreaticoduodenal artery
20 Dorsal pancreatic artery
21 Great pancreatic artery
22 Artery of tail of pancreas
23 Short gastric artery
24 Left gastroepiploic artery
25 Inferior pancreatic artery
26 Inferior phrenic artery
27 Inferior pancreaticoduodenal artery
28 Posterior inferior pancreaticoduodenal ramus
29 Anterior inferior pancreaticoduodenal ramus
30 Right gastroepiploic artery
31 Cystic artery
32 Common bile duct
33 Cystic duct
34 Common hepatic duct
35 Portal vein
36 Superior mesenteric vein
37 Superior mesenteric artery
38 Middle colic artery

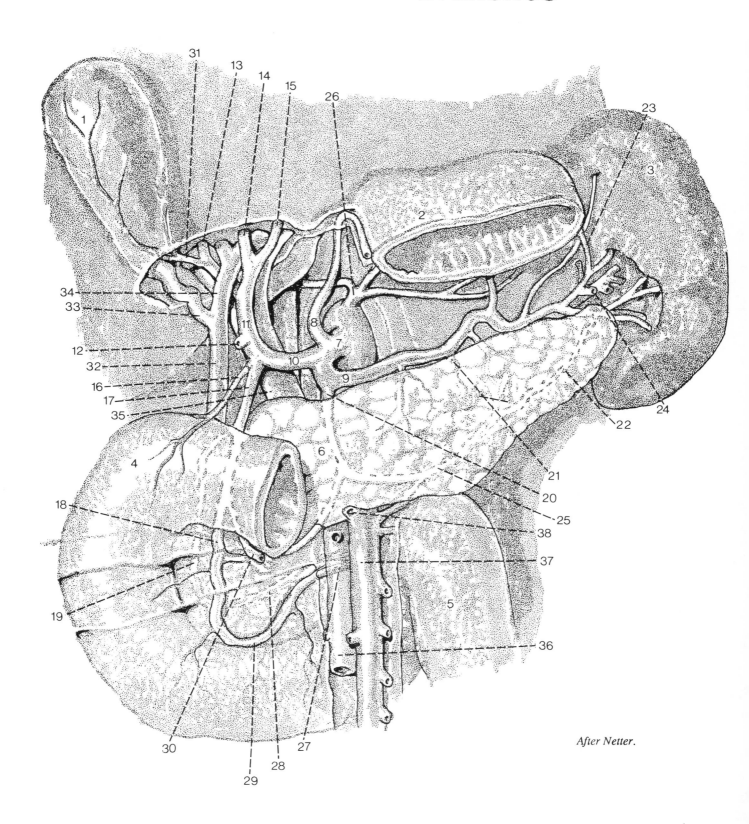

After Netter.

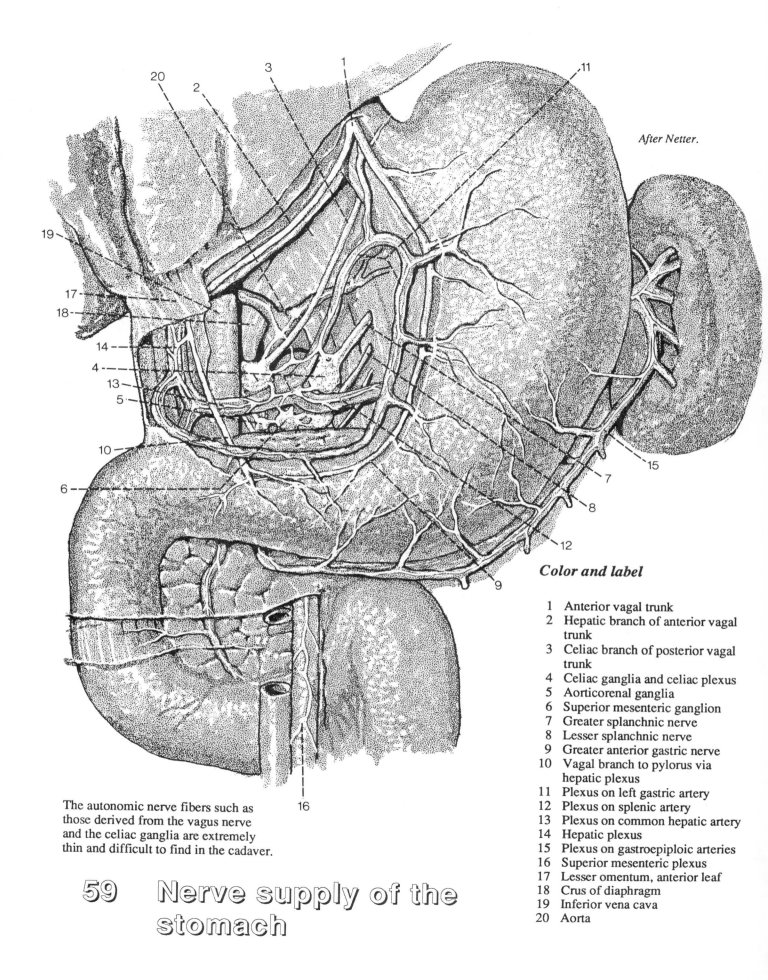

After Netter.

The autonomic nerve fibers such as those derived from the vagus nerve and the celiac ganglia are extremely thin and difficult to find in the cadaver.

Color and label

1 Anterior vagal trunk
2 Hepatic branch of anterior vagal trunk
3 Celiac branch of posterior vagal trunk
4 Celiac ganglia and celiac plexus
5 Aorticorenal ganglia
6 Superior mesenteric ganglion
7 Greater splanchnic nerve
8 Lesser splanchnic nerve
9 Greater anterior gastric nerve
10 Vagal branch to pylorus via hepatic plexus
11 Plexus on left gastric artery
12 Plexus on splenic artery
13 Plexus on common hepatic artery
14 Hepatic plexus
15 Plexus on gastroepiploic arteries
16 Superior mesenteric plexus
17 Lesser omentum, anterior leaf
18 Crus of diaphragm
19 Inferior vena cava
20 Aorta

59 Nerve supply of the stomach

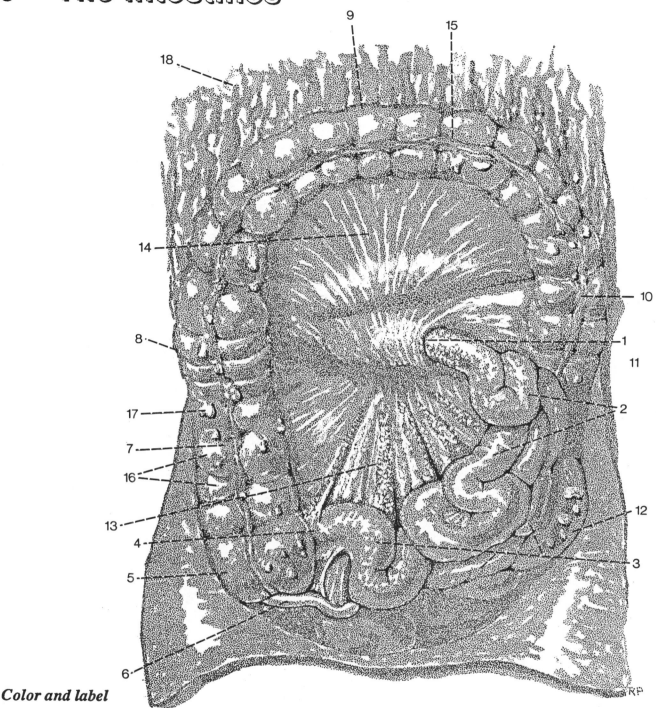

Color and label

1 Duodenojejunal flexure
2 Jejunum (second part of small intestine)
3 Ileum (third part of small intestine)
4 Ileocolic junction (end of small intestine)
5 Cecum
6 Vermiform (*Latin, worm-like*) appendix
7 Ascending colon
8 Right colic flexure
9 Transverse colon
10 Left colic flexure

11 Descending colon
12 Sigmoid colon
13 Mesentery (*attaches jejunum and
     ileum to posterior abdominal wall*)
14 Transverse mesocolon (*attaches
     transverse colon posteriorly*)
15 Taenia coli (*longitudinal strip of smooth muscle*)
16 Haustra coli (*outpouchings*)
17 Omental appendices (old name, epiploic appendices)
18 Greater omentum (*raised up*)

61 Blood supply of the jejunum

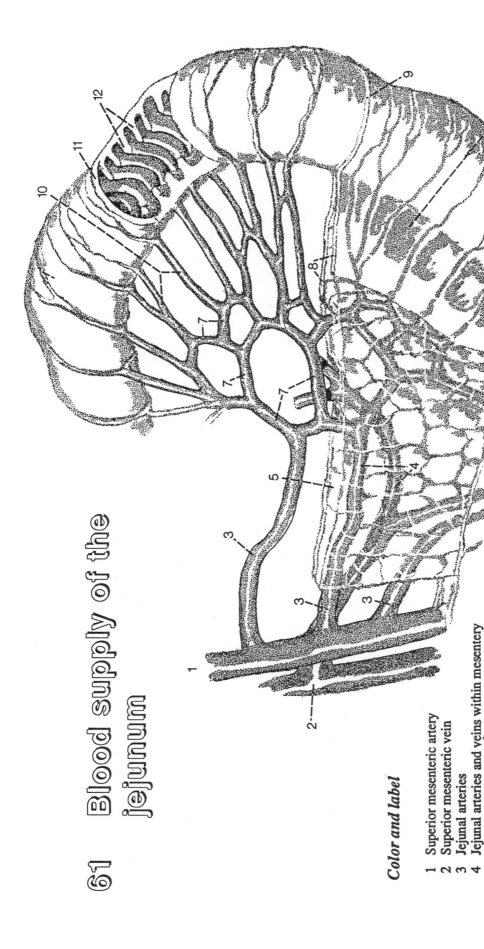

*In addition to fat and blood vessels, the mesentery carries lymphatic vessels, lymph nodes, sympathetic nerves, para-sympathetic nerves, and afferent nerves.

Color and label

1 Superior mesenteric artery
2 Superior mesenteric vein
3 Jejunal arteries
4 Jejunal arteries and veins within mesentery
5 Fat within mesentery *
6 Fat-free "windows" in mesentery next to jejunum impart a translucency to jejunal mesentery
7 Arcades (here there are three rows of arcades; the ileal part of the mesentery may have as many as five rows of arcades)
8 Peritoneum forming two walls of mesentery
9 Cut edge of peritoneum
10 Straight arteries (arteriae rectae; veins follow the same pattern, forming similar arcades and venae rectae, together forming vasae rectae with the arteries; the jejunal straight arteries tend to be longer than the ileal arteries)
11 Jejunum (cut open)
12 Circular folds (plicae circulares; old name: valves of Kerckrung)

62 Ileocecal junction

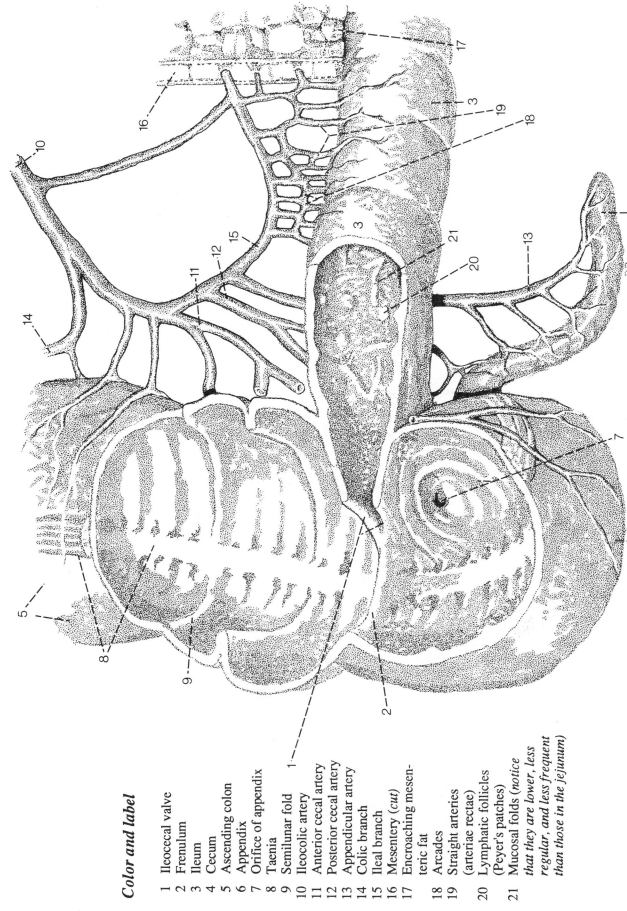

Color and label

1 Ileocecal valve
2 Frenulum
3 Ileum
4 Cecum
5 Ascending colon
6 Appendix
7 Orifice of appendix
8 Taenia
9 Semilunar fold
10 Ileocolic artery
11 Anterior cecal artery
12 Posterior cecal artery
13 Appendicular artery
14 Colic branch
15 Ileal branch
16 Mesentery (*cut*)
17 Encroaching mesen-
   teric fat
18 Arcades
19 Straight arteries
   (arteriae rectae)
20 Lymphatic follicles
   (Peyer's patches)
21 Mucosal folds (*notice
   that they are lower, less
   regular, and less frequent
   than those in the jejunum*)

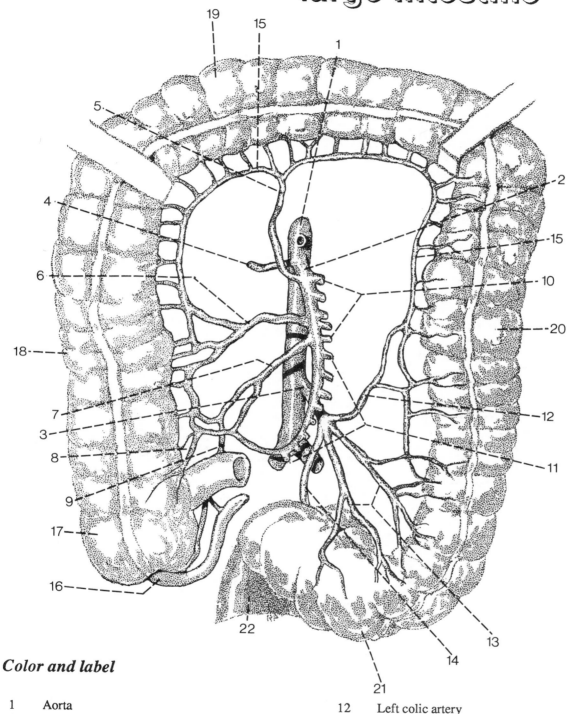

Color and label

1	Aorta	12	Left colic artery
2	Superior mesenteric artery	13	Sigmoid arteries
3	Inferior mesenteric artery	14	Superior rectal artery
4	Inferior pancreaticoduodenal artery	15	Marginal artery (of Drummond)
5	Middle colic artery	16	Appendix
6	Right colic artery	17	Cecum
7	Ileocolic artery	18	Ascending colon
8	Anterior cecal branch	19	Transverse colon
9	Posterior cecal branch	20	Descending colon
10	Jejunal arteries	21	Sigmoid colon
11	Ileal arteries	22	Rectum

64 The hepatic portal system

(See opposite page)

Color and label

1 Portal vein
2 Superior mesenteric vein
3 Splenic vein
4 Inferior mesenteric vein
5 Left gastric vein
6 Right gastric vein
7 Superior pancreaticoduodenal vein
8 Right gastroepiploic vein
9 Middle colic vein
10 Inferior pancreaticoduodenal vein
11 Right colic vein
12 Ileocolic vein
13 Appendicular vein
14 Jejunal veins
15 Ileal veins
16 Left colic vein
17 Sigmoid veins
18 Superior rectal vein
19 Dorsal pancreatic vein
20 Round ligament of liver *(obliterated umbilical vein)*
21 Falciform ligament
22 Coronary ligament
23 Duodenum
24 Stomach (*cut*)
25 Spleen
26 Right lobe of liver
27 Left gastroepiploic vein

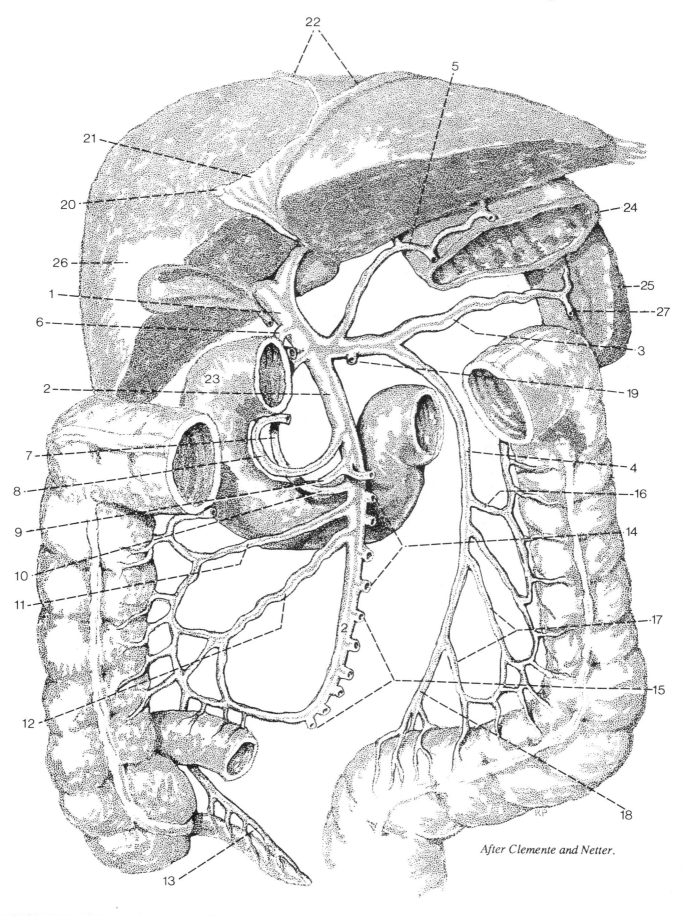

After Clemente and Netter.

(See opposite page)

Color and label

1 Esophagus
2 Diaphragm
3 Site of contact of bare area of liver on diaphragm
4 Coronary ligament of liver
5 Inferior vena cava
6 Hepatic veins
7 Aorta
8 Duodenum
9 Duodenojejunal flexure
10 Hepatoduodenal ligament (portal vein, proper hepatic artery, common bile duct)
11 Pancreas
12 Attachment of transverse mesocolon
13 Site of ascending colon
14 Site of descending colon
15 Root of mesentery
16 Superior mesenteric artery and vein
17 Inferior mesenteric artery
18 Gastrosplenic ligament
19 Gastrophrenic ligament
20 Attachment of sigmoid mesocolon
21 Rectum
22 Attachment of lesser omentum
23 Bifurcation of the aorta
24 Ureter
25 Testicular artery and vein

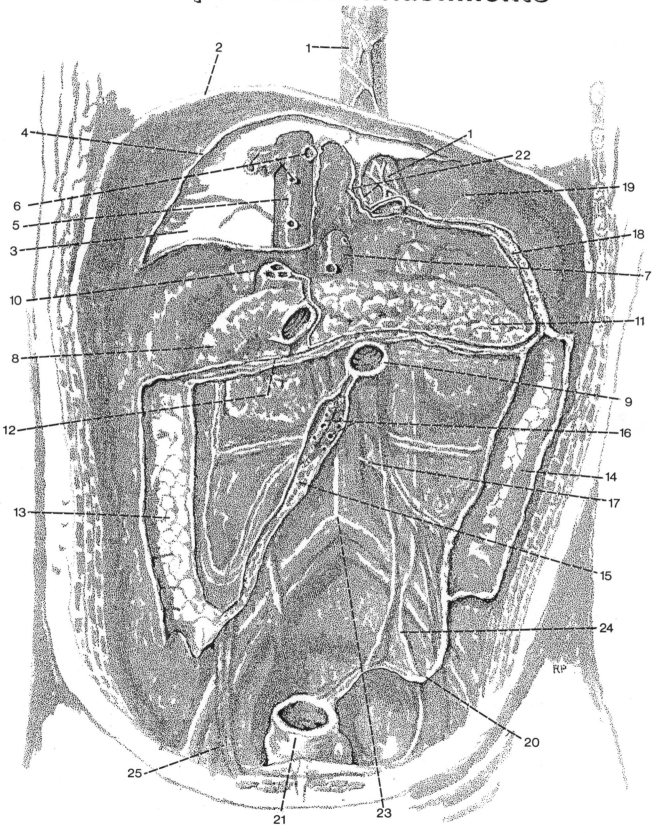

(See opposite page)

Color and label

  1   Inferior vena cava
  2   Aorta (abdominal part)
  3   Hepatic veins
  4   Inferior phrenic artery
  5   Superior suprarenal artery
  6   Suprarenal artery
  7   Inferior suprarenal artery
  8   Celiac trunk (*cut*)
  9   Superior mesenteric artery
10   Renal artery
11   Renal vein
12   Testicular artery
13   Testicular vein
14   Pampiniform plexus
15   Common iliac artery and vein
16   External iliac artery
17   Internal iliac artery
18   Middle sacral artery and vein
19   Inferior mesenteric artery
20   Superior rectal artery
21   Sigmoid arteries (*cut*)
22   Esophagus
23   Left vagus nerve
24   Suprarenal gland
25   Kidney
26   Ureter
27   Rectum
28   Sigmoid mesocolon
29   Urinary bladder
30   Pelvic peritoneum (*cut*)
31   Subcostal nerve (T12)
32   Iliohypogastric nerve
33   Ilioinguinal nerve
34   Lateral femoral cutaneous nerve
35   Femoral nerve
36   Genitofemoral nerve
37   Femoral branch
38   Genital branch

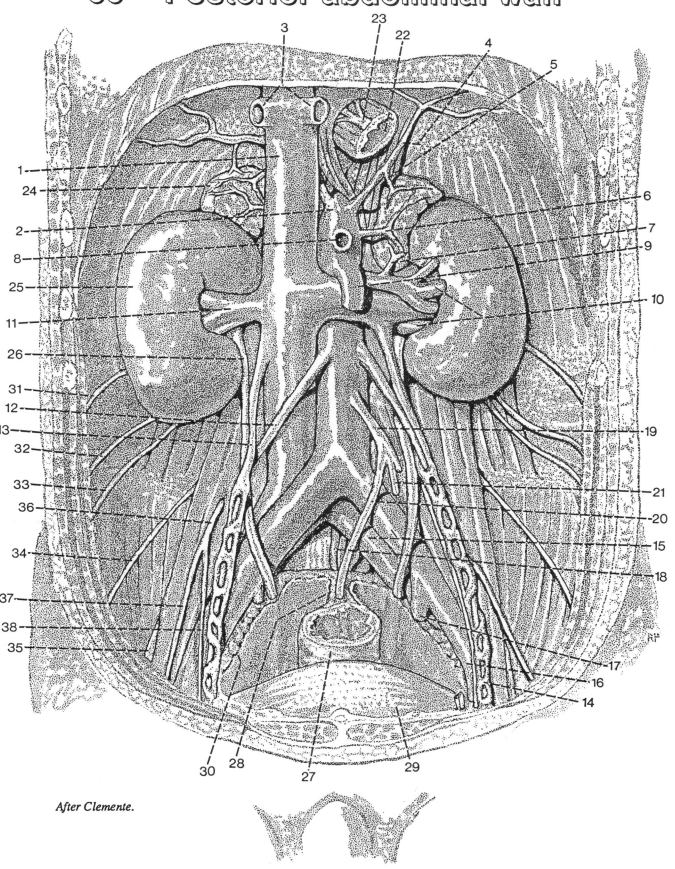

After Clemente.

**THE RIGHT KIDNEY,
ANTERIOR ASPECT**

Color and label

1 Renal artery
2 Renal vein
3 Ureter
4 Renal pelvis (*cut open*)
5 Major calix
6 Minor calix (*plural:* calices)
7 Renal pyramids (*lower four are whole, upper six are cut*)
8 Renal papillae
9 Renal sinus (*filled with renal blood vessels, fat, renal pelvis, and renal calices*)

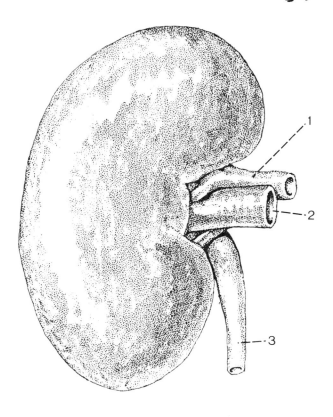

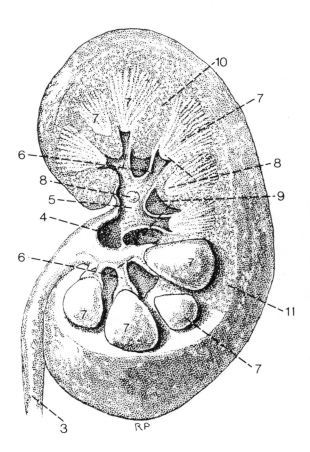

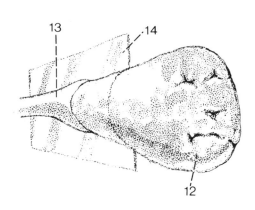

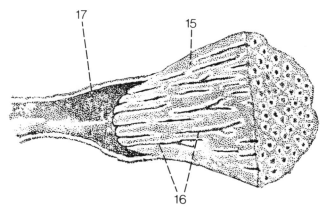

10 Renal columns (*cortical substance between renal pyramids; the medulla of the kidney consists of the renal pyramids and renal columns*)
11 Renal cortex
12 Single pyramid
13 Single minor calix
14 Plane of section
15 Portion of pyramid cut to show collecting ducts
16 Collecting ducts
17 Minor calix (*cut*)

Color and label

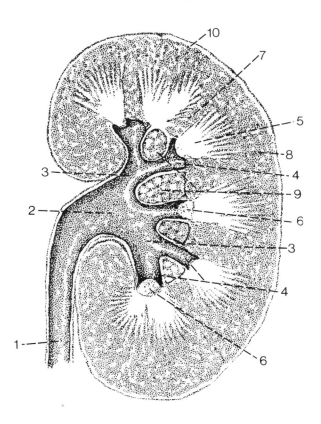

**LEFT KIDNEY
SECTIONED CORONALLY**

1 Ureter
2 Renal pelvis
3 Major calix
4 Minor calix
5 Renal pyramids
6 Renal papillae
7 Renal columns
8 Renal cortex
9 Fat in renal sinus
10 Capsule of kidney

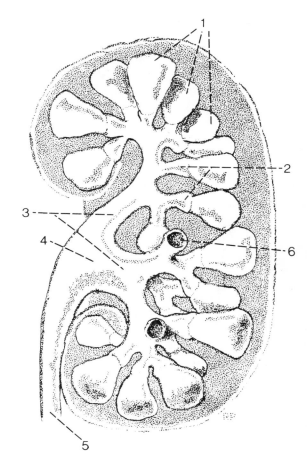

DETAIL OF CALIX AND PAPILLA

1 Minor calix enclosing papilla
2 Minor calix with papilla missing
3 Minor calix cut open to expose papilla with openings of renal duct
4 Cribriform area containing openings of renal ducts
5 Papilla
6 Pyramid

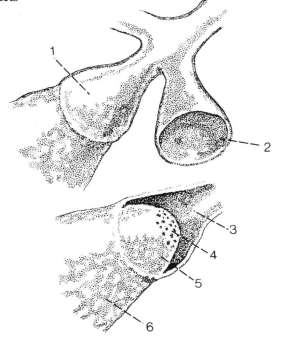

**LEFT KIDNEY
PYRAMIDS, CALICES, PELVIS,
AND URETER**

1 Renal pyramids
2 Minor calices
3 Major calices
4 Renal pelvis
5 Ureter
6 Opening of minor calix (pyramid missing)

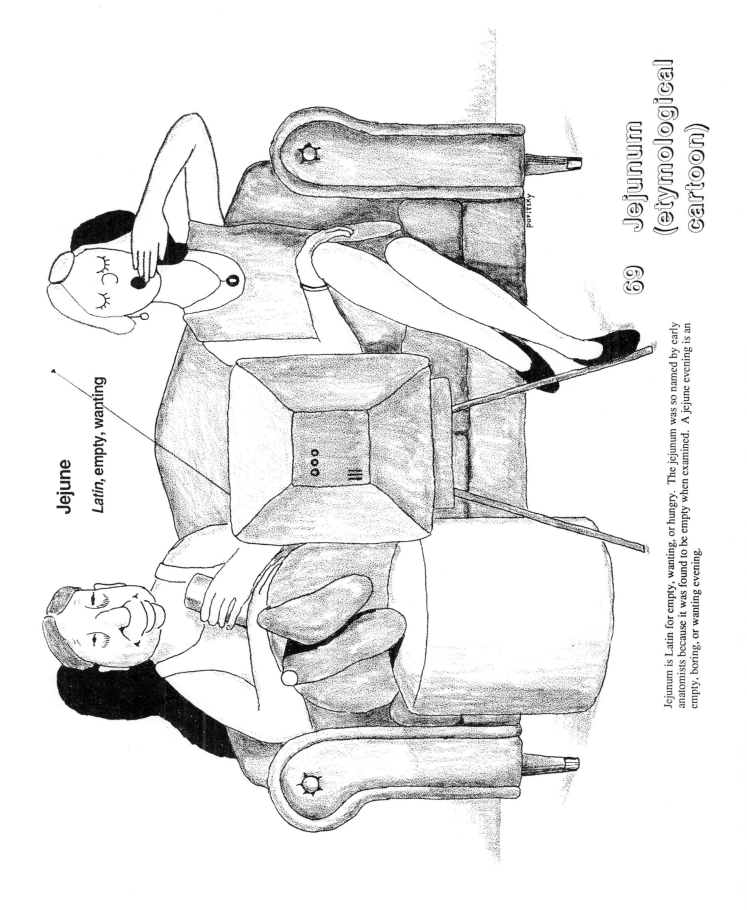

Jejune

Latin, empty, wanting

69   Jejunum
     (etymological
     cartoon)

Jejunum is Latin for empty, wanting, or hungry. The jejunum was so named by early anatomists because it was found to be empty when examined. A jejune evening is an empty, boring, or wanting evening.

PART III:

PELVIS AND PERINEUM

PLATES 70-105

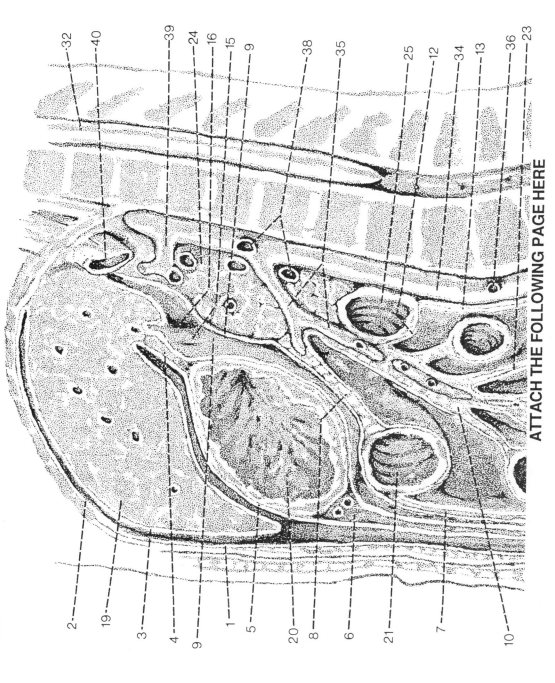

ATTACH THE FOLLOWING PAGE HERE

Trace the folding of the peritoneum and label

1   Parietal peritoneum lining inner surface of abdominal wall

2   Parietal peritoneum lining inferior surface of diaphragm

3   Peritoneum (visceral) covering most of liver

4   Lesser omentum formed by double layer of peritoneum extending from liver to stomach

5   Peritoneum covering stomach (serous layer)

6   Greater omentum suspended from greater curvature of stomach formed by outpouching and folding of embryonic dorsal mesentery (mesogastrium)

7   Greater omentum posterior layer that has secondarily fused with transverse colon and its mesentery (transverse mesocolon)

8   Transverse mesocolon

9   Peritoneum covering pancreas and lining posterior surface of omental bursa (lesser sac)

10   Mesentery of small intestine (*notice that it consists of two layers of peritoneum containing fat, blood vessels, nerves, lymphatics, and lymph nodes*)

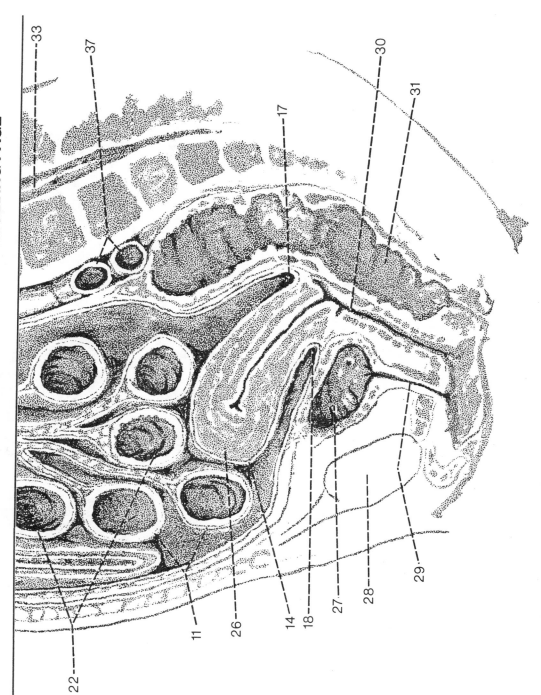

*The pancreas, duodenum, ascending colon, and descending colon orginally developed with an attached mesentery like that of the jejunum and ileum. Subsequent rotation and fusion of the gut with peritoneum of the posterior abdominal wall resulted in their losing their mesentery and becoming secondarily retroperitoneal.

After Netter and Clemente.

11 Peritoneum (visceral) surrounding jejunum and ileum except at mesenteric attachment
12 Peritoneum covering duodenum (organs behind the peritoneum such as the pancreas and duodenum do not have peritoneum on most of their surfaces and are referred to as retroperitoneal)
13 Peritoneum on posterior abdominal wall
14 Peritoneum on uterus (organs such as the stomach, transverse colon, jejunum, ileum, and uterus are almost completely covered with peritoneum, which forms their outermost tunic, the tunica serosa)
15 Omental bursa (lesser sac)
16 Omental foramen (former name: epiploic foramen)
17 Rectouterine pouch (of Douglas)
18 Vesicouterine pouch
19 Liver
20 Stomach
21 Transverse colon
22 Small intestine (jejunum and ileum)
23 Mesentery
24 Pancreas *
25 Duodenum *
26 Uterus
27 Urinary bladder
28 Pubic symphysis
29 Urethra
30 Vagina
31 Rectum
32 Spinal cord
33 Spinal canal
34 Aorta
35 Superior mesenteric artery
36 Inferior mesenteric artery
37 Common iliac artery and vein
38 Renal artery and vein
39 Celiac trunk
40 Esophagus

ANTERIOR VIEW

Color and label

1 Anterior superior iliac spine
2 Anterior inferior iliac spine
3 Iliopectineal eminence
4 Iliac fossa
5 Iliac crest
6 Ischial spine
7 Sacrospinal ligament
8 Sacrotuberous ligament
9 Greater sciatic foramen

10 Lesser sciatic foramen
11 Anterior longitudinal ligament
12 Anterior sacroiliac ligament
13 Iliolumbar ligament (superior band)
14 Iliolumbar ligament (inferior band)
15 Pectineal ligament (Cooper's)
16 Superior pubic ligament
17 Interpubic disc

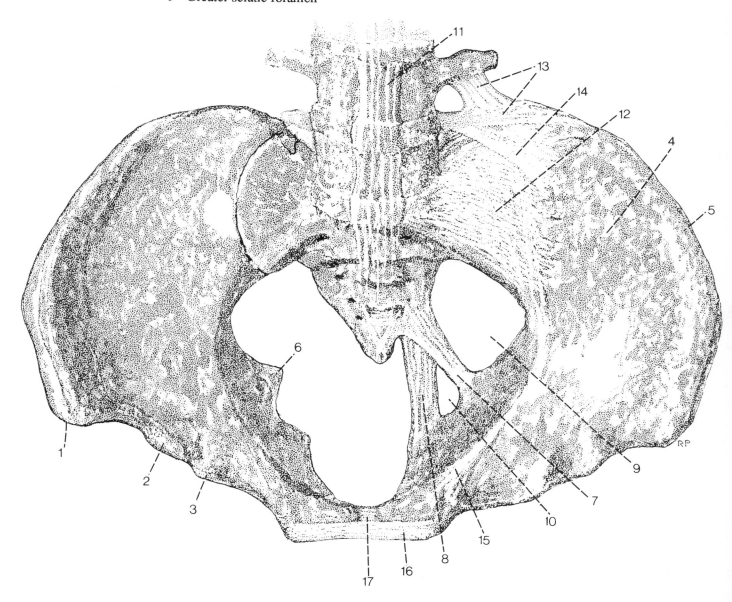

71 Pelvis and ligaments

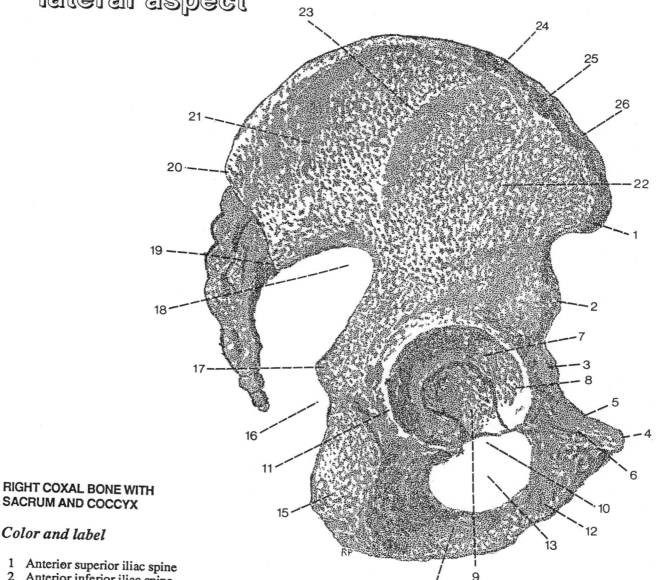

RIGHT COXAL BONE WITH SACRUM AND COCCYX

Color and label

1 Anterior superior iliac spine
2 Anterior inferior iliac spine
3 Ileopectineal eminence
4 Pubic tubercle
5 Pecten of pubic bone (pubis)
6 Superior ramus of pubic bone
7 Acetabulum *(Latin, vinegar cup)*
8 Lunate surface (covered with articular cartilage)
9 Acetabular fossa
10 Acetabular notch
11 Border (lumbus) of acetabulum
12 Inferior ramus of pubic bone
13 Obturator foramen *(Latin, obturo, to stop up; so named because it is stopped up by the two obturator muscles and membrane; however, the obturator canal pierces these three structures)*

14 Ramus of ischial bone (ischium)
15 Ischial tuberosity
16 Lesser sciatic notch
17 Ischial spine
18 Greater sciatic notch
19 Posterior inferior iliac spine
20 Posterior superior iliac spine
21 Posterior gluteal line
22 Ala *(Latin, wing)* of ilium
23 Anterior gluteal line
24 External lip of iliac crest
25 Intermediate lip of iliac crest
26 Internal lip of iliac crest

Color and label

1. Ilium *(present at birth)*
2. Ischium *(present at birth)*
3. Pubis *(present at birth)*
4. Acetabulum *(fuses at 15 years)*
5. Iliac crest *(appears at 16 years; fuses at 25 years)*

6. Anterior inferior iliac spine *(appears at 16 years; fuses at 25 years)*
7. Pubic tubercle *(appears at 16 years; fuses at 25 years)*
8. Ischial tuberosity *(appears at 16 years; fuses at 30 years)*

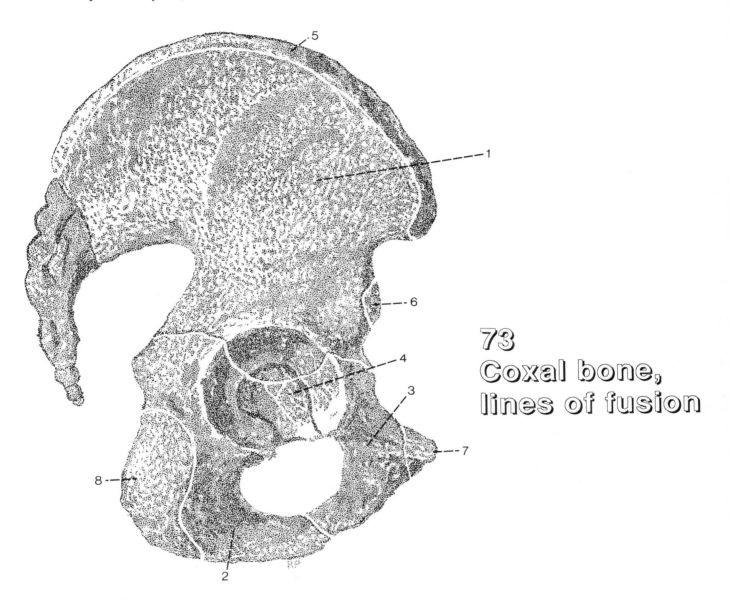

73
Coxal bone, lines of fusion

Notice how the coxal bone is formed by the ilium, pubis, and ischium as well as separate centers of ossification (epiphyses) that fuse with the main portion of bone. Notice how the ilium, ischium, and pubis each form part of the socket-like acetabulum. The ilium, ischium, and pubis are present at birth and fuse together at 15 years. However, at birth they are widely separated by cartilage. The iliac crest, anterior inferior iliac spine, pubic tubercle, and ischial tuberosity are formed as epiphyses and do not even appear as ossification centers until 16 years and fuse at 25-30 years.

Color the origins (O) red and the insertions (I) blue

1 Transversus abdominis (O)
2 Internal abdominal oblique (O)
3 External abdominal oblique (I)
4 Tensor fasciae latae (0)
5 Sartorius (O)
6 Rectus femoris (O)
7 Pectineus (O)
8 External abdominal oblique (I
   (*via inguinal ligament*)
9 Adductor longus (O)
10 Obturator externus (O)
11 Adductor brevis (O)

12 Gracilis (O)
13 Adductor magnus (O)
14 Quadratus femoris (O)
15 Semitendinosus (O) and biceps femoris (O)
16 Semimembranosus (O)
17 Gemellus inferioris (O)
18 Gemellus superioris (O)
19 Piriformis (O)
20 Gluteus minimus (O)
21 Gluteus medius (O)
22 Gluteus maximus (O)

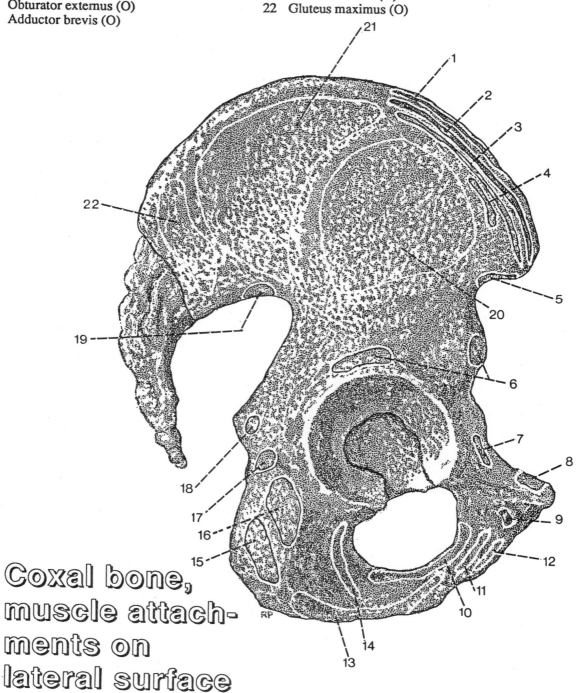

74 Coxal bone, muscle attachments on lateral surface

75 Coxal bone, medial view

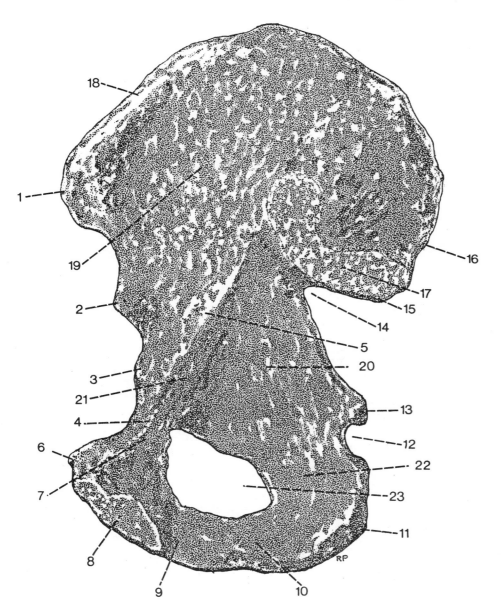

Color and label

1 Anterior superior iliac spine
2 Anterior inferior iliac spine
3 Iliopectineal eminence
4 Pecten of pubic bone
5 Arcuate line
6 Pubic tubercle
7 Superior ramus of pubic bone
8 Symphysis surface
9 Inferior ramus of pubic bone
10 Ramus of ischium
11 Ischial tuberosity

12 Lesser sciatic notch
13 Ischial spine
14 Greater sciatic notch
15 Posterior inferior iliac spine
16 Posterior superior iliac spine
17 Auricular surface for sacroiliac joint
18 Iliac crest
19 Iliac fossa
20 Body of ilium
21 Body of pubis
22 Body of ischium
23 Obturator foramen

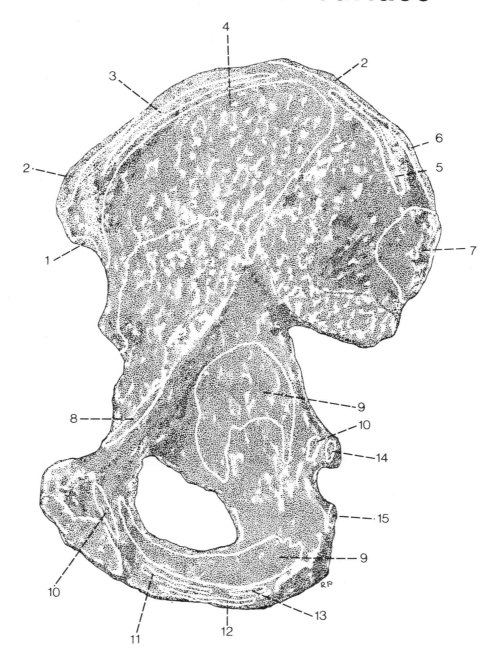

Color and label (all are origins, O)

1   Sartorius muscle (O)
2   Internal abdominal oblique
    muscle (O)
3   Transverse abdominal muscle (O)
4   Iliacus muscle (O)
5   Quadratus lumborum muscle (O)
6   Latissimus dorsi muscle (O)
7   Erector spinae muscle (O)

8   Pectineus muscle (O)
9   Obturator internus muscle (O)
10 Levator ani muscle (O)
11 Deep transverse perineus muscle (O)
12 Ischiocavernosus muscle (O)
13 Superficial transverse perineus muscle (O)
14 Coccygeus muscle (O)
15 Gemellus superior muscle (O)

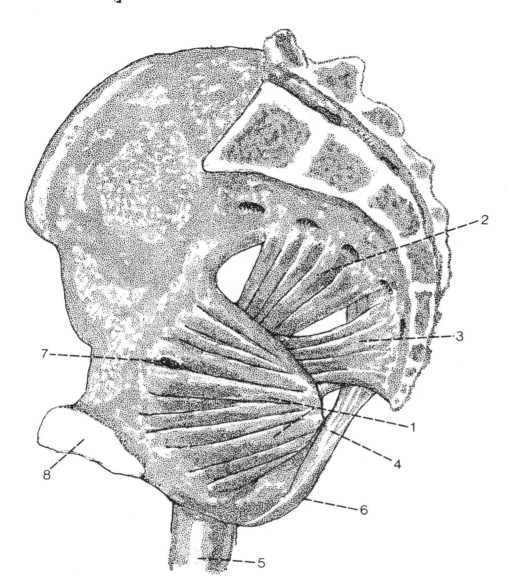

Color and label

1 Obturator internus muscle (notice it leaves the pelvis via the lesser sciatic foramen and inserts on the femur)
2 Piriformis muscle
3 Coccygeus muscle

4 Sacrotuberous ligament
5 Femur
6 Ischial tuberosity
7 Obturator canal
8 Pubic symphysis

After Spalterholz and Spanner.

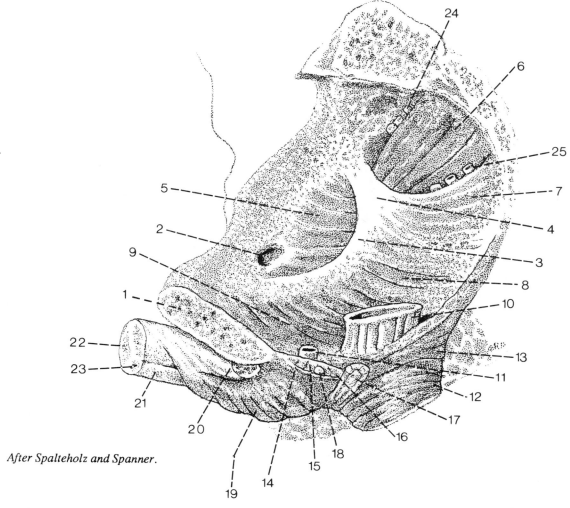

After Spalteholz and Spanner.

Viewed from the left; the pelvis has been sectioned sagittally to the left of the rectum and penis

Color and label

1 Pubic bone
2 Obturator canal
3 Tendinous arch of levator ani muscle
4 Ischial spine
5 Obturator internus muscle
6 Piriformis muscle
7 Coccygeus muscle (*coccygeus + levator ani = pelvic diaphragm*)
8 Iliococcygeus muscle (levator ani)
9 Pubococcygeus muscle (levator ani)
10 Rectum (*cut*)
11 Urethra (*cut*)
12 External anal sphincter
13 Puborectalis muscle (levator ani)

14 Inferior fascia of urogenital diaphragm (*also called perineal membrane; the upper fascia of the urogenital diaphragm does not exist; the urogenital diaphragm is not the commonly illustrated sandwich of muscle between two fascial layers*)
15 Sphincter urethrae muscle
16 Deep transverse perineus muscle
17 Superficial perineus muscle
18 Bulbourethral glands
19 Bulbospongiosus muscle
20 Crus of penis (*cut*)
21 Corpus spongiosum penis (*cut*)
22 Corpus cavernosum penis (*cut*)
23 Urethra (*cut*)
24 Superior gluteal nerve, artery, and vein
25 Inferior gluteal nerve, artery, and vein

Color and label

1 Skin
2 Superficial (fatty) layer of superficial fascia (Camper's)
3 Deep membranous layer of superficial fascia (Scarpa's)
4 Dartos tunic (*a sheet of smooth muscle comprising the superficial fascia of the scrotum*)
5 Skin of scrotum
6 Testis (*covered with tunica vaginalis*)
7 Epididymis
8 Cut edge of parietal layer of tunica vaginalis testis
9 Testicular vein forming pampiniform plexus
10 Ductus (vas) deferens
11 Superior ramus of pubic bone
12 Ramus of ischium

13 Membranous layer of superficial fascia (Colles')
14 Puborectalis muscle (*part of levator ani muscle*)
15 Levator ani
16 Rectum
17 Peritoneum (*cut edge*)
18 Prostate gland
19 Bladder
20 Seminal vesicle
21 Ureter (*cut*)
22 Superficial fascia of penis
23 Corpus cavernosus penis
24 Corpus spongiosum
25 Prepuce of penis
26 Glans
27 External anal sphincter

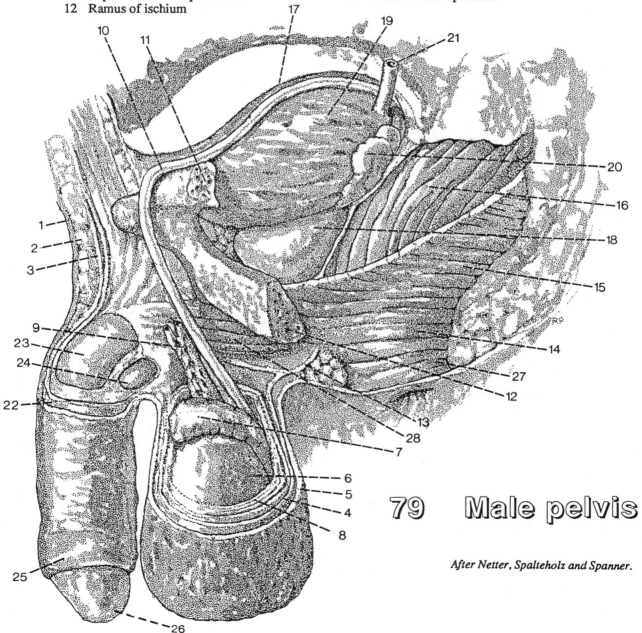

79 Male pelvis

After Netter, Spalteholz and Spanner.

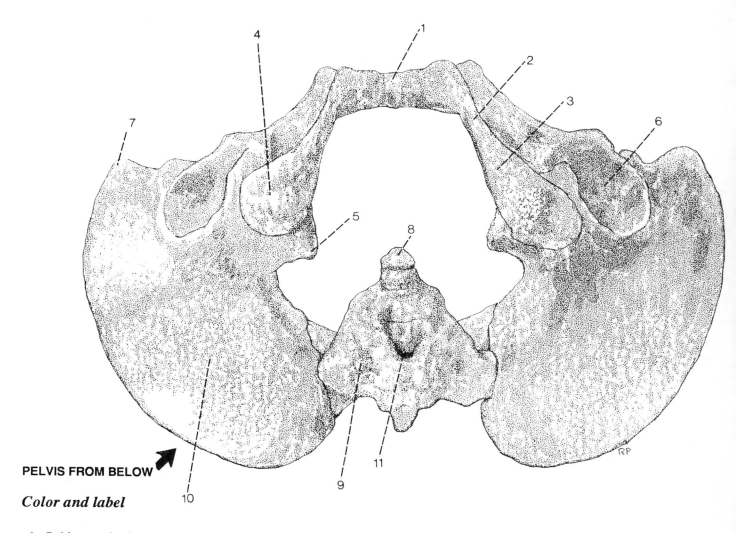

PELVIS FROM BELOW

Color and label

1 Pubic symphysis
2 Inferior ramus of pubic bone
3 Ramus of ischial bone
4 Ischial tuberosity
5 Ischial spine
6 Acetabulum
7 Anterior superior iliac spine
8 Coccyx
9 Sacrum
10 Ala of ilium
11 Sacral hiatus and sacral canal

OUTLINE AND TRIANGLES OF PERINEUM FROM BELOW

Connect the points

1 Pubic symphysis to
2 Ischial tuberosity *(right)* to
3 Coccyx to
4 Ischial tuberosity *(left)* to
1 Pubic symphysis
    *Connect right and left ischial tuberosities
    (2 and 4), thus dividing the perineum into
    an anterior urogenital triangle and a
    posterior anal triangle*
5 Urogenital triangle
6 Anal triangle

80   Pelvis and perineum

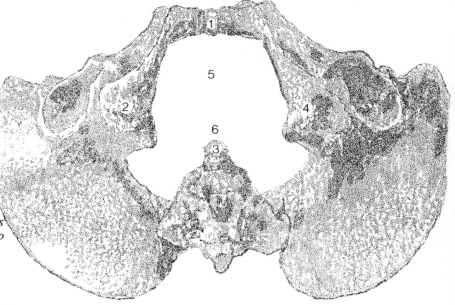

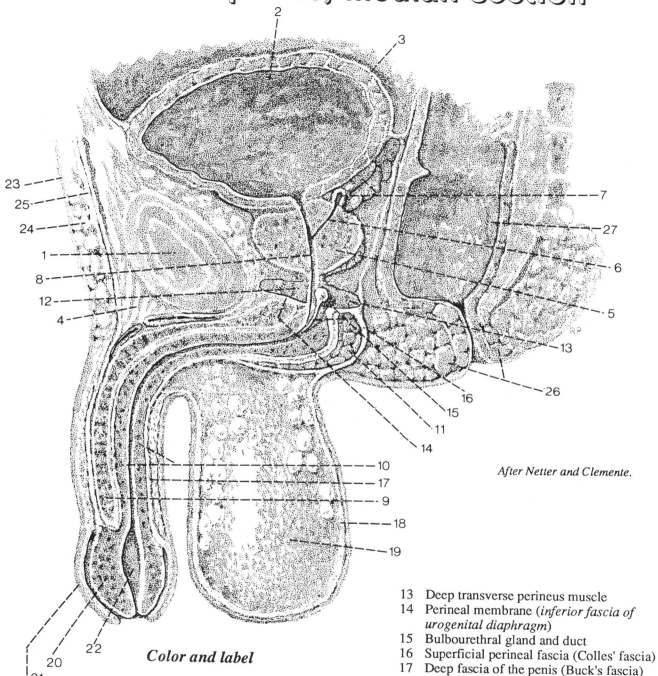

After Netter and Clemente.

Color and label

1 Pubic symphysis
2 Bladder
3 Peritoneum
4 Suspensory ligament of penis
5 Prostate gland
6 Ejaculatory duct
7 Ductus deferens (ampulla)
8 Urethra
9 Corpus cavernosum penis
10 Corpus spongiosum penis
11 Bulbospongiosus muscle
12 Sphincter urethrae muscle

13 Deep transverse perineus muscle
14 Perineal membrane (*inferior fascia of urogenital diaphragm*)
15 Bulbourethral gland and duct
16 Superficial perineal fascia (Colles' fascia)
17 Deep fascia of the penis (Buck's fascia)
18 Dartos tunic (*smooth muscle in the skin of the scrotum and penis*)
19 Septum of scrotum
20 Glans penis
21 Prepuce of penis (*a fold of skin that covers the glans penis; removed in circumcision*)
22 Navicular fossa of the urethra
23 Skin
24 Superficial layer of superficial fascia (Camper's)
25 Deep layer of superficial fascia (Scarpa's)
26 External anal sphincter
27 Rectum

THREE ERECTILE BODIES

Skin, superficial fascia, and muscles covering roots have been removed.

Color and label

1 Corpus spongiosum (*contains spongy party of urethra*)
2 Glans (*this is the expanded terminal portion of the corpus spongiosum*)
3 Corpus cavernosum penis (*plural: corpora cavernosa*)
4 Bulb of penis (*the bulbospongiosus muscle has been removed*)
5 Crus of penis (*the two crura are each attached to the ischiopubic ramus and to the perineal membrane*)
6 Perineal membrane*

Although most books call this the inferior fascial layer of the urogenital diaphragm, it should be called the perineal membrane since there is no superior fascial layer.

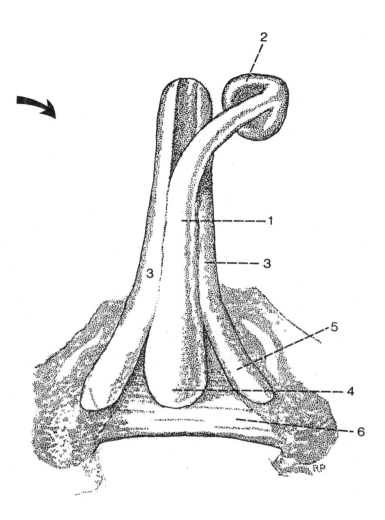

82 Penis

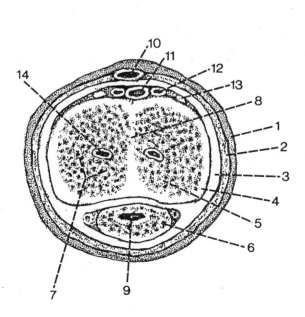

BODY OF PENIS IN CROSS SECTION

Color and label

1 Skin
2 Loose connective tissue (superficial fascia)
3 Deep fascia of penis (Buck's fascia)
4 Tunica albuginea
5 Corpus cavernosum penis
6 Corpus spongiosum penis
7 Erectile tissue with cavernous spaces*
8 Septum
9 Urethra (*spongy part*)
10 Superficial dorsal vein of penis
11 Deep dorsal vein of penis
12 Dorsal artery of penis
13 Dorsal nerve of penis**
14 Deep artery of penis

The penis becomes erect and enlarged by blood filling the cavernous spaces in the erectile tissue.
**Notice that the dorsal artery and deep dorsal vein and the dorsal nerve of the penis are deep to the deep fascia (below Buck's fascia).*

Color and label

1 Spermatic cord
2 Ductus deferens
3 Epididymis (head)
4 Pampiniform plexus (*drains into testicular vein; acts as counter-current heat exchanger with testicular artery, thus cooling arterial blood*)
5 Testicular artery
6 Ductus deferens artery (*arises from patent part of umbilical artery*)
7 Testis (*covered with visceral layer of tunica vaginalis*)
8 Superficial inguinal ring

9 Ilioinguinal nerve
10 Genitofemoral nerve (*genital branch; supplies cremaster muscle*)
11 Tunica vaginalis (*parietal layer*)
12 External spermatic fascia
13 Cremasteric fascia and muscle
14 Internal spermatic fascia
15 Epididymis (*isolated with efferent ductules*)
16 Testis (*sectioned with lobules*)
17 Skin of scrotum
18 Dartos tunic (*smooth muscle*)
19 Septum of scrotum

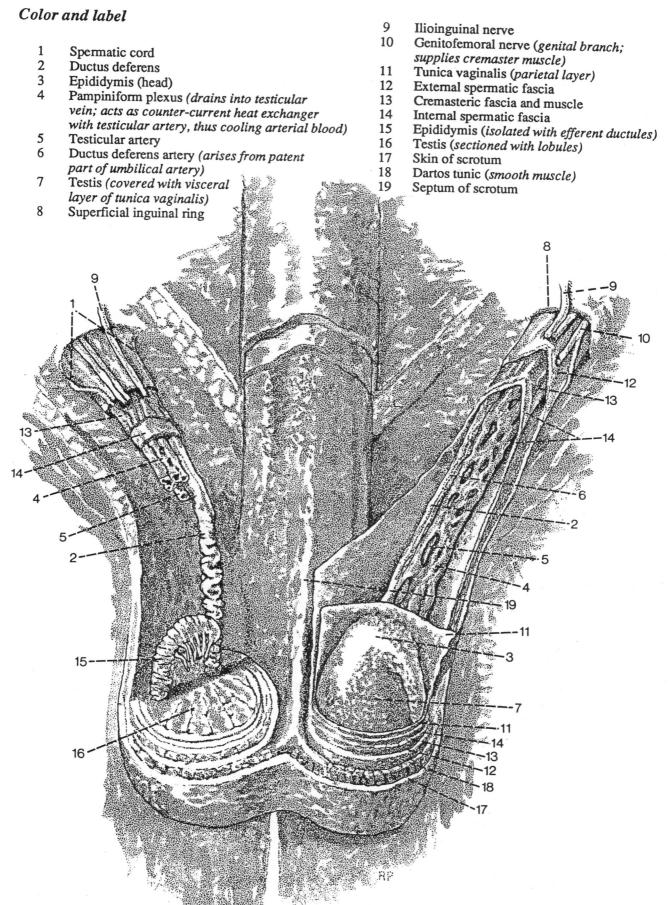

83 Scrotum and spermatic cord

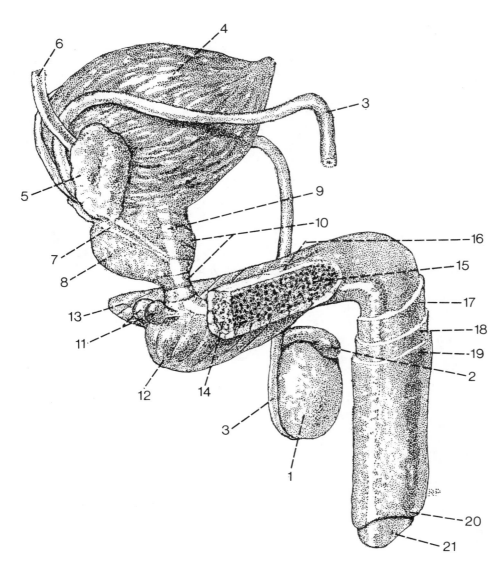

Color and label

1 Testis
2 Epididymis *(Greek, upon the twin, i.e., the testes)*
3 Ductus deferens
4 Bladder
5 Seminal vesicle
6 Ureter *(cut)*
7 Ejaculatory duct *(common duct for ductus deferens and seminal vesicle; conveys semen to urethra)*
8 Prostate gland
9 Prostatic urethra
10 Urethral spincter muscle
11 Bulbourethral glands
12 Bulb of penis and bulbospongiosus muscle
13 Left crus of penis and ischiocavernosus muscle
14 Right crus of penis *(cut showing cavernous spaces in erectile tissue)*
15 Site of attachment to ischipubic ramus
16 Site of attachment to perineal membrane
17 Deep fascia of penis
18 Superficial fascia of penis
19 Skin of penis
20 Prepuce (foreskin)
21 Glans

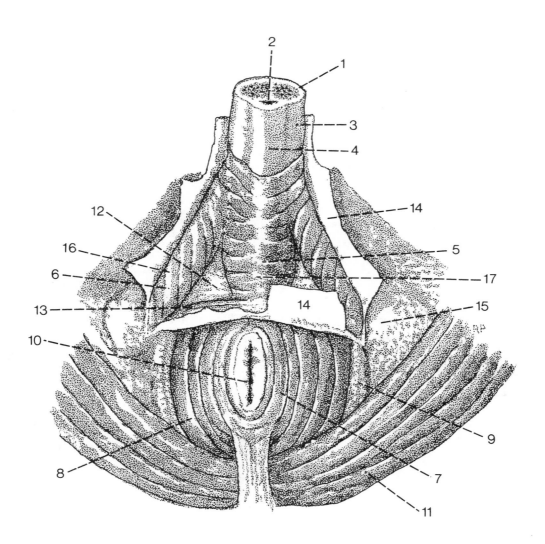

INFERIOR VIEW

Color and label

1 Penis (*cut*)
2 Urethra
3 Corpus cavernosum penis
4 Corpus spongiosum penis
5 Bulbospongiosus muscle
6 Ischiocavernosus muscle
7 External anal sphincter
8 Levator ani (*normally this wedge shaped space is filled with fat and is called ischiorectal fossa and ischiorectal fat pad*)
9 Pudendal canal
10 Anus

11 Gluteus maximus muscle
12 Perineal membrane
13 Superficial transverse perineus muscle
14 Superficial perineal fascia (Colles', *cut and partially reflected*)
15 Ischial tuberosity
16 Crus of penis (*that portion of the corpus cavernosus that is attached to both the inferior pubic ramus and the perineal membrane; covered by ischiocavernosus muscle*)
17 Bulb of penis (*enlarged proximal part of of the corpus spongiosum; covered by bulbospongiosus muscle*)

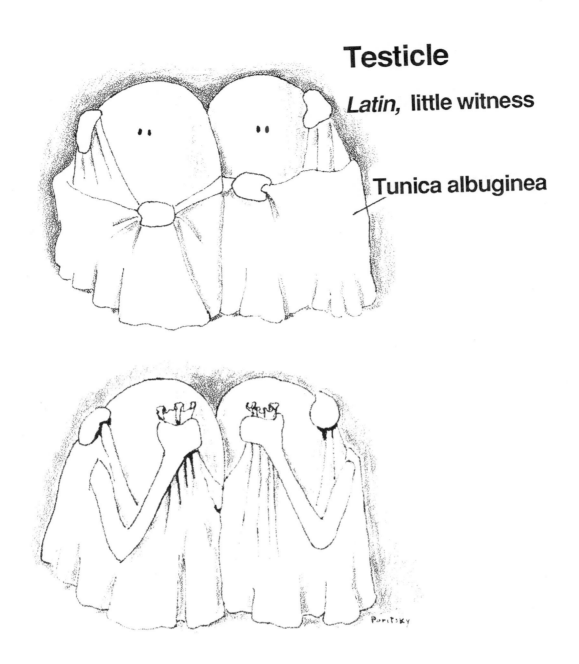

Testicle

Latin, **little witness**

Tunica albuginea

86 Testicle (etymological cartoon)

Testis, which means witness in Latin — testicle being little witness — is probably derived from the Romans' allowing only men to testify in court. Thus, having and displaying testes would prove one to be male, and hence, qualified to testify (or to give testimony). Another somewhat different origin may be the ancient Israelites' custom of holding one another's scrotum (and testes) when swearing an oath. A third explanation could be the Romans' referring to the testes as "peepers" or "lookers-on" since the testes would be in a position to witness the sexual act close up.

Top figure: Normal testes   Bottom figure: Embarrassed testes

Tunica albuginea, white tunic, one of the coverings of the testis

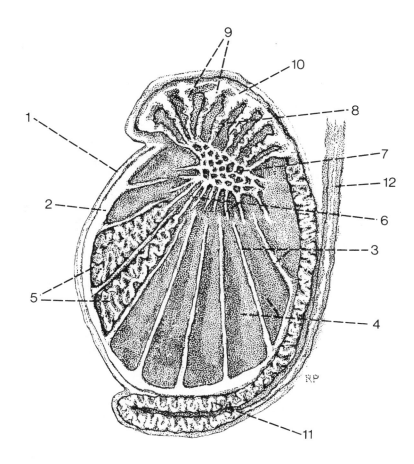

Sectioned to show internal structure

Color and label

1   Tunica vaginalis (*visceral layer; the tunica vaginalis is derived from the peritoneum when the testis descends into the scrotum during development*)
2   Tunica albuginea
3   Septula (septums) testis
4   Lobules of testis (*shown empty*)
5   Seminiferous tubules (*contorted part*)
6   Seminiferous tubules (*straight part*)
7   Rete (*Latin, net*) testis
8   Efferent ductules of testis
9   Lobules of epididymis
10 Head of epididymis
11 Tail of epididymis (*the epididymis is extremely coiled; unraveled, its total length is about 3 meters*)
12 Ductus deferens

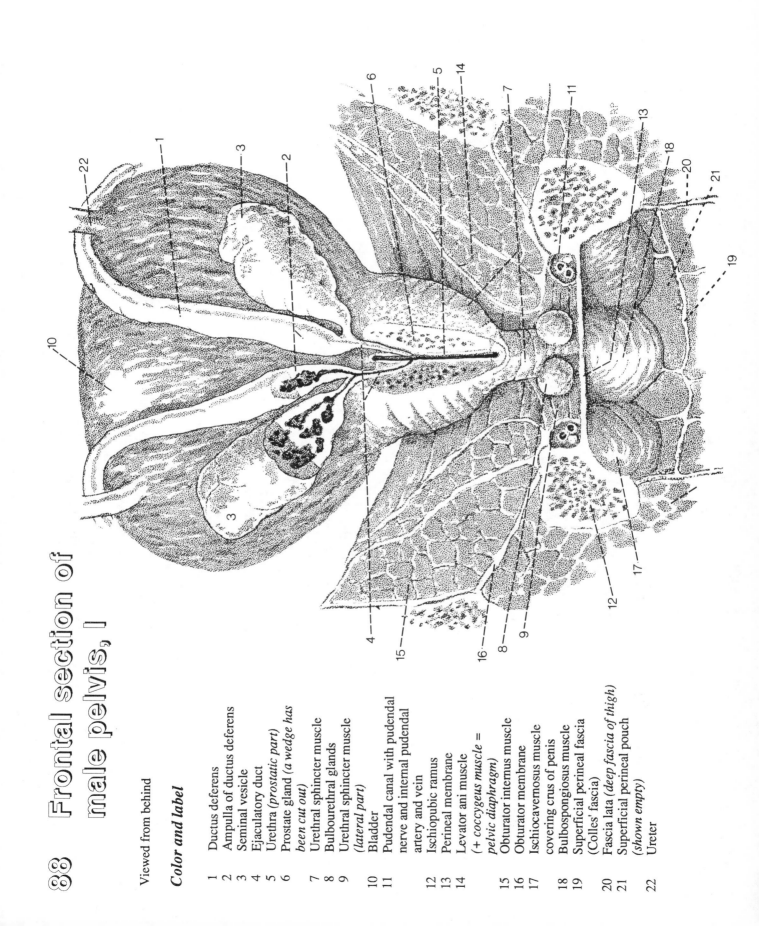

88 Frontal section of male pelvis, I

Viewed from behind

Color and label

1   Ductus deferens
2   Ampulla of ductus deferens
3   Seminal vesicle
4   Ejaculatory duct
5   Urethra *(prostatic part)*
6   Prostate gland *(a wedge has been cut out)*
7   Urethral sphincter muscle
8   Bulbourethral glands
9   Urethral sphincter muscle *(lateral part)*
10 Bladder
11 Pudendal canal with pudendal nerve and internal pudendal artery and vein
12 Ischiopubic ramus
13 Perineal membrane
14 Levator ani muscle *(+ coccygeus muscle = pelvic diaphragm)*
15 Obturator internus muscle
16 Obturator membrane
17 Ischiocavernosus muscle covering crus of penis
18 Bulbospongiosus muscle
19 Superficial perineal fascia (Colles' fascia)
20 Fascia lata *(deep fascia of thigh)*
21 Superficial perineal pouch *(shown empty)*
22 Ureter

Frontal section of male pelvis, II

(See opposite page)

FIGURE ON RIGHT:
Cut at right angle to the perineal membrane
(after Oelrich); looking dorsally

Color and label

1 Perineal membrane
2 Urethra (*membranous part*)
3 Urethral sphincter mucle
4 Ejaculatory duct
5 Prostate gland
6 Ductus deferens (ampulla)
7 Seminal vesicle
8 Pelvic diaphragm
9 Obturator internus muscle
10 Inferior pubic ramus
11 Corpus cavernosus penis
12 Ischiocavernosus muscle
13 Corpus spongiosum penis
14 Bulbospongiosus muscle
15 Superficial perineal fascia (Colles')
16 Deep perineal fascia (Buck's)
17 Obturator membrane
18 Pudendal canal with internal pudendal
   artery, vein, and pudendal nerve
19 Fascia lata (*deep fascia of thigh*)
20 Ilium
21 Sheath of prostate
22 Transversalis fascia
23 Puboprostatic ligament

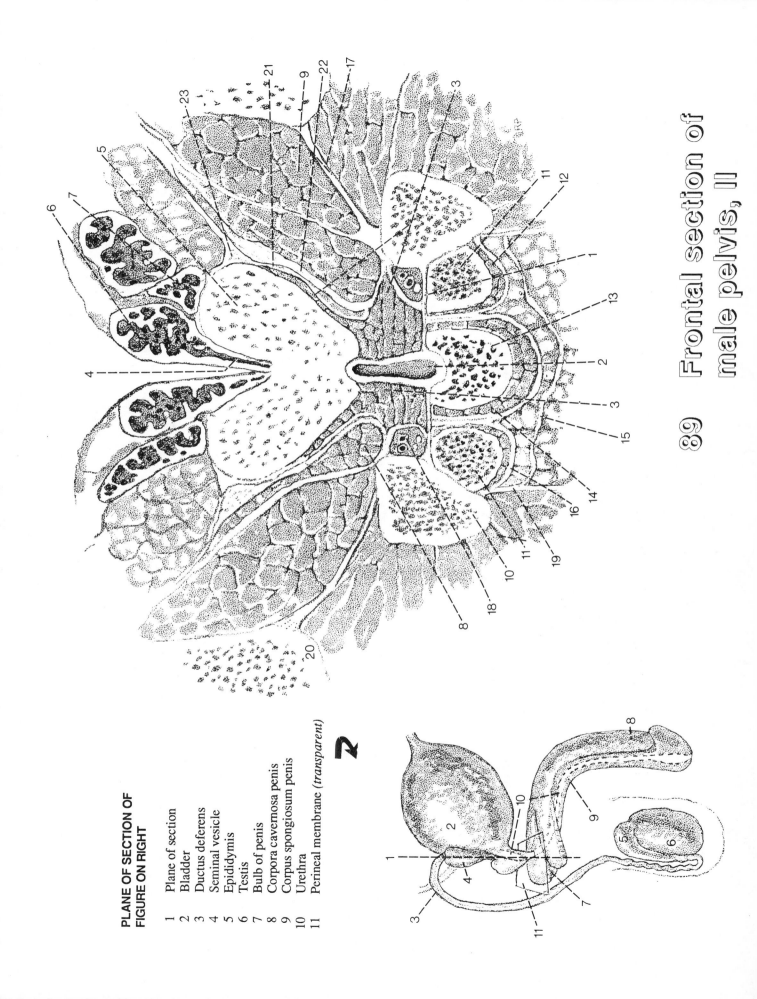

PLANE OF SECTION OF FIGURE ON RIGHT

1 Plane of section
2 Bladder
3 Ductus deferens
4 Seminal vesicle
5 Epididymis
6 Testis
7 Bulb of penis
8 Corpora cavernosa penis
9 Corpus spongiosum penis
10 Urethra
11 Perineal membrane (*transparent*)

89   Frontal section of male pelvis, II

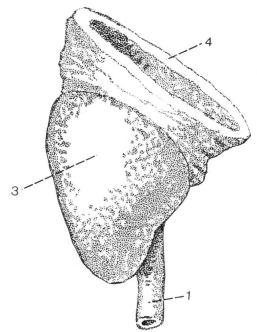

**LATERAL VIEW WITH URETHRAL
SPHINCTER MUSCLE REMOVED**

Color and label

1   Urethra
2   Urethral sphincter muscle
3   Prostate gland
4   Bladder (lower part)
5   Lateral part of urethral
     sphincter muscle

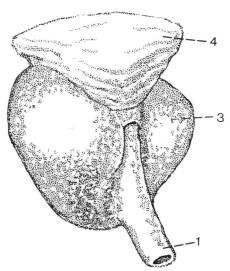

**OBLIQUE VIEW WITH URETHRAL
SPHINCTER MUSCLE REMOVED**

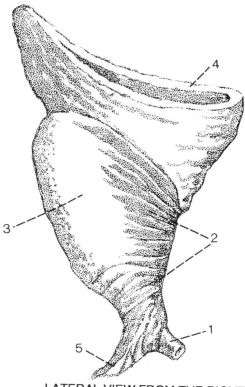

LATERAL VIEW FROM THE RIGHT

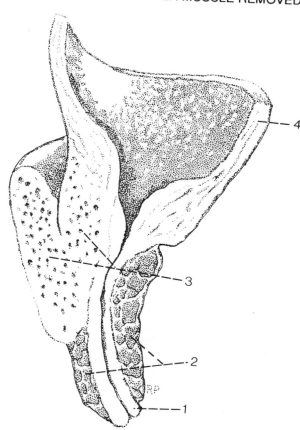

**MEDIAN SECTION SHOWING EXTENT OF CONTACT
BETWEEN URETHRA AND URETHRAL SPHINCTER**

Notice that the urethral sphincter is vertical rather than flat as pictured in most anatomy books. It encircles the front and sides of the urethra and spreads dorsally and laterally. The concept of a urogenital diaphragm of muscle sandwiched between two horizontal membranes of fascia is not correct. The inferior fascia layer of perineal membrane does exist. However, there is not a superior fascia and the urethral sphincter and deep transverse perineus muscle do not form a flat diaphragm, but are as pictured here (after Oelrich, 1980).

Color and label

1 Uterus (body)
2 Cervix of uterus
3 Vagina
4 Rectouterine pouch (of Douglas)
5 Bladder
6 Urethra
7 Anus
8 Rectum
9 Round ligament of uterus
10 Transverse vesical fold
11 Uterine tube (ampulla)
12 Ovary
13 Fimbriae
14 Infundibulum
15 Suspensory ligament of the ovary
16 Ligament of the ovary
17 Posterior lip of the uterus
18 Glans of clitoris and prepuce
19 Pubic symphysis
20 Posterior fornix of vagina
21 Vesicouterine pouch

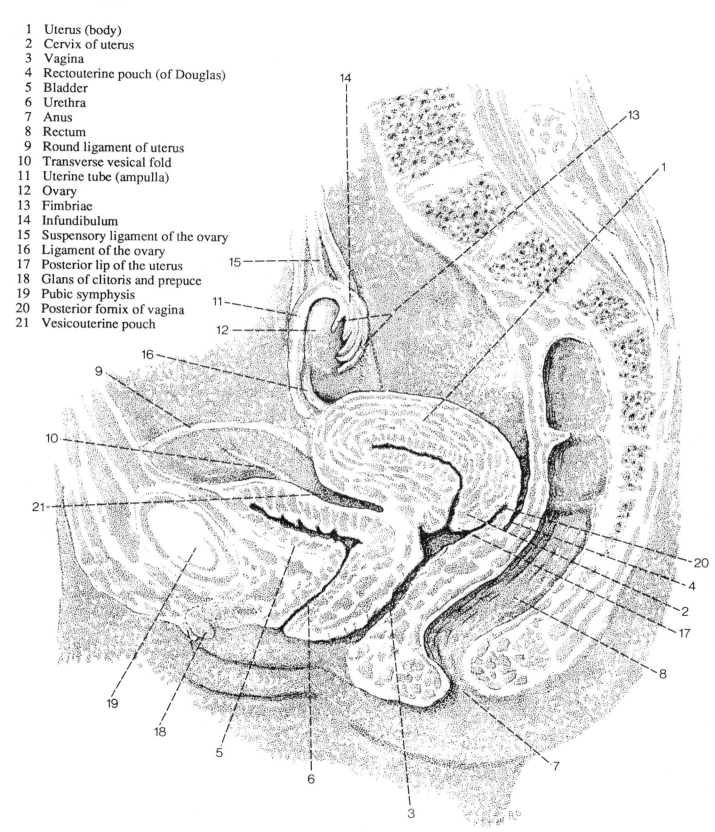

91   Female pelvis, median section

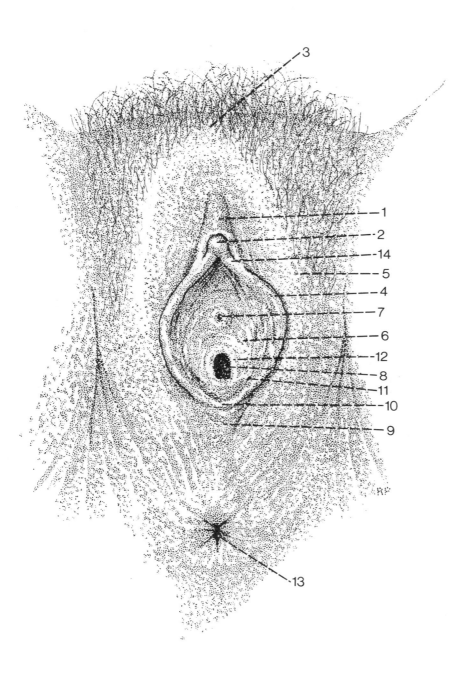

Color and label

1	Prepuce of clitoris	8	Ostium of vagina
2	Glans of clitoris	9	Posterior labial commissure
3	Mons pubis	10	Frenulum of labia minora (Forchet)
4	Labium minus pudendi	11	Opening of greater vestibular glands
5	Labium majus pudendi	12	Hymen
6	Vestibule of vagina	13	Anus
7	External urethral ostium	14	Frenulum of clitoris

Color and label

1 Suspensory ligament of clitoris
2 Body of crus of clitoris
3 Bulbospongiosus muscle *(covering bulb of vestibule and greater vestibular gland)*
4 Ischiocavernosus muscle *(covering crus of clitoris)*
5 Gland of clitoris
6 External urethral orifice

7 Vagina
8 Labium minus *(cut)*
9 Perineal membrane
10 Superficial transverse perineus muscle
11 Levator ani
12 External anal sphincter muscle
13 Anus
14 Gluteus maximus muscle

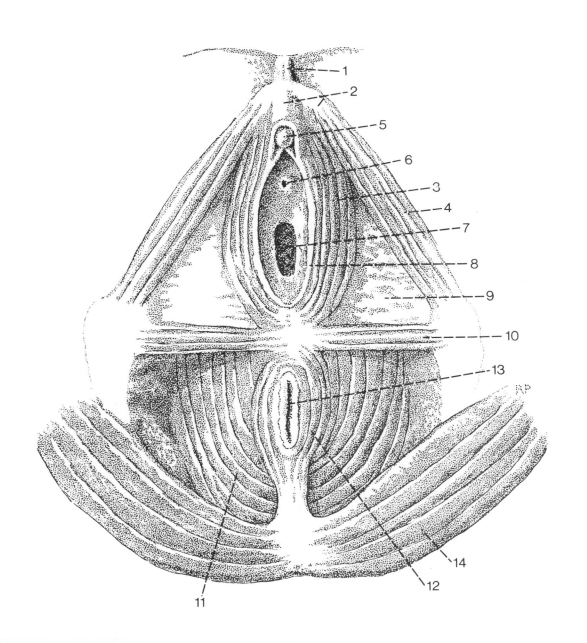

Color and label

1 Suspensory ligament of clitoris
2 Body of clitoris
3 Glans of clitoris
4 Vestibular bulb (*the clitoris and vestibular bulb consist of erectile tissue and become tumescent during sexual arousal*)
5 Commissure of vestibular bulb (*joins the two vestibular bulbs to the underside of the clitoris; the clitoris is richly supplied with nerves and its stimulation plays a dominant role in sexual response*)

6 Left crus of clitoris
7 Greater vestibular gland and duct (*Bartholin's gland; secretes a lubricating mucus*)
8 External urethral orifice
9 Labium minus (*cut*)
10 Orifice of greater vestibular glands

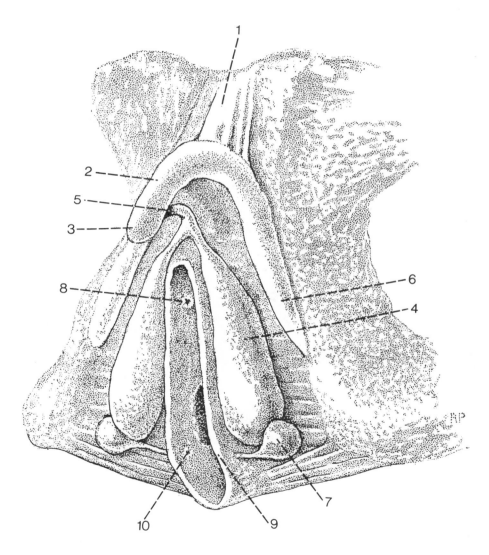

94   Female erectile tissue

Color and label

1   Clitoris (*prepuce removed*)
2   Vestibule of vagina
3   Anus
4   Superficial transverse perineus muscle (*cut on viewer's right*)
5   Gluteus maximus muscle
6   Labium majus pudendi (*cut*)

7   Perineal nerve (*a branch of the pudendal nerve, gives off posterior labial nerves and supplies bulbospongiosus and and ischiocavernosus muscles and the bulb of the vestibule*)
8   Posterior labial nerves
9   Inferior rectal nerves
10   Dorsal nerve of clitoris
11   Posterior femoral cutaneous nerve
12   Perineal branch of posterior femoral cutaneous nerve
13   Inferior clunial nerve

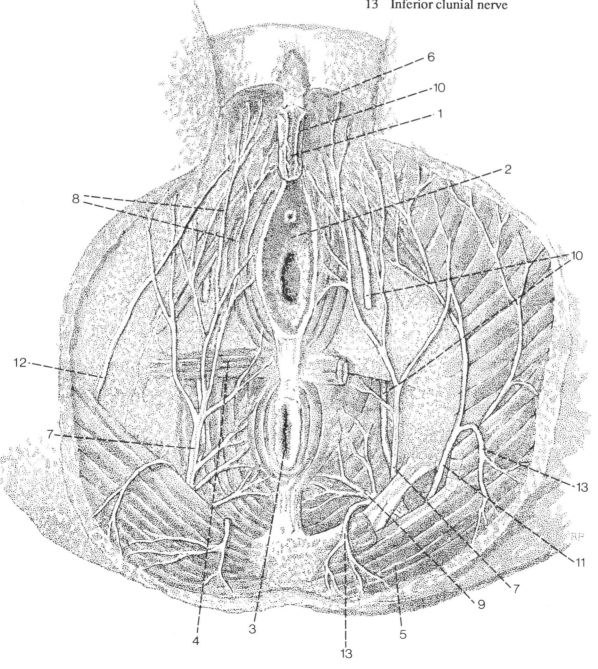

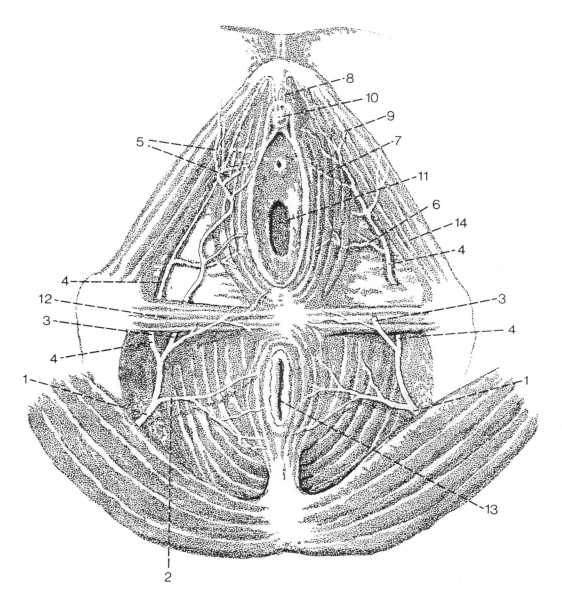

Color and label

1 Internal pudendal artery
2 Inferior rectal artery
3 Perineal artery (*cut on left side*)
4 Artery of clitoris*
5 Posterior labial arteries
6 Artery of vestibular bulb
7 Urethral artery

8 Dorsal artery of the clitoris
9 Deep artery of the clitoris
10 Glans of clitoris
11 Vagina
12 Superficial transverse perineus muscle
13 Anus
14 Ischiocavernosus muscle

*Partly exposed deep to perineal membrane; not listed in Nomina Anatomica.

Blood supply of male pelvis

(See opposite page)

Color and label

1 Abdominal aorta
2 Left common iliac artery and vein *(cut)*
3 Inferior mesenteric artery
4 Right common iliac artery
5 Right external iliac artery and vein
6 Inferior epigastric artery
7 Deep circumflex iliac artery
8 Right internal iliac artery
9 Anterior trunk of internal iliac artery *
10 Posterior trunk of internal iliac artery *
11 Umbilical artery
12 Superior vesical artery *(right; left cut)*
13 Obturator artery
14 Inferior vesical artery *(right; left cut)*
15 Middle rectal artery
16 Inferior gluteal artery
17 Internal pudendal artery
18 Iliolumbar artery
19 Lateral sacral artery
20 Superior gluteal artery
21 Middle sacral artery
22 Inferior rectal artery
23 Perineal artery
24 Dorsal artery of penis
25 Deep artery of penis
26 Obturator nerve
27 Lumbosacral trunk
28 First sacral nerve
29 Obturator internus muscle
30 Coccygeus muscle
31 Ductus deferens
32 Bladder
33 Prostate gland
34 Ureter

*These trunks are often not present.

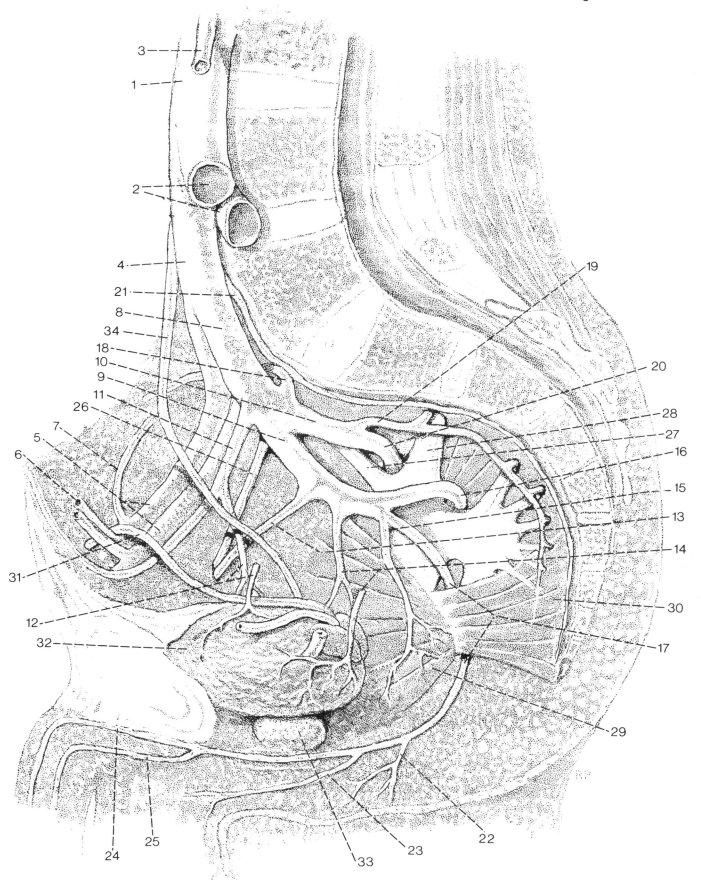

Blood supply of female pelvis

(See opposite page)

VIEW FROM LEFT SIDE; PART OF HIP BONE REMOVED

Color and label

1　Aorta
2　Inferior mesenteric artery
3　Right common iliac artery
4　Right external iliac artery and vein
5　Left common iliac artery and vein
6　Left external iliac artery and vein *(cut)*
7　Internal iliac artery
8　Superior gluteal artery
9　Inferior gluteal artery
10　Internal pudendal artery
11　Inferior rectal artery
12　Obturator artery
13　Umbilical artery
14　Superior vesical artery
15　Obliterated part of umbilical artery
　　(medial umbilical fold)
16　Uterine artery
17　Vaginal artery
18　Piriformis muscle
19　Coccygeus muscle
20　Levator ani muscle
21　Obturator internus muscle
22　External anal sphincter
23　Labia minora
24　Glans of clitoris
25　Ureter
26　Uterus
27　Bladder

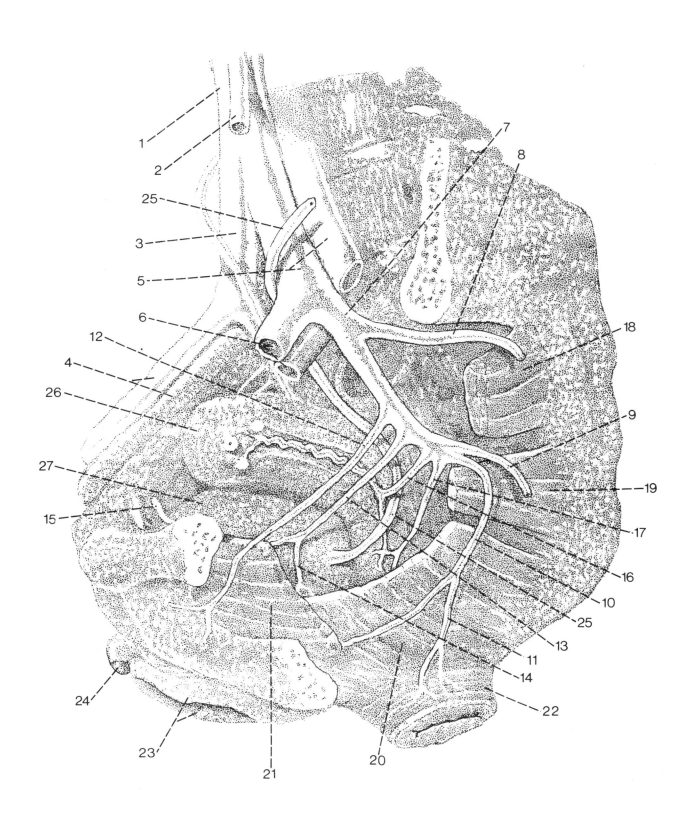

Color and label

1 Urethra
2 Vagina
3 Rectum
4 Pubococcygeus muscle (levator ani)
5 Iliococcygeus muscle (levator ani)
6 Coccygeus muscle
7 Piriformis muscle

8 Obturator internus muscle
9 Tendinous arch of levator ani
10 Pubovaginals (levator ani)
11 Ischial spine
12 Obturator canal
13 Dorsal vein of clitoris
14 Pubic symphysis

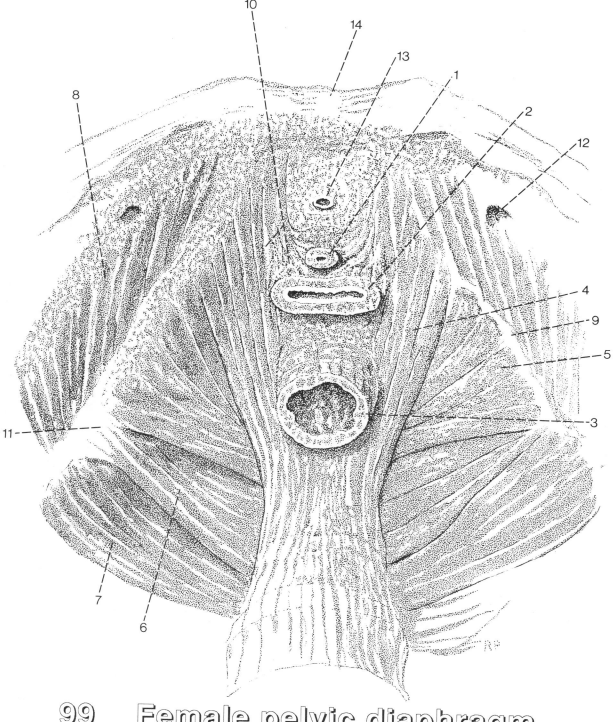

99 Female pelvic diaphragm from above

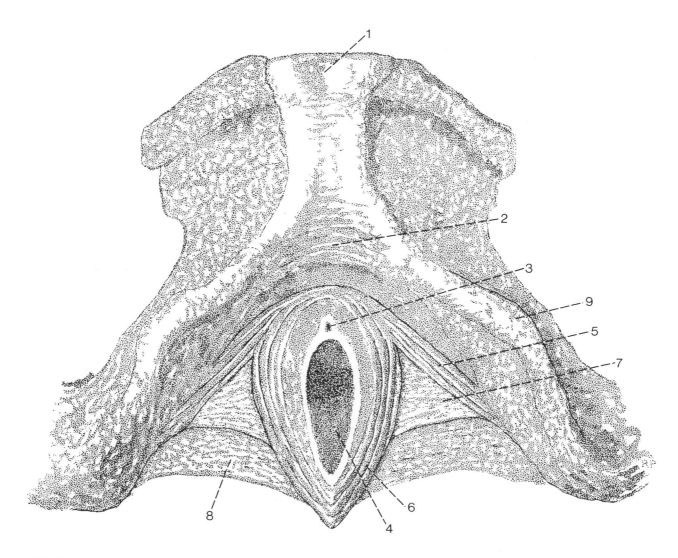

PERINEAL VIEW

**Perineal membrane and superficial musculature
and clitoris removed (after Oelrich, 1983)**

Color and label

1 Pubic symphysis
2 Arcuate pubic ligament
3 Urethra
4 Vagina
5 Urethral compressor muscle*
6 Urethrovaginal sphincter muscle*
7 Transverse vaginal muscle*
8 Smooth muscle of urethrovaginal
   compartment*
9 Ischiopubic ramus

100   Female urogenital
sphincter, I

*Oelrich's thorough investigation of the striated
urogential sphincter musculature in the female
(1983) calls for a revision of the traditional
description and terminology of these structures,
which unfortunately have been incompletely and
erroneously described in anatomy textbooks.
According to Oelrich's findings, the traditional–
and erroneous–view of a urogential diaphragm
consisting of two muscles, the urethral sphincter
muscle and the deep transverse perineus muscle,
sandwiched between a superior and an inferior
fascial layer, must be modified. Oelrich's work
shows that the striated urogential sphincter
muscle of the female consists of 1) a sphincter
surrounding the middle third of the urethra
(urethral sphincter); 2) a urethrovaginal sphincter
surrounding the urethra and vaginal vestibule; and
3) a compressor of the urethra arching across the
ventral side of the urethra (compressor urethrae
muscle). Other, variable, striated fibers may
occur, including a transverse vaginal muscle.
*Oelrich, TM: The striated urogenital sphincter
muscle in the female. Anatomical Record,
205:223-232, 1983.*

Portion of bladder and pubic symphysis removed (after Oelrich, 1983)

Color and label

1 Bladder
2 Vagina
3 Urethra
4 Vaginal wall
5 Urethral sphincter muscle
6 Urethral compressor muscle

7 Urethrovaginal sphincter
8 Transverse vaginal muscle
9 Smooth muscle of urethrovaginal compartment
10 Ischiopubic ramus (*cut and partially removed*)
11 Uterus

The transverse vaginal muscle fibers are thin and delicate and have been confused with the so-called deep transverse perineus muscle, which Oelrich could not find in the female. Oelrich reports the deep transverse perineus muscle is primarily missing in the female (personal communication).

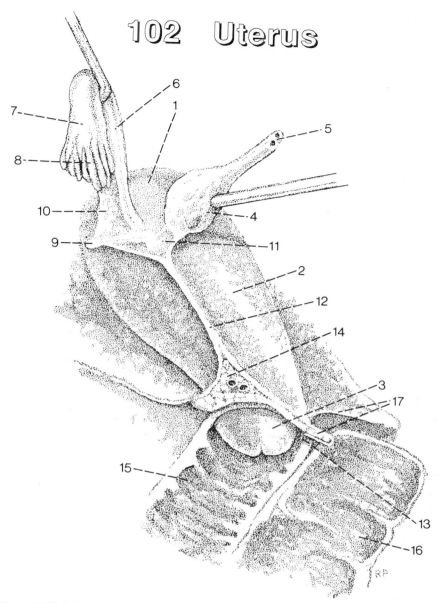

VIEWED FROM THE LEFT

Color and label

1 Uterus (fundus)
2 Uterus (body)
3 Cervix of uterus (*vaginal part*)
4 Ovary
5 Suspensory ligament of ovary with ovarian artery and vein (*cut*)
6 Uterine tube (fallopian tube; oviduct; salpinx; *salpinx is Greek for trumpet or tube*)
7 Infundibulum of uterine tube
8 Fimbriae of uterine tube
9 Round ligament of uterus
10 Mesosalpinx (*part of broad ligament attached to uterine tube*)

11 Mesovarium (*part of broad ligament attached to ovary*)
12 Mesometrium (*part of broad ligament attached to uterus*)
13 Posterior fornix of vagina
14 Lateral cervical ligament (cardinal ligament; Mackenrodt's ligament) and uterine vessels
15 Vagina (*cut, showing rugae*)
16 Rectum (*cut*)
17 Uterosacral ligament and fold

103

Female pelvic diaphragm and related structures (*See opposite page*)

VIEWED FROM BELOW

Color and label

1 Anus
2 External anal sphincter
3 Puborectalis muscle (levator ani)
4 Iliococcygeus muscle (levator ani)
5 Coccygeus muscle (+ *levator ani = pelvic diaphragm*)
6 Superficial transverse perineus muscle
7 Bulbospongiosus muscle (*cut on left side*)
8 Ischiocavernosus muscle
9 Piriformis muscle
10 Obturator internus muscle
11 Sciatic nerve (*cut*)
12 Pudendal nerve (*with internal pudendal vessels*)
13 Perineal membrane
14 Glans of clitoris
15 Urethra
16 Vagina
17 Greater vestibular gland and duct opening
18 Bulb of the vestibule (*erectile tissue*)
19 Obturator membrane
20 Obturator nerve, artery, and vein
21 Acetabulum
22 Ischial tuberosity
23 Sacrotuberous ligament
24 Dorsal sacroiliac ligament
25 Superficial dorsal sacrococcygeal ligament
26 Coccyx
27 Anococcygeal ligament

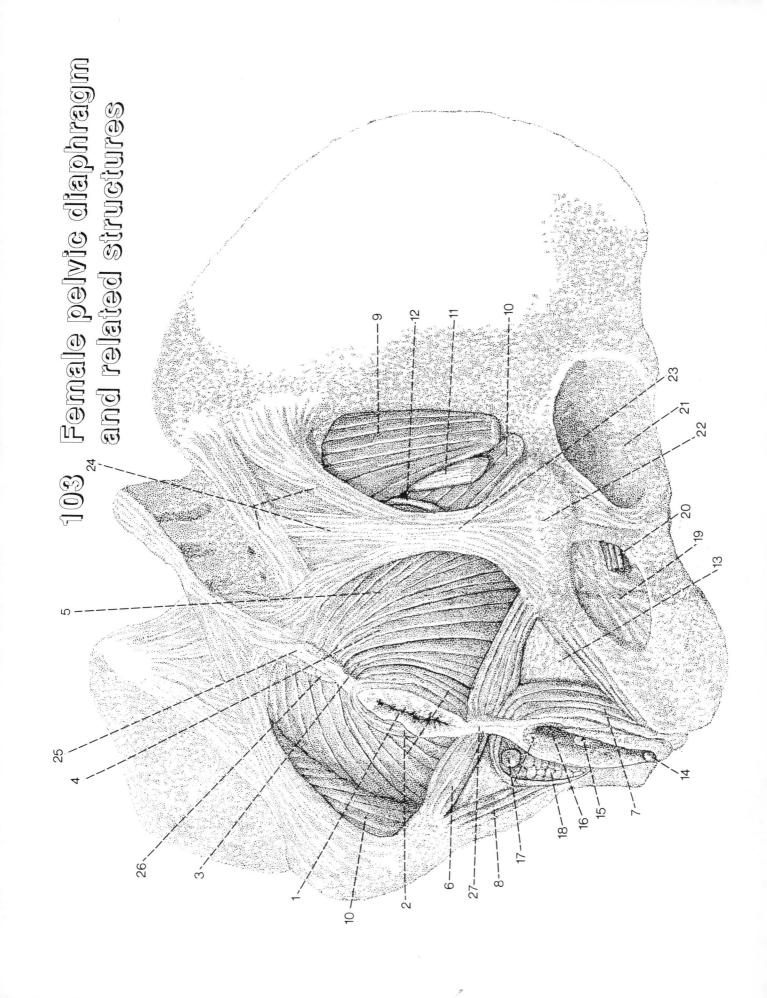

103 Female pelvic diaphragm and related structures

104 Female pelvis from the front and above

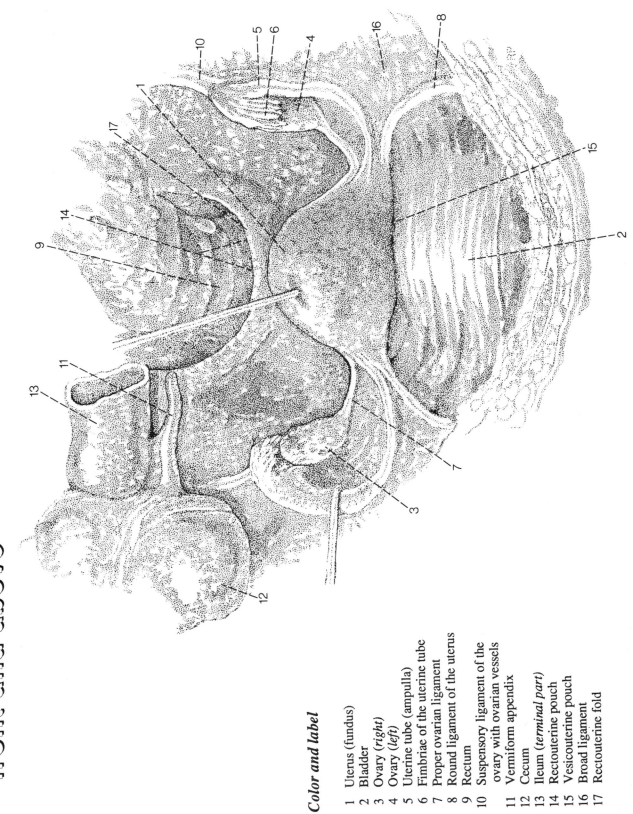

Color and label

1 Uterus (fundus)
2 Bladder
3 Ovary (*right*)
4 Ovary (*left*)
5 Uterine tube (ampulla)
6 Fimbriae of the uterine tube
7 Proper ovarian ligament
8 Round ligament of the uterus
9 Rectum
10 Suspensory ligament of the ovary with ovarian vessels
11 Vermiform appendix
12 Cecum
13 Ileum (*terminal part*)
14 Rectouterine pouch
15 Vesicouterine pouch
16 Broad ligament
17 Rectouterine fold

Uterus and related structures

(See opposite page)

FROM THE BACK

Color and label

1 Fundus of uterus
2 Cavity of uterus
3 Body of uterus
4 Cervix of uterus (*supravaginal part*)
5 Cervix of uterus (*vaginal part*)
6 Cervical canal
7 Vagina
8 Opening of uterus (ostium uteri)
9 Anterior lip of cervix
10 Lateral fornices of vagina
11 Isthmus of uterus
12 Endometrium (*mucosal lining*)
13 Myometrium (*smooth muscle*)
14 Perimetrium (peritoneum; tunica serosa)
15 Broad ligament of uterus (mesometrium)
16 Mesovarium (broad ligament)
17 Mesosalpinx (broad ligament)
18 Uterine tube
19 Infundibulum (of uterine tube)
20 Ampulla (of uterine tube)
21 Fimbriae (of uterine tube)
22 Ureter
23 Uterine artery
24 Rectouterine (ureterosacral) ligament
25 Lateral cervical ligament (cardinal ligament; Mackenrodt's ligament)
26 Ovary
27 Proper ligament of ovary
28 Ovarian artery

105　Uterus and related structures

PART IV: ARM AND HAND

PLATES 106-139

POSTERIOR ASPECT

Color and label

1 Clavicle (collar bone)
2 Sternal *(medial)* end
3 Acromial *(lateral)* end
4 Most frequent site of fracture *(the clavicle is the most frequently broken bone)*
5 Scapula (shoulder blade)
6 Medial (vertebral) border
7 Lateral (axillary) border
8 Superior border
9 Superior angle
10 Inferior angle
11 Lateral angle *(forms glenoid cavity)*
12 Spine of scapula
13 Acromion
14 Scapular notch
15 Coracoid process
16 Supraspinatus fossa *(for supraspinatus muscle)*
17 Infraspinatus fossa *(for infraspinatus muscle)*
18 Infraglenoid tubercle *(for triceps long head origin)*
19 Neck of scapula
20 Head of humerus
21 Anatomical neck *(rarely fractured)*
22 Surgical neck *(site of usual fracture at proximal humerus)*
23 Deltoid tuberosity
24 Medial epicondyle
25 Lateral epicondyle
26 Radial groove for radial nerve
27 Olecranon fossa under olecranon
28 Sulcus for ulnar nerve
29 Olecranon
30 Head of radius
31 Neck of radius
32 Styloid process of ulna
33 Styloid process of radius
34 Pisiform bone
35 Triquetral bone
36 Lunate bone *(most frequently dislocated wrist bone)*
37 Scaphoid bone *(most frequently fractured wrist bone)*
38 Hamate bone
39 Capitate bone
40 Trapezoid bone
41 Trapezium bone
42 Metacarpal bones
43 Proximal phalanx
44 Middle phalanx
45 Distal phalanx

106
Bones of the
upper extremity

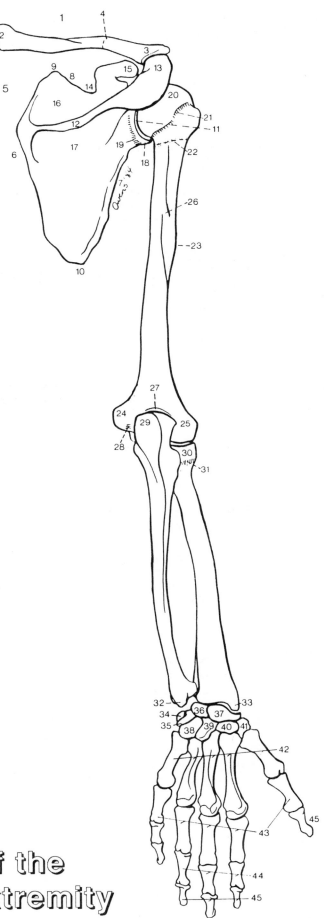

Dissection of the posterior shoulder and arm *(See opposite page)*

Color and label

1   Trapezius muscle upper fibers
2   Trapezius insertion of upper fibers on spine and acromion of scapula
3   Trapezius lower fibers
4   Trapezius insertion of lower fibers on spine of scapula
5   Outline of trapezius muscle
6   Sternocleidomastoid muscle
7   Levator scapulae muscle
8   Rhomboid minor muscle
9   Rhomboid major muscle
10   Accessory nerve (cranial nerve XI) supplying sternocleidomastoid and trapezius
11   Transverse cervical artery
12   Superficial branch of transverse cervical artery
13   Ascending branch of superficial branch of transverse cervical artery
14   Descending branch of superficial branch of transverse cervical artery
15   Deep branch of transverse cervical artery
16   Supraspinatus muscle *(cut)*
17   Insertion of supraspinatus on greater tubercle of humerus
18   Infraspinatus muscle *(cut)*
19   Insertion of infraspinatus on greater tubercle of humerus
20   Suprascapular nerve innervating supraspinatus and infraspinatus
21   Teres minor
22   Teres major
23   Axillary nerve passing through quadrangular space and supplying teres minor and deltoid muscle
24   Deltoid muscle origin on spine of scapula and acromion
25   Deltoid muscle *(cut longitudinally)*
26   Deltoid muscle insertion
27   Triceps brachii muscle, long head
28   Triceps brachii, lateral head *(cut)*
29   Treceps brachii, medial head
30   Radial nerve innervating three heads of triceps *(radial nerve supplies all extensor muscles of arm)*
31   Insertion of three heads of triceps brachii on olecranon of ulna
32   Outline of deltoid muscle
33   Deep brachial (profunda brachii) artery

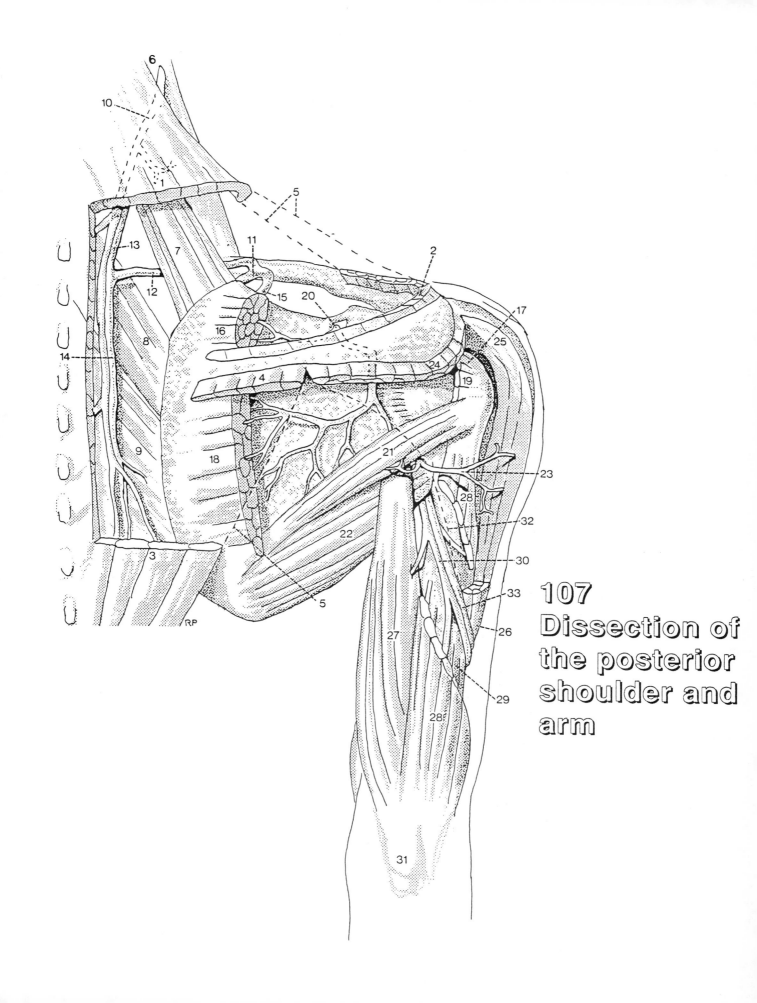

107
Dissection of the posterior shoulder and arm

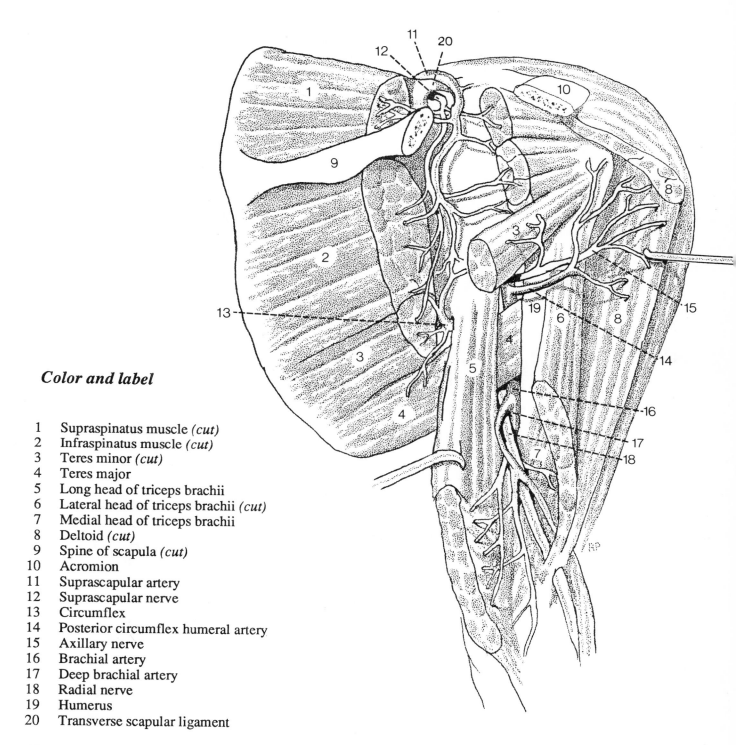

Color and label

1   Supraspinatus muscle *(cut)*
2   Infraspinatus muscle *(cut)*
3   Teres minor *(cut)*
4   Teres major
5   Long head of triceps brachii
6   Lateral head of triceps brachii *(cut)*
7   Medial head of triceps brachii
8   Deltoid *(cut)*
9   Spine of scapula *(cut)*
10   Acromion
11   Suprascapular artery
12   Suprascapular nerve
13   Circumflex
14   Posterior circumflex humeral artery
15   Axillary nerve
16   Brachial artery
17   Deep brachial artery
18   Radial nerve
19   Humerus
20   Transverse scapular ligament

After Wolf-Heidegger.

108   Nerves and arteries of the posterior shoulder

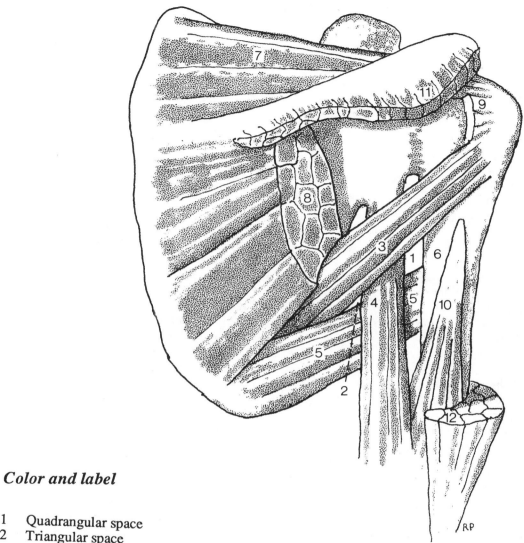

Color and label

1 Quadrangular space
2 Triangular space
3 Teres minor *(superior border)*
4 Long head of triceps brachii *(medial border)*
5 Teres major *(inferior border)*
6 Humerus *(lateral border)*
7 Supraspinatus
8 Infraspinatus
9 Insertion of infraspinatus
10 Lateral end of triceps brachii
11 Origin of deltoid on spine of scapula and acrmion
12 Deltoid

109 Quadrangular space

Color and label

SC-1   First part of
       subclavian artery
SC-2   Second part of
       subclavian artery
SC-3   Third part of
       subclavian artery

1   Brachiocephalic artery
2   Common carotid artery
3   Right vagus nerve (X)
4   Recurrent laryngeal nerve
5   Vertebral artery
6   Thyrocervical trunk *(on ventral side)*
7   Inferior thyroid artery
8   Ascending cervical artery
9   Transverse cervical artery
10 Superficial branch of transverse
    cervical artery *(supplies trapezius)*
11 Ascending branch
12 Descending branch *accompanies
    accessory nerve XI; notice it lies
    deep to trapezius but superficial to
    rhomboids)*
13 Deep branch of transverse cervical artery
    (it accompanies dorsal scapular nerve)
14 Dorsal scapular nerve *(a small section)*
15 Suprascapular artery *(notice it goes over
    the superior transverse scapular ligament)*
16 Suprascapular nerve *(notice it goes under
    the superior transverse scapular ligament
    and through the scapular foramen)*
17 Arterial plexus in supraspinatus fossa
    and within infraspinatus muscle
18 Arterial plexus in infraspinatus fossa
    and within infraspinatus muscle

19 Axillary artery *(on ventral side of scapula;
    a continuation of subclavian artery)*
20 Internal thoracic (mammary) artery
21 Costocervical trunk
22 Supreme or highest intercostal artery
23 Deep cervical artery
24 Subscapular artery
25 Circumflex scapular artery
26 Thoracodorsal artery
27 Posterior circumflex humeral artery
28 Anterior circumflex humeral artery
29 Brachial artery *(a continuation of
    axillary artery)*
30 Deep brachial artery (profunda brachii)
31 Deltoid *(ascending branch)*
32 Superior ulnar collateral artery
33 Inferior ulnar collateral artery
34 Posterior ulnar recurrent artery
35 Radial collateral branch of deep brachial artery
36 Middle collateral branch of deep brachial artery
37 Ulnar artery
38 Radial artery
39 Interosseous artery
40 Posterior interosseous artery
41 Anterior interosseous artery
43 Axillary nerve
44 Radial nerve *(cut)*
45 Ulnar nerve *(a small section)*

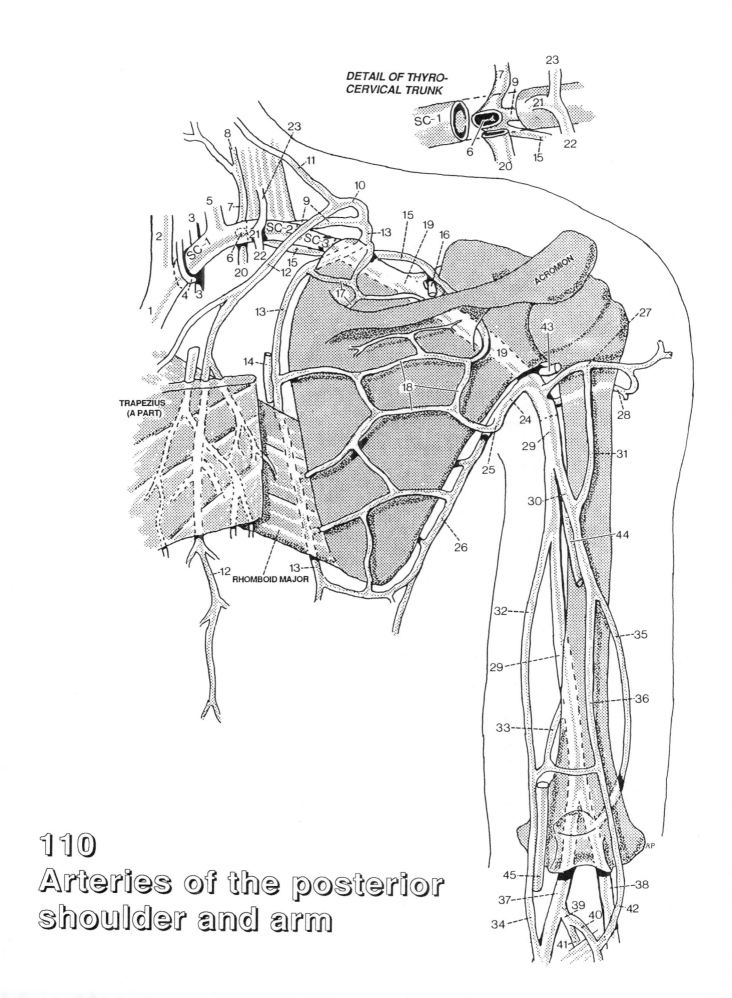

DETAIL OF THYRO-CERVICAL TRUNK

SC-1

TRAPEZIUS
(A PART)

ACROMION

RHOMBOID MAJOR

110
Arteries of the posterior shoulder and arm

Subclavian, axillary, and brachial arteries *(See opposite page)*

VIEWED FROM THE FRONT (ANTERIOR ASPECT)

Color and label

1 Ascending aorta
2 Brachiocephalic artery
3 Left common carotid artery
4 Right common carotid artery
5 Subclavian artery
6 Vertebral artery
7 Thyrocervical artery
8 Inferior thyroid artery
9 Ascending cervical artery
10 Inferior laryngeal artery
11 Transverse cervical artery
12 Superficial branch of transverse cervical artery
13 Deep branch of transverse cervical artery
14 Ascending branch of superficial branch of transverse cervical artery
15 Descending branch of superficial branch of transverse cervical artery
16 Suprascapular artery
17 Internal thoracic (mammary) artery
18 Anterior intercostal arteries
19 Perforating branches
20 Musculophrenic artery
21 Superior epigastric artery
22 Deep cervical artery *(branch of costocervical trunk)*
23 Axillary artery
24 Supreme thoracic artery
25 Thoracoacromial artery
26 Clavicular branch of thoracoacromial artery
27 Acromial branch
28 Deltoid branch
29 Pectoral branch(es)
30 Lateral thoracic artery *(usually it arises from thoracoacromial artery or from subscapular artery and not from axillary artery as shown here)*
31 Subscapular artery
32 Circumflex scapular artery
33 Thoracodorsal artery
34 Anterior humeral circumflex artery
35 Posterior humeral circumflex artery
36 Brachial artery
37 Profunda brachii (deep brachii) artery
38 Radial collateral artery of deep brachial artery
39 Middle collateral artery of deep brachial artery
40 Superior ulnar collateral artery
42 Anterior ulnar recurrent artery
43 Posterior ulnar recurrent artery
44 Radial recurrent artery
45 Interosseous recurrent artery
46 Posterior interosseous artery
47 Anterior interosseous artery
48 Interosseous artery

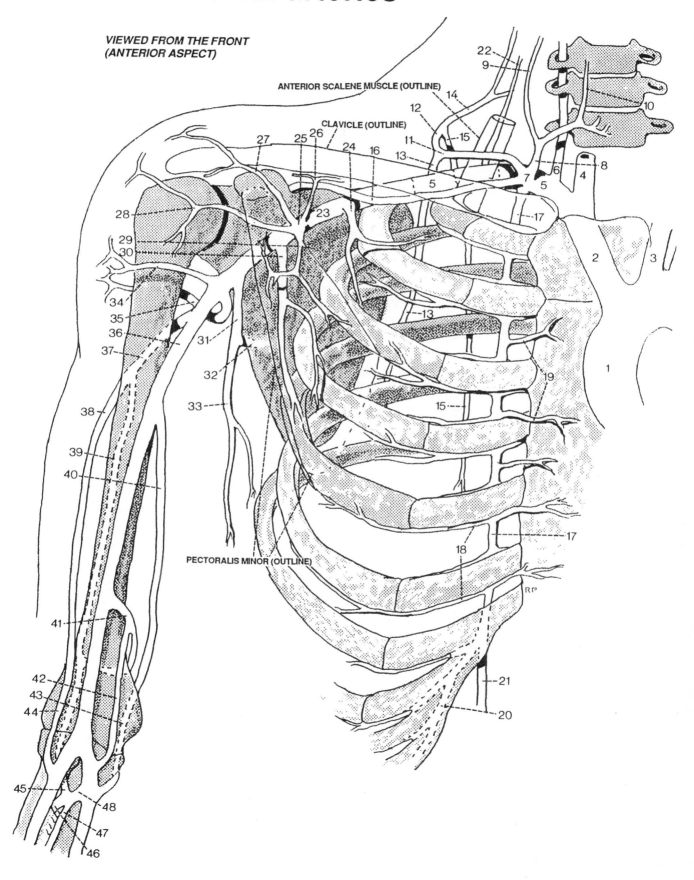

VIEWED FROM THE FRONT
(ANTERIOR ASPECT)

ANTERIOR SCALENE MUSCLE (OUTLINE)

CLAVICLE (OUTLINE)

PECTORALIS MINOR (OUTLINE)

Label and color the origins (O) RED and the insertions (I) BLUE

1 Sternocleidomastoid (O)
2 Pectoralis major (O)
3 Deltoid (O)
4 Trapezius (I)
5 Omohyoid (O)
6 Supraspinatus (O)
7 Levator scapulae (I)
8 Rhomboid minor (I)
9 Rhomboid major (I)
10 Infraspinatus (O)
11 Teres major (O)
12 Teres minor (O)
13 Deltoid (I)
14 Infraspinatus (I)
15 Teres minor (I)
16 Triceps brachii lateral head (O)
17 Triceps brachii long head (O)
18 Triceps brachii medial head (O)
19 Anconeus (O)
20 Flexor carpi ulnaris (O)
21 Triceps brachii (I)
22 Anconeus (I)
23 Flexor digitorum superficialis (O)
24 Flexor digitorum profundus (O)
25 Supinator (O)
26 Abductor pollicis longus (O)
27 Extensor pollicis longus (O)
28 Extensor indicis (O)
29 Supinator (I)
30 Pronator teres (I)
31 Extensor pollicis brevis (I)
32 Common aponeurosis for origin of extensor carpi ulnaris, flexor carpi ulnaris, flexor digitorum profundus
33 Extensor carpi ulnaris (I)
34 Extensor carpi radialis longus (I)
35 Extensor carpi radialis brevis (I)
36 First dorsal interosseous (O)
37 Second dorsal interosseous (O)
38 Third dorsal interosseous (O)
39 Fourth dorsal interosseous (O)
40 Extensor pollicis brevis (I)
41 Extensor pollicis longus (I)
42 First dorsal interosseous (I)
43 Second dorsal interosseous (O)
44 Third dorsal interosseous (I)
45 Fourth dorsal interosseous (I)
46 Extensor digitorum (I)
47 Extensor indicis (I) *(common insertion)*
48 Extensor digiti minimi *(common insertion)*

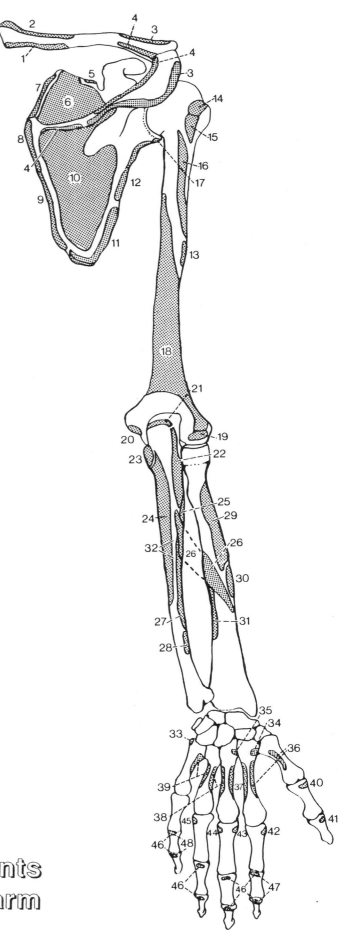

112 Muscle attachments of the posterior arm

Color and label

Rami

Trunks
    UT, upper trunk
    MT, middle trunk
    LT, lower trunk

Divisions
    VENT, ventral divisions
    DORS, dorsal divisions

Cords
    LT, lateral cord
    PC, posterior cord
    MC, medial cord

Terminal nerves
    AX, axillary nerves
    MUSC, musculocutaneous nerve
    MED, median nerve
    RAD, radial nerve
    UL, ulnar nerve

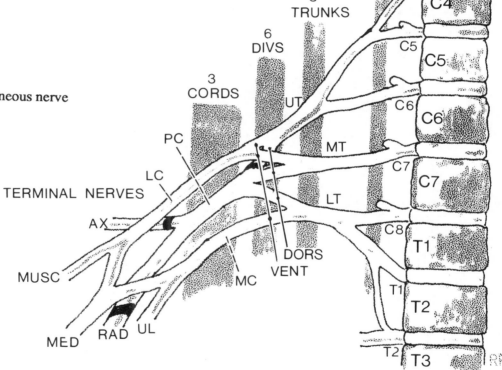

The brachial plexus forms and reforms into 5 stages: rami, trunks, divisions, cords, and terminal nerves. It begins with the 5 anterior RAMI or cervical nerves C5-T1, with C4 contributing fibers to C5. These rami coalesce into 3 TRUNKS, an upper, middle, and lower trunk. Each of the 3 trunks divides into an interior and a posterior DIVISION. The 6 divisions regroup into 3 CORDS, a lateral cord, a medial cord, and a posterior cord. Most of the nerves of the arm arise from the 3 cords. However, other essential arm nerves arise higher up in the plexus as well.

Color and label

1 Phrenic nerve *(mainly from C4)*
2 Dorsal scapular nerve *(to levator scapulae and rhomboids)*
3 Suprascapular nerve *(to supraspinatus and infraspinatus)*
4 Nerve to subclavius muscle
5 Upper trunk
6 Lateral pectoral nerve *(to pectoralis major)*
7 Communicating link between pectoral nerves
8 Lateral cord
9 Musculocutaneous nerve
10 Lateral root of median nerve
11 Median nerve
12 Medial root of median nerve
13 Ulnar nerve
14 Radial nerve
15 Axillary nerve
16 Medial cord
17 Medial antebrachial cutaneous nerve
18 Medial brachial cutaneous nerve
19 Medial pectoral nerve *(to pectoralis major and minor)*
20 Posterior cord
21 Inferior subscapular nerve *(to subscapularis and teres major)*
22 Thoracodorsal nerve *(to latissimus dorsi)*
23 Superior subscapular nerve *(to subscapularis)*
24 Anterior and posterior divisions
25 Middle trunk
26 Lower trunk
27 Long thoracic nerve *(to serratus anterior)*
28 Nerves to prevertebral muscles and scalene muscles

114 Brachial plexus and its nerves

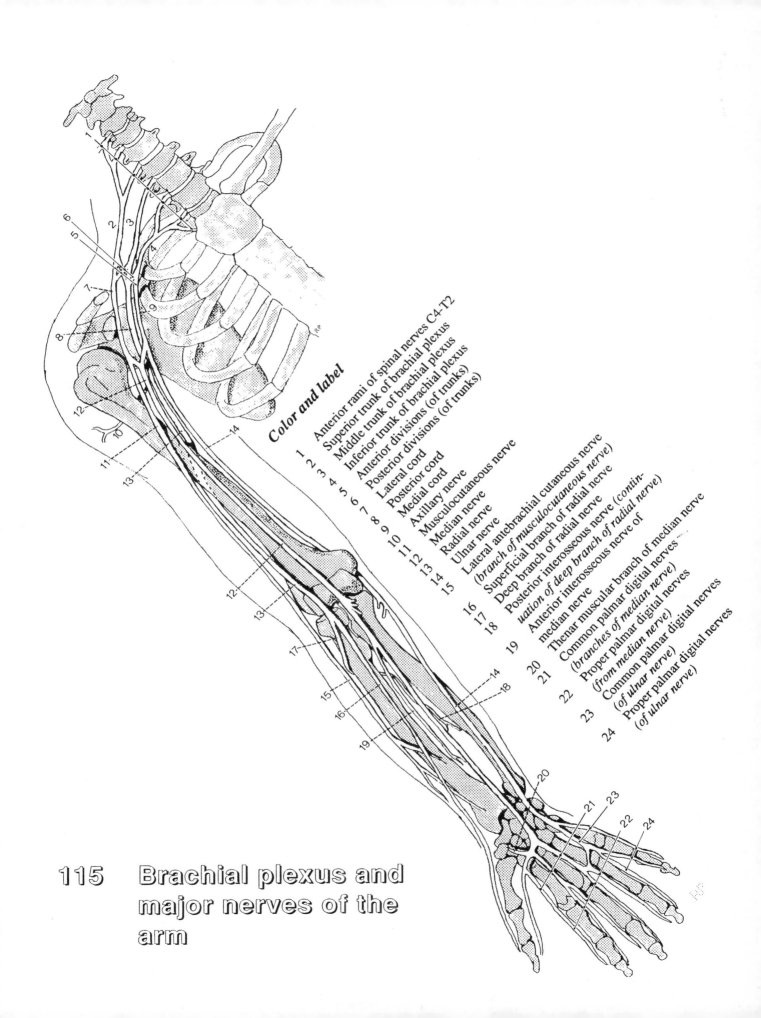

Color and label

1. Anterior rami of spinal nerves C4-T2
2. Superior trunk of brachial plexus
3. Middle trunk of brachial plexus
4. Inferior trunk of brachial plexus
5. Anterior divisions (of trunks)
6. Posterior divisions (of trunks)
7. Lateral cord
8. Posterior cord
9. Medial cord
10. Axillary nerve
11. Musculocutaneous nerve
12. Median nerve
13. Radial nerve
14. Ulnar nerve
15. Lateral antebrachial cutaneous nerve *(branch of musculocutaneous nerve)*
16. Superficial branch of radial nerve
17. Deep branch of radial nerve *(continuation of deep branch of radial nerve)*
18. Posterior interosseous nerve
19. Anterior interosseous nerve of median nerve
20. Thenar muscular branch of median nerve
21. Common palmar digital nerves *(branches of median nerve)*
22. Proper palmar digital nerves *(from median nerve)*
23. Common palmar digital nerves *(of ulnar nerve)*
24. Proper palmar digital nerves *(of ulnar nerve)*

115   Brachial plexus and major nerves of the arm

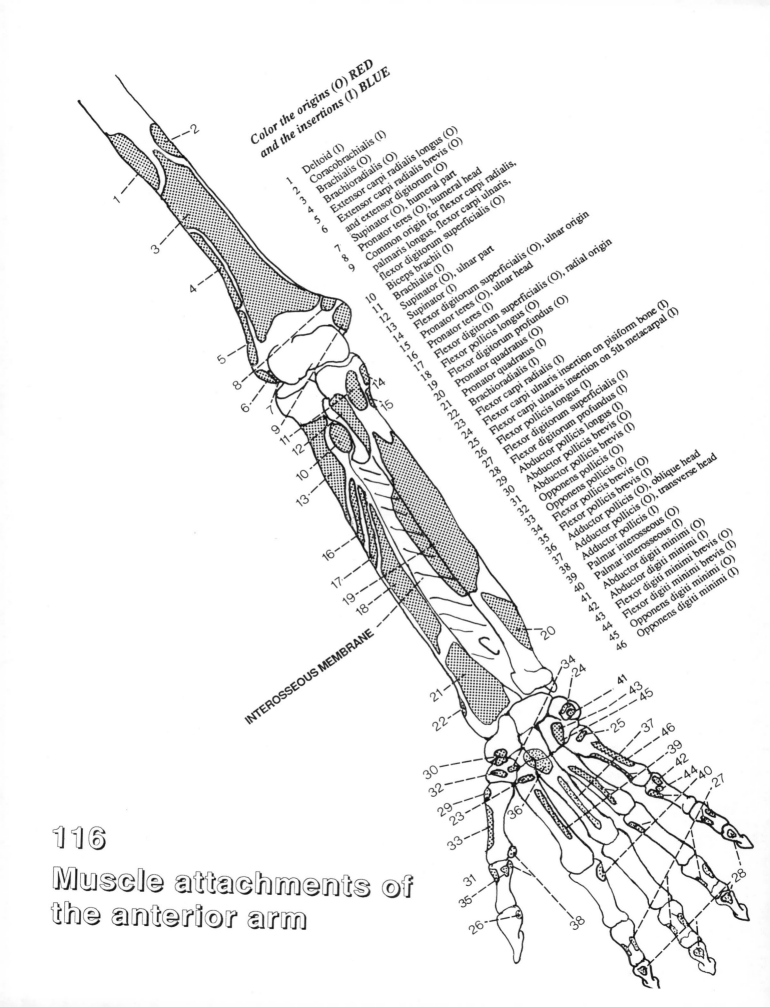

Color the origins (O) RED
and the insertions (I) BLUE

1 Deltoid (I)
2 Coracobrachialis (I)
3 Brachialis (O)
4 Brachioradialis (O)
5 Extensor carpi radialis longus (O)
6 Extensor carpi radialis brevis (O)
   and extensor digitorum (O)
7 Supinator (O), humeral part
8 Pronator teres (O)
9 Common origin for flexor carpi radialis,
   palmaris longus, flexor carpi ulnaris,
   flexor digitorum superficialis (O)
10 Biceps brachii (I)
11 Brachialis (I)
12 Supinator (O), ulnar part
13 Supinator (I)
14 Flexor digitorum superficialis (O), ulnar origin
15 Pronator teres (O), ulnar head
16 Pronator teres (I)
17 Flexor digitorum superficialis (O), radial origin
18 Flexor pollicis longus (O)
19 Flexor digitorum profundus (O)
20 Pronator quadratus (O)
21 Pronator quadratus (I)
22 Brachioradialis (I)
23 Flexor carpi radialis (I)
24 Flexor carpi ulnaris insertion on pisiform bone (I)
25 Flexor carpi ulnaris insertion on 5th metacarpal (I)
26 Flexor pollicis longus (I)
27 Flexor digitorum superficialis (I)
28 Flexor digitorum profundus (I)
29 Abductor pollicis longus (I)
30 Abductor pollicis brevis (I)
31 Opponens pollicis (O)
32 Opponens pollicis (I)
33 Flexor pollicis brevis (O)
34 Flexor pollicis brevis (I)
35 Adductor pollicis (O), oblique head
36 Adductor pollicis (O), transverse head
37 Adductor pollicis (I)
38 Palmar interosseous (O)
39 Palmar interosseous (I)
40 Abductor digiti minimi (O)
41 Abductor digiti minimi (I)
42 Flexor digiti minimi brevis (O)
43 Flexor digiti minimi brevis (I)
44 Opponens digiti minimi (O)
45 Opponens digiti minimi (O)
46 Opponens digiti minimi (I)

INTEROSSEOUS MEMBRANE

116

Muscle attachments of
the anterior arm

THE BICEPS IS ALSO A SUPINATOR

SHORT HEAD
ORIGIN ON CORACOID PROCESS

Color the biceps brachii and the radius and ulna

LONG HEAD
ORIGIN ON
SUPRAGLENOID TUBERCLE

ORIGIN USUALLY
DOES NOT MOVE
AND IS PROXIMAL

LONG HEAD

SHORT HEAD

Notice that the biceps brachii does two things: it flexes the elbow and it supinates the forearm so the palm of the hand is up and the radius and ulna are parallel. This is the SUPINE position. In the PRONE position, the radius is crossed in front of the ulna and the palm faces down. Notice also that the biceps brachii has two heads, each with its own origin. Origins of muscles are usually nearer the trunk (proximal) and usually do not move, whereas insertions of muscles are usually further from the trunk (distal) and the insertions usually move.

INSERTION ON
RADIAL TUBEROSITY

INSERTION USUALLY
MOVES AND IS DISTAL

ULNA

RADIUS

RADIUS

ULNA

BONES CROSSED
PALM DOWN

BONES PARALLEL
PALM UP

PRONATION

SUPINATION

117 Biceps brachii muscle

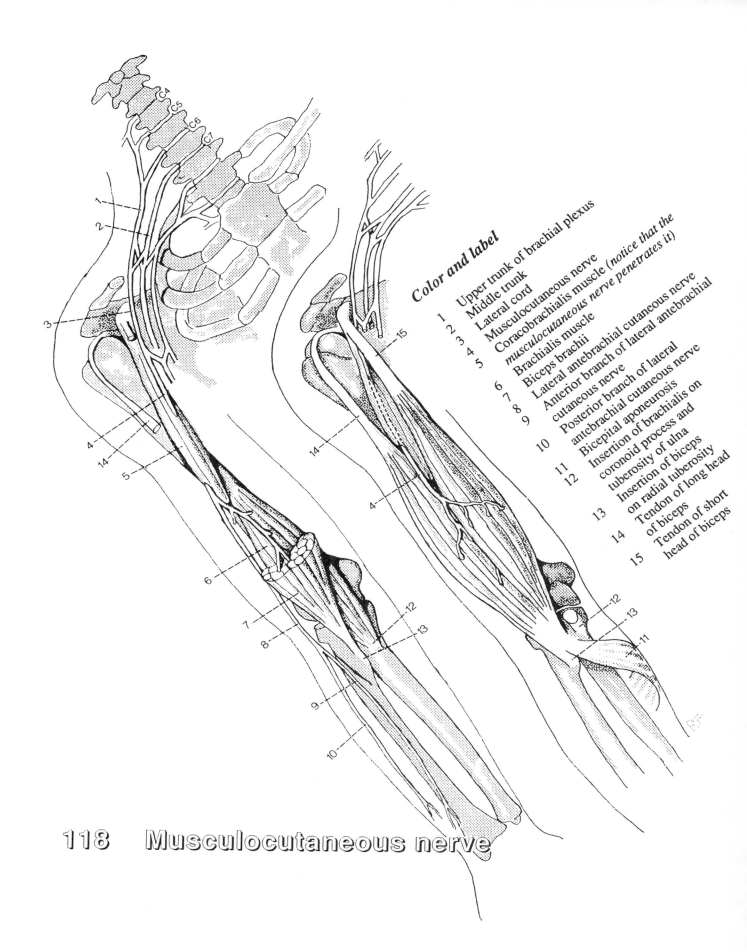

Upper trunk of brachial plexus
Middle trunk

1   Lateral cord
2   Musculocutaneous nerve (notice that the
3   Coracobrachialis muscle *musculocutaneous nerve penetrates it*)
4   Brachialis muscle
5   Biceps brachii
6   Lateral antebrachial cutaneous nerve
7   Anterior branch of lateral antebrachial
8   cutaneous nerve
9   Posterior branch of lateral
    antebrachial cutaneous nerve
10 Bicepital aponeurosis
    Insertion of brachialis on
11 coronoid process and
    tuberosity of ulna
12 Insertion of biceps
13 on radial tuberosity
    Tendon of long head
14 of biceps
    Tendon of short
15 head of biceps

118   Musculocutaneous nerve

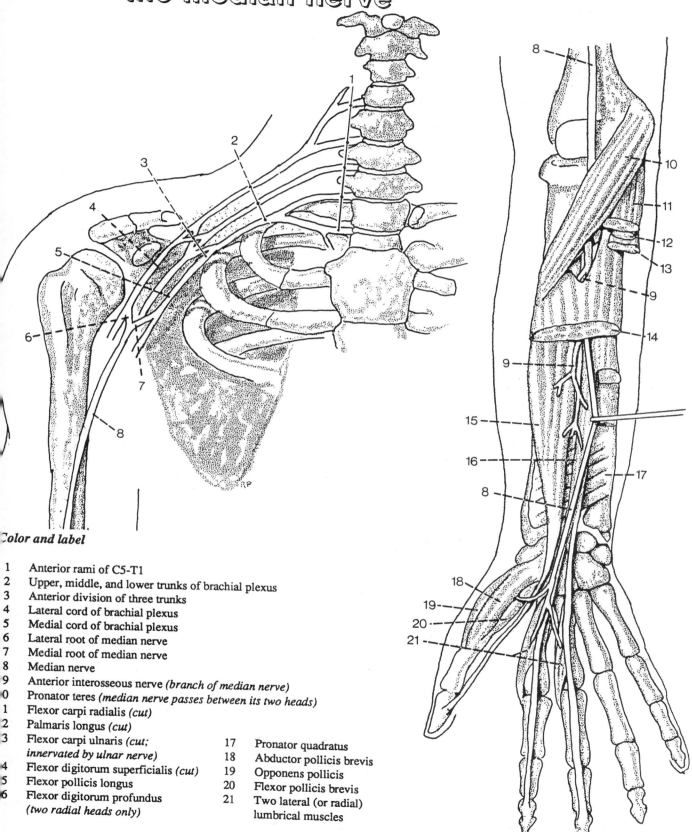

Color and label

1 Anterior rami of C5-T1
2 Upper, middle, and lower trunks of brachial plexus
3 Anterior division of three trunks
4 Lateral cord of brachial plexus
5 Medial cord of brachial plexus
6 Lateral root of median nerve
7 Medial root of median nerve
8 Median nerve
9 Anterior interosseous nerve *(branch of median nerve)*
10 Pronator teres *(median nerve passes between its two heads)*
11 Flexor carpi radialis *(cut)*
12 Palmaris longus *(cut)*
13 Flexor carpi ulnaris *(cut; innervated by ulnar nerve)*
14 Flexor digitorum superficialis *(cut)*
15 Flexor pollicis longus
16 Flexor digitorum profundus *(two radial heads only)*

17 Pronator quadratus
18 Abductor pollicis brevis
19 Opponens pollicis
20 Flexor pollicis brevis
21 Two lateral (or radial) lumbrical muscles

1   Median nerve
2   Pronator teres *(humeral head)*
3   Pronator teres *(ulnar head)*
4   Flexor carpi radialis
5   Palmaris longus
6   Palmar aponeurosis
7   Flexor carpi ulnaris
    (ulnar nerve innervated)
8   Pisiform bone
9   Flexor retinaculum
10 Brachioradialis
    (radial nerve)
11 Extensor carpi
    radialis longus
    (radial nerve)

120   Pronator teres and superficial wrist flexors

121 Flexor digitorum superficialis muscle

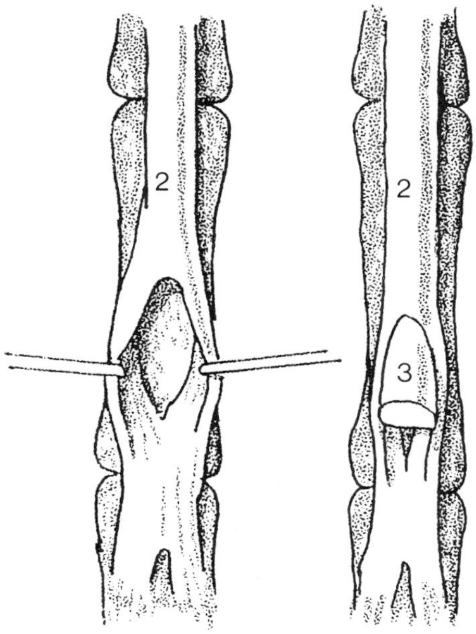

Color and label

1 Flexor digitorum superficialis
2 Flexor digitorum superficialis tendon
3 Flexor digitorum profundus tendon
4 Short vinculum
5 Long vinculum

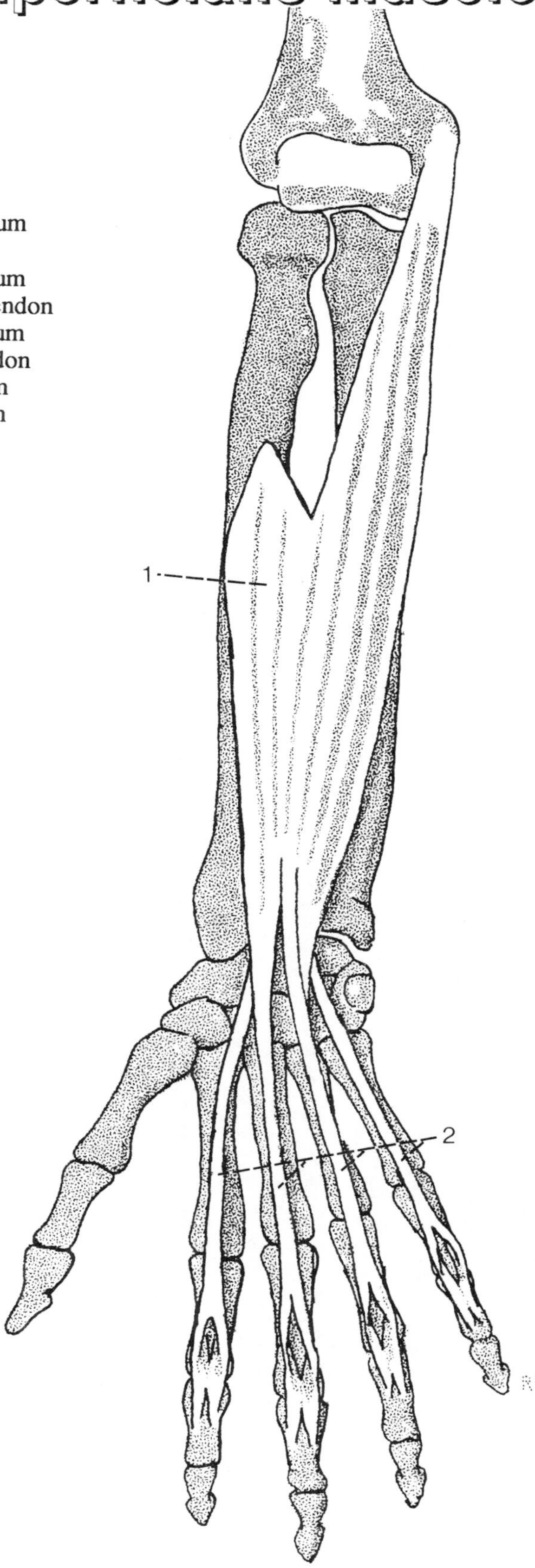

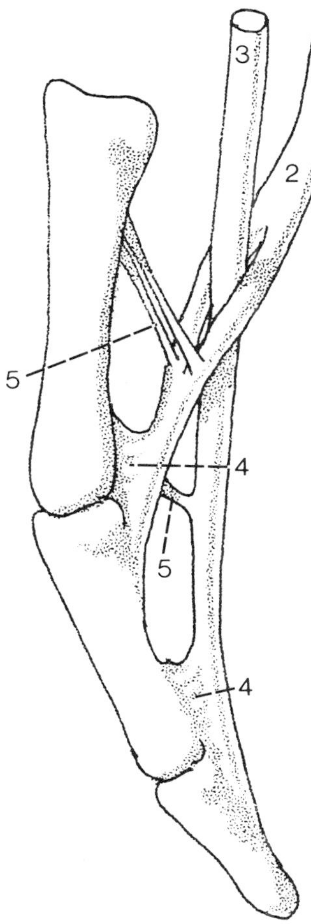

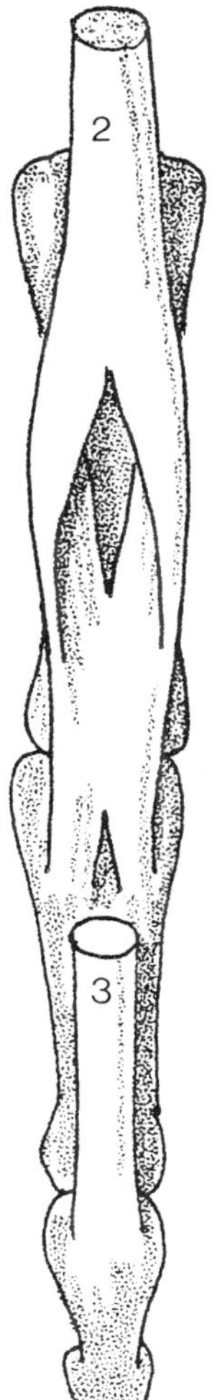

Notice that the median nerve supplies all the flexor muscles of the hand and fingers except the flexor carpi ulnaris and the medial two heads of the flexor digitorum profundus, which are both supplied by the ulnar nerve. Thus, making a fist and a strong grasp depend on a strong median nerve.

Color and label

1   Median nerve
2   Anterior interosseous nerve
3   Ulnar nerve
4   Flexor pollicis longus *(long flexor of the thumb)*
5   Flexor digitorum profundus *(deep flexor of the fingers)*
6   Lumbrical muscles
7   Pronator teres *(humeral superficial head)*
8   Pronator teres *(ulnar deep head)*
9   Flexor carpi radialis
10 Palmaris longus
11 Flexor carpi ulnaris
12 Flexor digitorum superficialis
13 Pronator quadratus

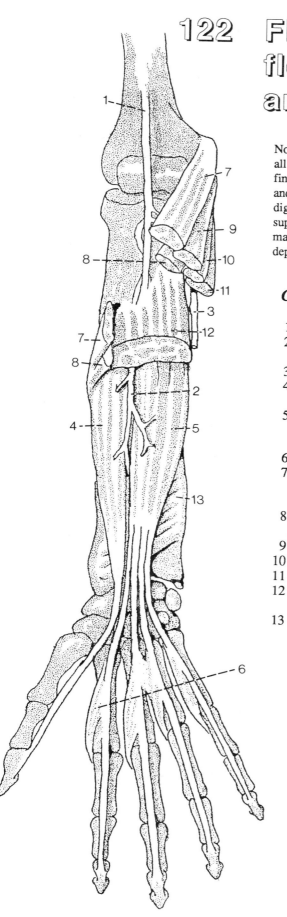

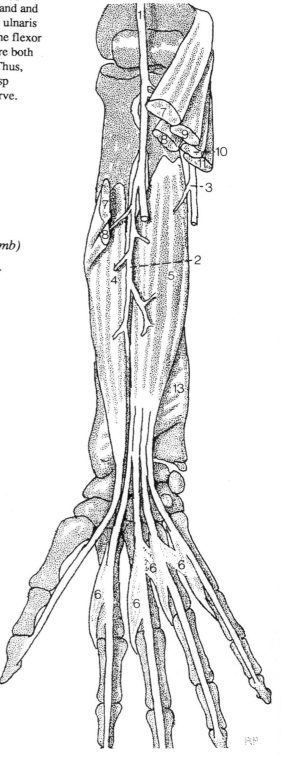

Color and label

1 Median nerve
2 Anterior interosseous nerve
3 Ulnar nerve
4 Flexor pollicis longus
5 Flexor digitorum profundus
6 Lumbrical muscles
7 Pronator teres (humeral superficial head)
8 Pronator teres (ulnar deep head)
9 Flexor carpi radialis
10 Palmaris longus
11 Flexor carpi ulnaris
12 Flexor digitorum superficialis
13 Pronator quadratus
14 Opponens pollicis
15 Abductor pollicis brevis
16 Flexor pollicis brevis
17 Motor branch of median nerve
   to thenar muscles (*recurrent branch*)
18 Common digital nerves
19 Proper digital nerves

Notice that the median nerve supplies the three thenar muscles, which are responsible for opposing the thumb to the other fingers. Opposition of the thumb is a test for median nerve function.

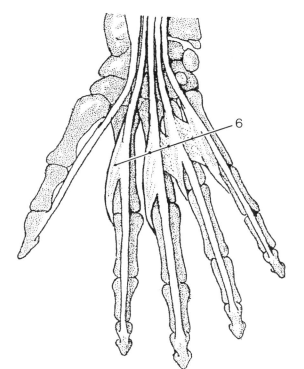

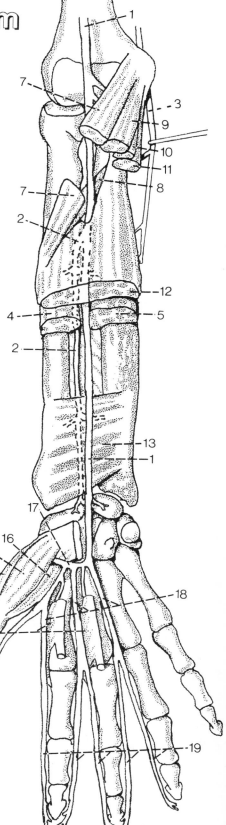

The ulnar nerve supplies most of the intrinsic hand muscles. Because it supplies all seven interosseous muscles, which abduct (spread) and adduct (bring together) digits 2-5, abducting and adducting these fingers is a test for ulnar nerve function.

Color and label

1 Upper trunk of brachial plexus
2 Middle trunk of brachial plexus
3 Lower trunk of brachial plexus
   *(notice that this trunk is made
   up of fibers from C8 and T1)*
4 Medial cord of brachial plexus
5 Posterior cord of brachial plexus
6 Lateral cord of brachial plexus

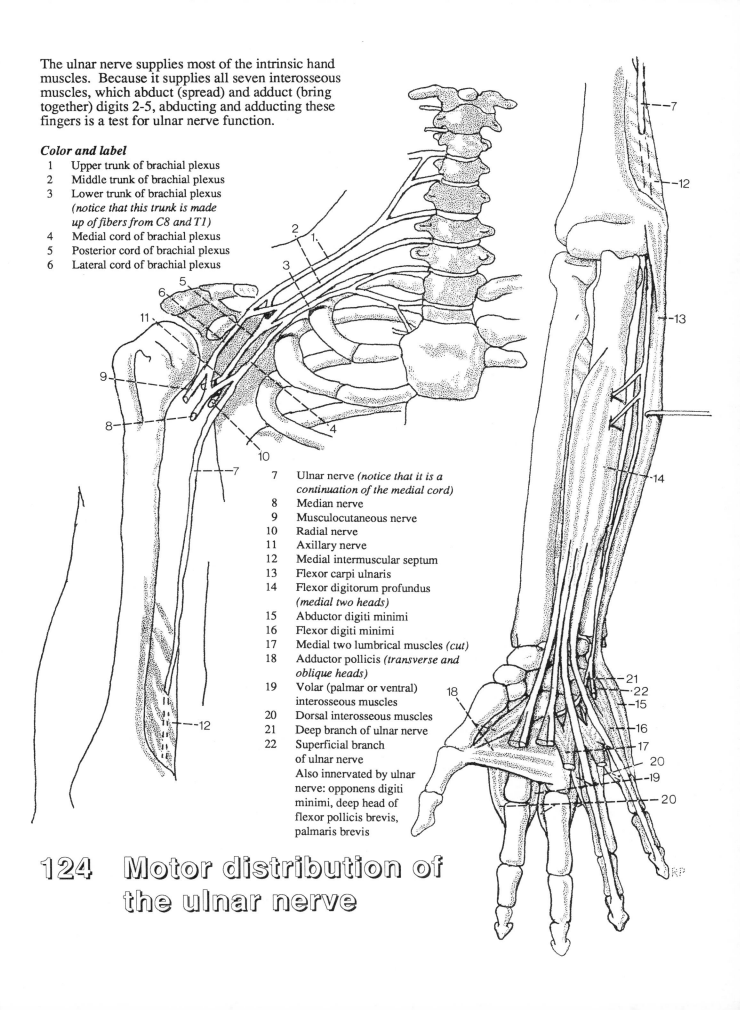

7 Ulnar nerve *(notice that it is a
   continuation of the medial cord)*
8 Median nerve
9 Musculocutaneous nerve
10 Radial nerve
11 Axillary nerve
12 Medial intermuscular septum
13 Flexor carpi ulnaris
14 Flexor digitorum profundus
   (medial two heads)
15 Abductor digiti minimi
16 Flexor digiti minimi
17 Medial two lumbrical muscles *(cut)*
18 Adductor pollicis *(transverse and
   oblique heads)*
19 Volar (palmar or ventral)
   interosseous muscles
20 Dorsal interosseous muscles
21 Deep branch of ulnar nerve
22 Superficial branch
   of ulnar nerve
   Also innervated by ulnar
   nerve: opponens digiti
   minimi, deep head of
   flexor pollicis brevis,
   palmaris brevis

124   Motor distribution of
the ulnar nerve

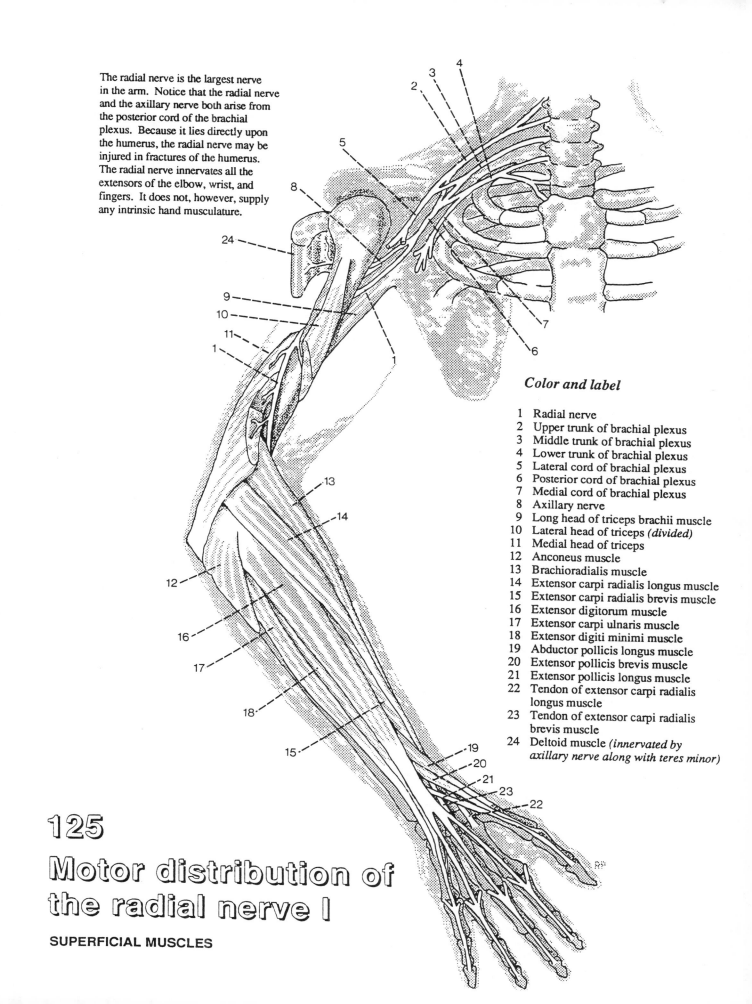

The radial nerve is the largest nerve in the arm. Notice that the radial nerve and the axillary nerve both arise from the posterior cord of the brachial plexus. Because it lies directly upon the humerus, the radial nerve may be injured in fractures of the humerus. The radial nerve innervates all the extensors of the elbow, wrist, and fingers. It does not, however, supply any intrinsic hand musculature.

Color and label

1 Radial nerve
2 Upper trunk of brachial plexus
3 Middle trunk of brachial plexus
4 Lower trunk of brachial plexus
5 Lateral cord of brachial plexus
6 Posterior cord of brachial plexus
7 Medial cord of brachial plexus
8 Axillary nerve
9 Long head of triceps brachii muscle
10 Lateral head of triceps *(divided)*
11 Medial head of triceps
12 Anconeus muscle
13 Brachioradialis muscle
14 Extensor carpi radialis longus muscle
15 Extensor carpi radialis brevis muscle
16 Extensor digitorum muscle
17 Extensor carpi ulnaris muscle
18 Extensor digiti minimi muscle
19 Abductor pollicis longus muscle
20 Extensor pollicis brevis muscle
21 Extensor pollicis longus muscle
22 Tendon of extensor carpi radialis longus muscle
23 Tendon of extensor carpi radialis brevis muscle
24 Deltoid muscle *(innervated by axillary nerve along with teres minor)*

125
Motor distribution of the radial nerve I
SUPERFICIAL MUSCLES

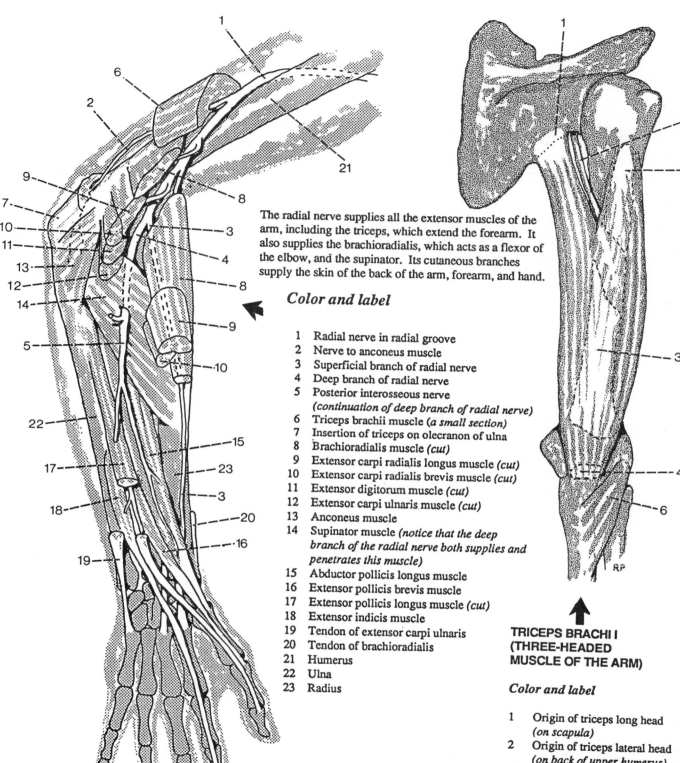

The radial nerve supplies all the extensor muscles of the arm, including the triceps, which extend the forearm. It also supplies the brachioradialis, which acts as a flexor of the elbow, and the supinator. Its cutaneous branches supply the skin of the back of the arm, forearm, and hand.

Color and label

1   Radial nerve in radial groove
2   Nerve to anconeus muscle
3   Superficial branch of radial nerve
4   Deep branch of radial nerve
5   Posterior interosseous nerve
    (*continuation of deep branch of radial nerve*)
6   Triceps brachii muscle (*a small section*)
7   Insertion of triceps on olecranon of ulna
8   Brachioradialis muscle (*cut*)
9   Extensor carpi radialis longus muscle (*cut*)
10 Extensor carpi radialis brevis muscle (*cut*)
11 Extensor digitorum muscle (*cut*)
12 Extensor carpi ulnaris muscle (*cut*)
13 Anconeus muscle
14 Supinator muscle (*notice that the deep
    branch of the radial nerve both supplies and
    penetrates this muscle*)
15 Abductor pollicis longus muscle
16 Extensor pollicis brevis muscle
17 Extensor pollicis longus muscle (*cut*)
18 Extensor indicis muscle
19 Tendon of extensor carpi ulnaris
20 Tendon of brachioradialis
21 Humerus
22 Ulna
23 Radius

**TRICEPS BRACHI I
(THREE-HEADED
MUSCLE OF THE ARM)**

Color and label

1   Origin of triceps long head
    (*on scapula*)
2   Origin of triceps lateral head
    (*on back of upper humerus*)
3   Origin of triceps medial head
    (*on back of lower humerus*)
4   Insertion of three heads of
    triceps on olecranon of ulna
5   Radial nerve
6   Anconeus muscle

126   Motor distribution of
the radial nerve II   **DEEP MUSCLES**

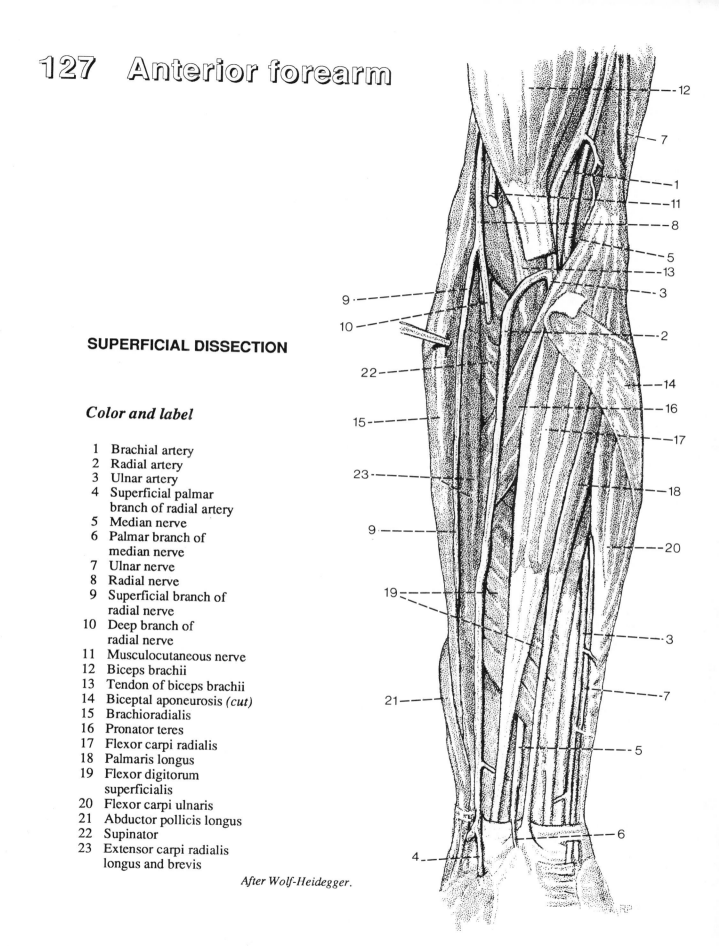

SUPERFICIAL DISSECTION

Color and label

1 Brachial artery
2 Radial artery
3 Ulnar artery
4 Superficial palmar
  branch of radial artery
5 Median nerve
6 Palmar branch of
  median nerve
7 Ulnar nerve
8 Radial nerve
9 Superficial branch of
  radial nerve
10 Deep branch of
  radial nerve
11 Musculocutaneous nerve
12 Biceps brachii
13 Tendon of biceps brachii
14 Biceptal aponeurosis *(cut)*
15 Brachioradialis
16 Pronator teres
17 Flexor carpi radialis
18 Palmaris longus
19 Flexor digitorum
  superficialis
20 Flexor carpi ulnaris
21 Abductor pollicis longus
22 Supinator
23 Extensor carpi radialis
  longus and brevis

After Wolf-Heidegger.

Color and label

1 Brachial artery
2 Ulnar artery
3 Radial artery
4 Ulnar recurrent artery
5 Common interosseous artery
6 Anterior interosseous artery
7 Posterior interosseous artery
8 Recurrent radial artery
9 Radial collateral artery
10 Inferior ulnar collateral artery
11 Superior ulnar collateral artery
12 Superficial palmar branch of ulnar artery
13 Deep palmar branch of ulnar artery
14 Superficial palmar branch of radial artery
15 Radial nerve
16 Median nerve
17 Anterior interosseous nerve
18 Palmar branch of median nerve
19 Ulnar nerve
20 Superficial branch of median nerve
21 Deep branch of ulnar nerve
22 Lateral antebrachial cutaneous nerve (musculocutaneous nerve) *(cut)*
23 Deep branch of radial nerve
24 Superficial branch of radial nerve
25 Biceps brachii
26 Tendon of biceps brachii
27 Aponeurosis of biceps brachii
28 Common head of forearm flexors *(cut)*
29 Brachioradialis *(cut)*
30 Flexor carpi ulnaris *(cut)*
31 Abductor pollicis longus
32 Flexor pollicis longus
33 Pronator quadratus
34 Flexor digitorum profundus

After Wolf-Heidegger.

Notice that the median nerve gives off the anterior interosseous nerve, which supplies the deeper flexor muscles of the forearm.

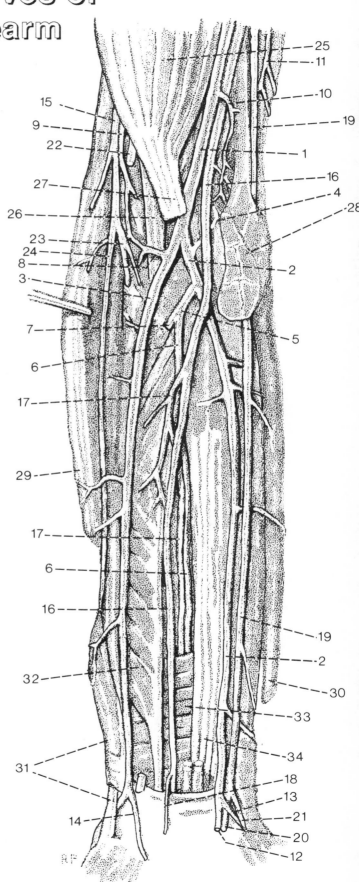

PALMAR (VENTRAL) VIEW OF THE RIGHT HAND

Color and label

1   Scaphoid *(boat-shaped)*
2   Lunate *(moon-shaped)*
3   Triquetral *(three-cornered)*
4   Pisiform *(pea-shaped)*
5   Trapezium *(the Greeks had a small table called a trapezion)*
6   Trapezoid *(a quadrilateral figure with two parallel sides)*
7   Capitate *(having a head or enlargement)*
8   Hamate *(shaped like a hook; hamus, Latin)*
9   First metacarpal bone *(of thumb)*
10 Base of fifth metacarpal
11 Body of fifth metacarpal
12 Head of fifth metacarpal
13 Base of proximal phalanx of index finger
14 Body of proximal phalanx of index finger
15 Head of proximal phalanx of index finger
16 Middle phalanx
17 Distal phalanx *(each phalanx has a base, body, and head)*
18 Proximal phalanx of thumb
19 Distal phalanx of thumb *(notice that the thumb, which is the most mobile and useful finger, has only two phalanges, whereas the other four digits each have three phalanges, resulting in a total of 14 phalanges)*
20 Radial sesamoid bone *(resembling a sesame seed)*
21 Ulnar sesamoid bone *(sesamoid bones develop and remain within tendons)*
22 Tuberosity of distal phalanx
23 Hamulus *(little hook) of hamate*
24 Tubercle of scaphoid
25 Tubercle of trapezium
26 Carpometacarpal joint *(that of the thumb is a saddle joint)*
27 Metacarpophalangeal joint *(abbreviated MP or MCP)*
28 Proximal interphalangeal joint *(PIP)*
29 Distal interphalangeal joint *(DIP)*

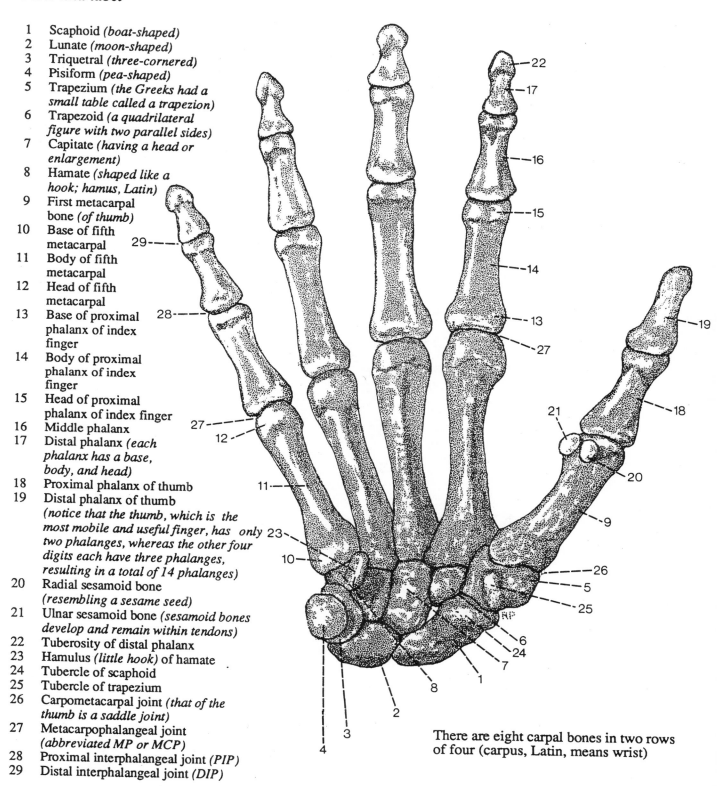

There are eight carpal bones in two rows of four (carpus, Latin, means wrist)

129   Bones of the hand

Color and label

1 Palmar aponeurosis
2 Palmaris longus tendon inserting on palmar aponeurosis
3 Thenar eminence (*abductor pollicis brevis, flexor pollicis brevis, opponens pollicis*)

4 First lumbrical muscle (*notice that the four lumbrical muscles lie on the radial or lateral side of the deep flexor tendons from which they arise*)
5 Lumbricals 2, 3, 4
6 Palmaris brevis
7 Hypothenar eminence (*flexor digiti minimi, abductor digiti minimi, opponens digiti minimi*)
8 Longitudinal fasciculi of palmar aponeurosis
9 Transverse fasciculi of palmar aponeurosis

After Wolf-Heidegger.

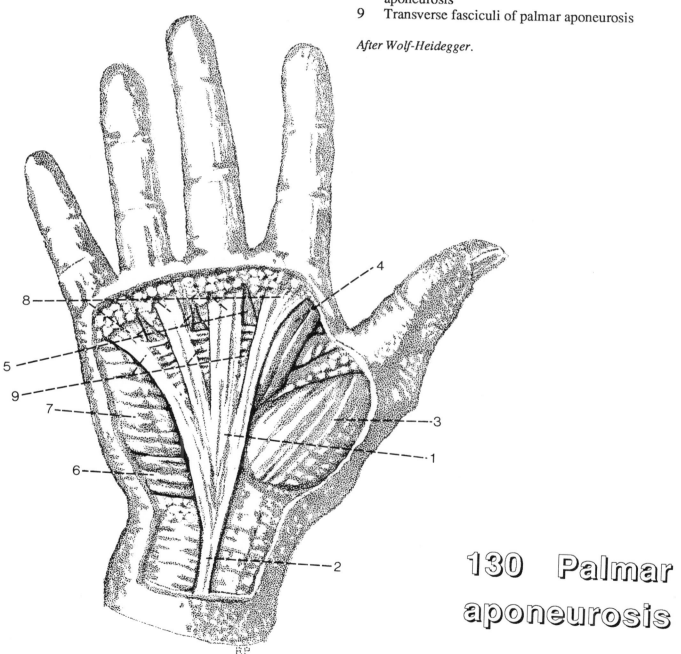

130   Palmar aponeurosis

Flexor retinaculum and superficial hand muscles

AFTER REMOVAL OF PALMAR APONEUROSIS

Color and label

1 Flexor retinaculum
2 Tendons of flexor digitorum superficialis to digits 2, 3, 4, 5
3 Tendon of flexor carpi radialis
4 Tendon of flexor pollicis longus
5 Tendon of abductor pollicis longus
6 Tendon of flexor carpi ulnaris
7 Pisiform bone
8 Abductor pollicis brevis
9 Flexor pollicis brevis
10 Opponens pollicis
11 Adductor pollicis
12 Lumbricals 1, 2, 3, 4
13 First dorsal interosseous
14 Flexor digiti minimi
15 Abductor digiti minimi
16 Opponens digiti minimi
17 Fibrous tendon sheath
18 Fibrous and synovial tendon sheaths of middle finger *(opened)*
19 Tendon of flexor digitorum profundus
20 Carpal tunnel

After Wolf-Heidegger

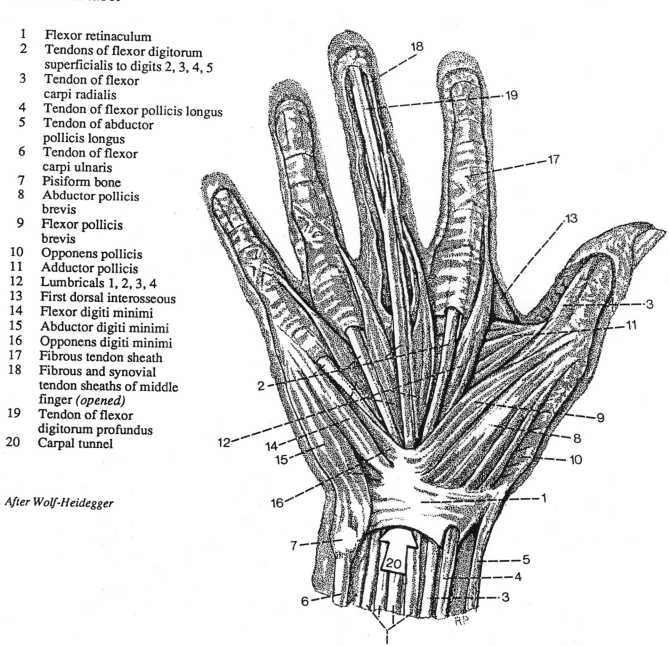

OPENED; DEEP FLEXOR TENDONS AND RELATED STRUCTURES

Color and label

1 Tendons of flexor digitorum profundus within carpal tunnel (*flexor digitorum superficialis tendons cut and removed*)
2 Flexor pollicis longus tendon within carpal tunnel
3 Flexor retinaculum (*cut and reflected*)
4 Abductor pollicis (*cut*)
5 Opponens pollicis
6 Flexor pollicis brevis (*superficial head*)
7 Adductor pollicis
8 First dorsal interosseous muscle
9 Lumbrical muscles (1, 2, 3, 4) (*notice their arising on the four profundus tendons*)
10 Flexor digitorum superficialis tendons (*cut and reflected*)
11 Opponens digiti minimi
12 Flexor digiti minimi
13 Abductor digiti minimi (*cut*)
14 Pisiform bone
15 Fibrous and synovial tendon sheaths (*cut open*)
16 Tendon of flexor carpi ulnaris
17 Tendon of flexor carpi radialis
18 Tendon of abductor pollicis
19 Tendon of flexor pollicis longus
20 Pronator quadratus
21 Radius
22 Ulna
23 Antebrachial interosseous membrane

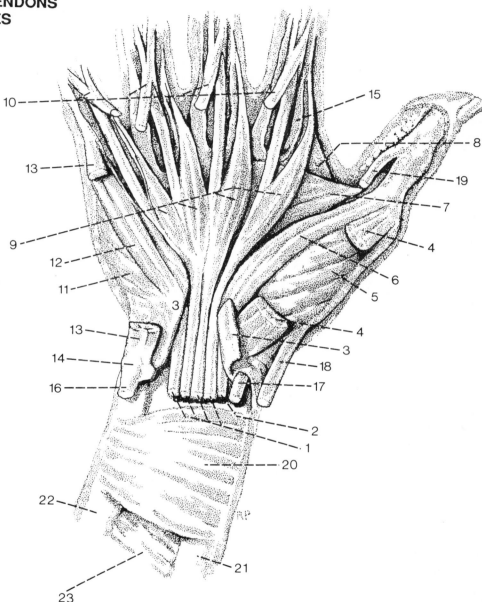

After Wolf-Heidegger.

Notice that nine tendons pass through the carpal tunnel, four from the flexor digitorum superficialis, four from the flexor digitorum profundus, and the ninth from the flexor pollicis longus. The median nerve, not shown here, also passes through the carpal tunnel. The two lateral lumbrical muscles are usually supplied by the median nerve and the two medial lumbricals by the ulnar nerve.

133 Deep thenar, hypothenar, and interosseous muscles

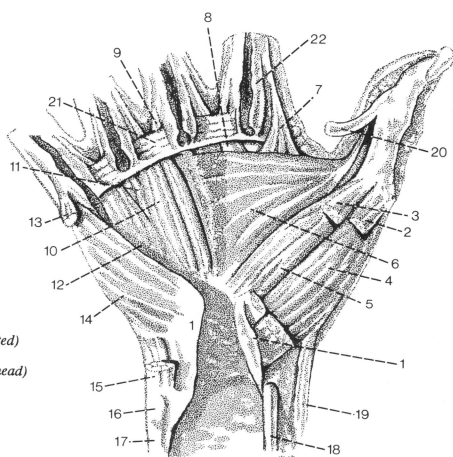

Color and label

1   Flexor retinaculum *(cut and reflected)*
2   Abductor pollicis brevis
3   Flexor pollicis brevis *(superficial head)*
4   Opponens pollicis
5   Flexor pollicis brevis *(deep head*)*
6   Adductor pollicis
7   First dorsal interosseous
8   First palmar interosseous
9   Third dorsal interosseous
10   Second palmar interosseous
11   Fourth dorsal interosseous
12   Third palmar interosseous
13   Abductor digiti minimi and
      flexor digiti minimi *(common
      insertion)*
14   Opponens digiti minimi
15   Abductor digiti minimi
16   Pisiform bone
17   Tendon of flexor carpi ulnaris
18   Tendon of flexor carpi radialis
19   Tendon of abductor pollicis longus
20   Tendon of flexor pollicis longus
21   Deep transverse metacarpal ligament
22   Fibrous sheath *(cut open and super-
      ficial and deep tendons removed)*

After Wolf-Heidegger.

**The deep head of the flexor pollicis brevis is
usually supplied by the ulnar nerve, and the
superficial head by the median nerve. Thus,
the median nerve usually supplies two and a
half of the three thenar muscles.*

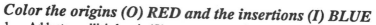

Color the origins (O) RED and the insertions (I) BLUE

1 Adductor pollicis brevis (O)
2 Opponens pollicis (O)
3 Opponens pollicis (I)
4 Flexor pollicis brevis (O)
5 Flexor pollicis brevis and adductor pollicis brevis common sesamoid bone and insertion (I)

6 Adductor pollicis *(oblique head)* (O)
7 Adductor pollicis *(transverse head)* (O)
8 Adductor pollicis sesamoid bone and insertion (I)
9 Dorsal interosseous (1, 2, 3, 4) (O)
10 Dorsal interosseous (1, 2, 3, 4) inserts on "hood" of extensor tendons (I)
11 Palmar (ventral) interosseous (1, 2, 3) (O)
12 Palmar (ventral) interosseous (1, 2, 3) (I)
13 Flexor digiti minimi (O) and pisohamate ligament
14 Abductor digiti minimi (O)
15 Opponens digiti minimi (O)
16 Opponens digiti minimi (I)
17 Abductor digiti minimi (I)
18 Flexor digiti minimi (I)

19 Abductor pollicis longus (I)
20 Flexor carpi radialis (I)
21 Flexor carpi ulnaris (I)
22 Flexor pollicis longus (I)

23 Flexor digitorum superficialis (I
24 Flexor digitorum profundus (I)
25 Extensor carpi ulnaris (I) and pisometacarpal ligament

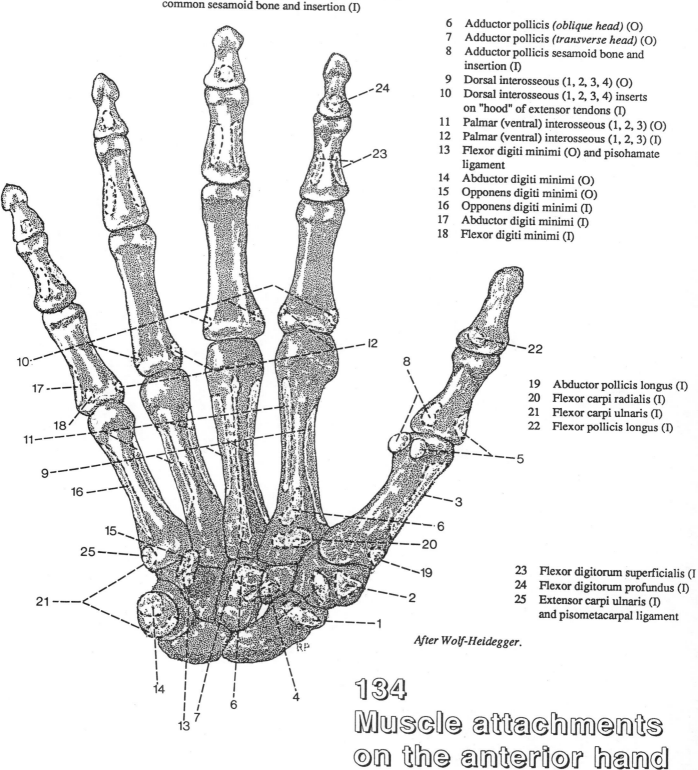

After Wolf-Heidegger.

134
Muscle attachments
on the anterior hand

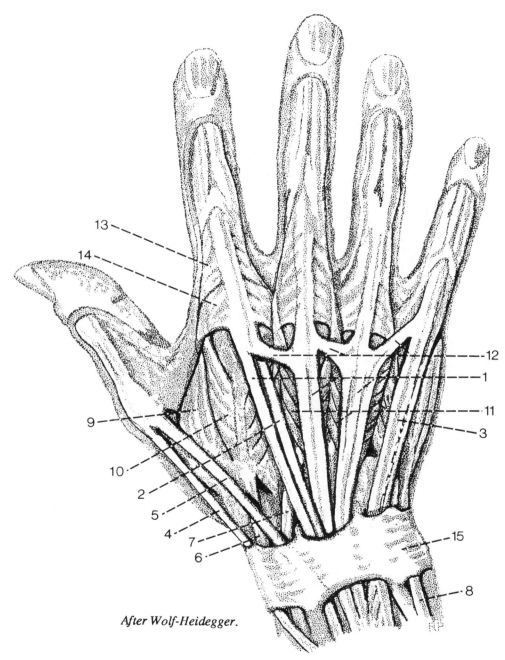

After Wolf-Heidegger.

Color and label

1 Tendons of extensor digitorum
  going to digits 2, 3, 4, 5
2 Tendon of extensor indicis
3 Tendon of extensor digiti minimi
4 Tendon of extensor pollicis brevis
5 Tendon of extensor pollicis longus
6 Tendon of extensor carpi radialis longus
7 Tendon of extensor carpi radialis brevis

8 Tendon of extensor carpi ulnaris
9 First dorsal interosseous muscle
  superficial head
10 First dorsal interosseous muscle deep head
11 Dorsal interosseous muscles 2, 3, 4
12 Intertendinous connections
13 Extensor expansion
14 Extensor hood
15 Extensor retinaculum

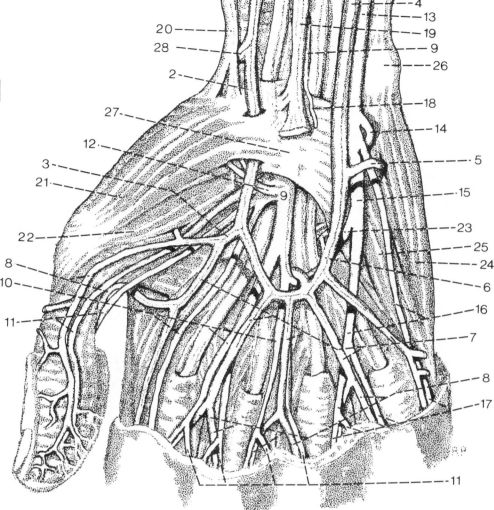

Color and label

1 Radial artery
2 Superficial palmar ramus
  of radial artery
3 Principal thumb artery
  (princeps pollicis)
4 Ulnar artery
5 Deep branch of ulnar artery
6 Superficial palmar arch
7 Common palmar digital arteries
8 Proper palmar digital arteries
9 Median nerve
10 Common palmar digital nerves
   (from median nerve)
11 Proper palmar digital nerves
   (from median nerve)
12 Thenar muscular branch of median
   nerve *(recurrent branch)*
13 Ulnar nerve

14 Deep branch of ulnar nerve
15 Superficial branch of ulnar nerve
16 Common palmar digital nerves
   (from ulnar nerve)
17 Proper palmar digital nerves
   (from ulnar nerve)
18 Palmar ramus of median nerve
19 Tendon of palmaris longus
20 Tendon of abductor pollicis longus
21 Abductor pollicis brevis
22 Flexor pollicis brevis
23 Communicating branch between
   median and ulnar nerves
24 Abductor digiti minimi
25 Flexor digiti minimi
26 Pisiform bone
27 Flexor retinaculum
28 Deep palmar branch (ramus) of
   radial artery

After Spalteholz and Spanner

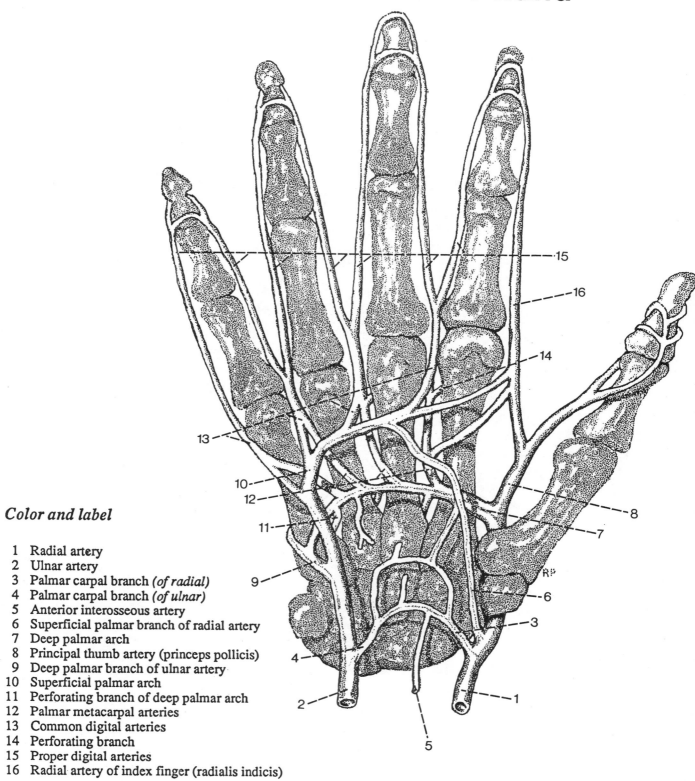

Color and label

1   Radial artery
2   Ulnar artery
3   Palmar carpal branch *(of radial)*
4   Palmar carpal branch *(of ulnar)*
5   Anterior interosseous artery
6   Superficial palmar branch of radial artery
7   Deep palmar arch
8   Principal thumb artery (princeps pollicis)
9   Deep palmar branch of ulnar artery
10 Superficial palmar arch
11 Perforating branch of deep palmar arch
12 Palmar metacarpal arteries
13 Common digital arteries
14 Perforating branch
15 Proper digital arteries
16 Radial artery of index finger (radialis indicis)

After Hollinshead and Rosse.

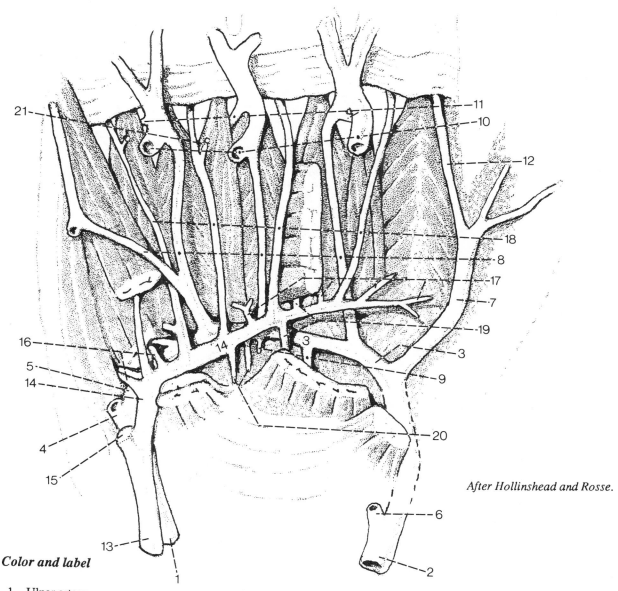

After Hollinshead and Rosse.

Color and label

1 Ulnar artery
2 Radial artery
3 Deep palmar arch
4 Superficial palmar arch *(cut)*
5 Deep palmar branch of ulnar artery
6 Superficial palmar branch of radial artery *(cut)*
7 Princeps pollicis artery
8 Palmar metacarpal arteries
9 Perforating branches from deep palmar arch
10 Common digital arteries *(cut)*
11 Perforating branches of metacarpal arteries

12 Radialis indicis artery
13 Ulnar nerve
14 Deep branch of ulnar nerve
15 Superficial branch of ulnar nerve *(cut)*
16 Ulnar nerve branches to hypothenar muscles
17 Branches to interosseous muslces
18 Articular branches *(to metacarpophalangeal joints)*
19 Branches to two heads of adductor pollicis
20 Carpal twigs *(to carpal bones and joints)*
21 Nerves to two medial lumbricals

Notice that usually the ulnar nerve supplies the three hypothenar muscles, all seven interosseous muscles, the two heads of the adductor pollicis, the two medial (or ulnar) lumbrical muscles, and the deep head of the flexor pollicis (not shown).

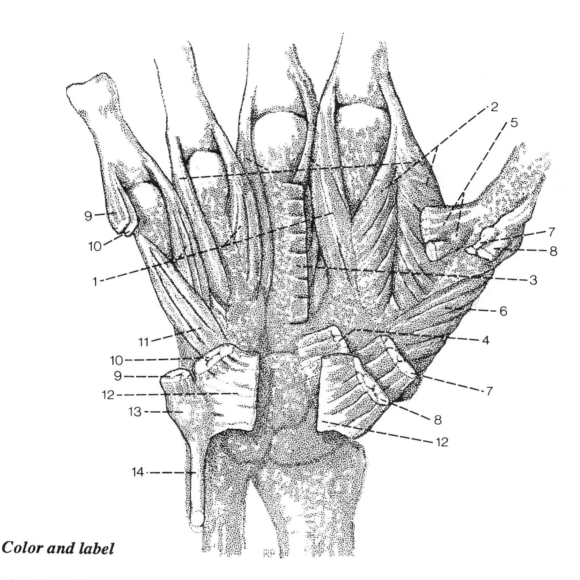

Color and label

1 Ventral interosseous muscles
2 Dorsal interosseous muscles
3 Adductor pollicis *(transverse head, cut)*
4 Adductor pollicis *(oblique head, cut)*
5 Adductor pollicis insertion with ulnar sesamoid bone
6 Opponens pollicis

7 Flexor pollicis brevis *(cut)*
8 Abductor pollicis brevis *(cut)*
9 Abductor digiti minimi *(cut)*
10 Flexor digiti minimi *(cut)*
11 Opponens digiti minimi
12 Flexor retinaculum *(cut)*
13 Pisiform bone
14 Tendon of flexor carpi ulnaris

The dorsal interosseous muscles abduct (spread apart) digits 2-5. The ventral interosseous muscles adduct (bring together) the same digits.

PART V: BACK

PLATES 140-153

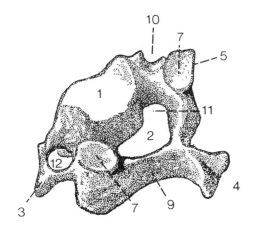

CERVICAL VERTEBRA

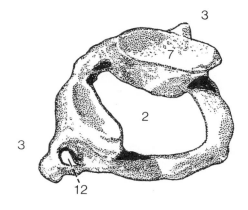

FIRST CERVICAL (C1) VERTEBRA (ATLAS)

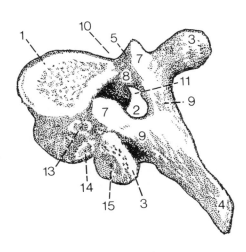

THORACIC VERTEBRA

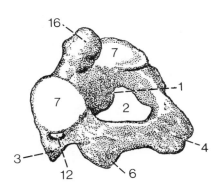

SECOND CERVICAL (C2) VERTEBRA (AXIS)

Color each vertebra and label

1 Body of vertebra
2 Vertebral foramen
3 Transverse process
4 Spinous process
5 Superior articular process
6 Inferior articular process
7 Superior articular facet
8 Pedicle
9 Lamina
10 Superior vertebral notch
11 Inferior vertebral notch
12 Foramen transversarium (cervical vertebrae)
13 Superior demifacet for head of rib (thoracic vertebra)
14 Inferior demifacet for head of rib (thoracic vertebra)
15 Facet on transverse process for tubercle of rib (thoracic vertebra)
16 Dens of axis
17 Mamillary process (lumbar vertebra)

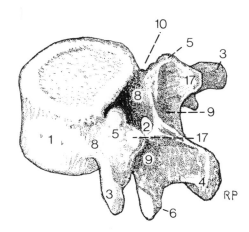

LUMBAR VERTEBRA

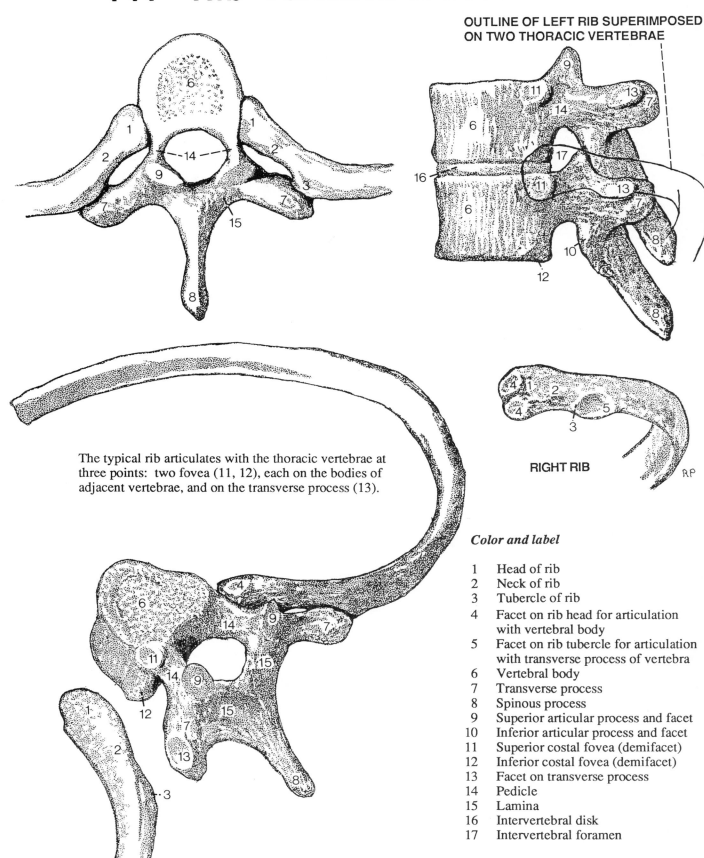

OUTLINE OF LEFT RIB SUPERIMPOSED
ON TWO THORACIC VERTEBRAE

The typical rib articulates with the thoracic vertebrae at three points: two fovea (11, 12), each on the bodies of adjacent vertebrae, and on the transverse process (13).

RIGHT RIB

Color and label

1   Head of rib
2   Neck of rib
3   Tubercle of rib
4   Facet on rib head for articulation with vertebral body
5   Facet on rib tubercle for articulation with transverse process of vertebra
6   Vertebral body
7   Transverse process
8   Spinous process
9   Superior articular process and facet
10 Inferior articular process and facet
11 Superior costal fovea (demifacet)
12 Inferior costal fovea (demifacet)
13 Facet on transverse process
14 Pedicle
15 Lamina
16 Intervertebral disk
17 Intervertebral foramen

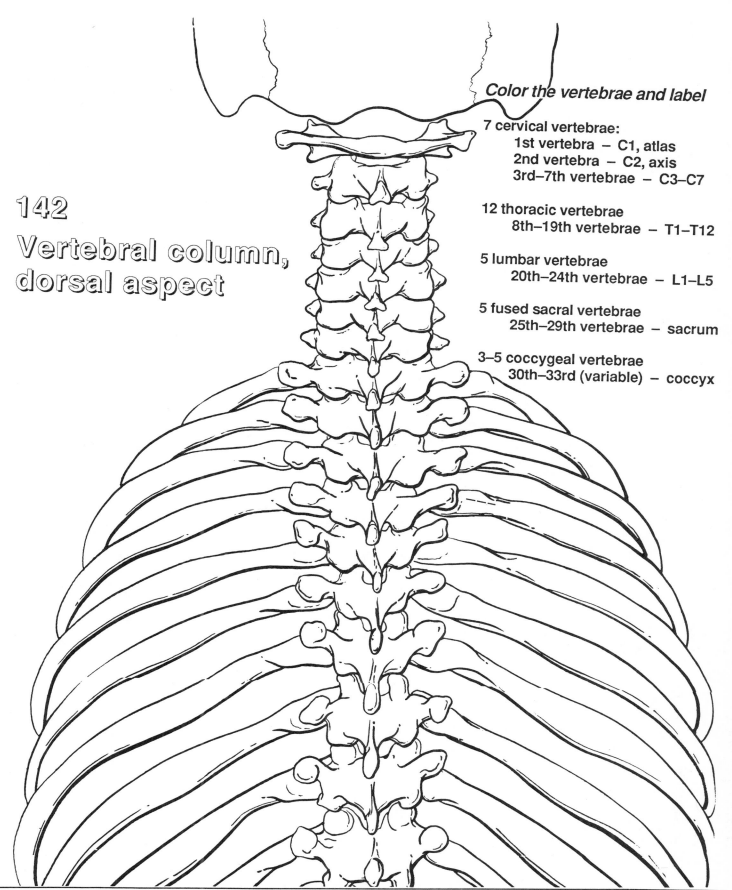

142

Vertebral column, dorsal aspect

Color the vertebrae and label

7 cervical vertebrae:
    1st vertebra — C1, atlas
    2nd vertebra — C2, axis
    3rd–7th vertebrae — C3–C7

12 thoracic vertebrae
    8th–19th vertebrae — T1–T12

5 lumbar vertebrae
    20th–24th vertebrae — L1–L5

5 fused sacral vertebrae
    25th–29th vertebrae — sacrum

3–5 coccygeal vertebrae
    30th–33rd (variable) — coccyx

ATTACH THE FOLLOWING PAGE HERE

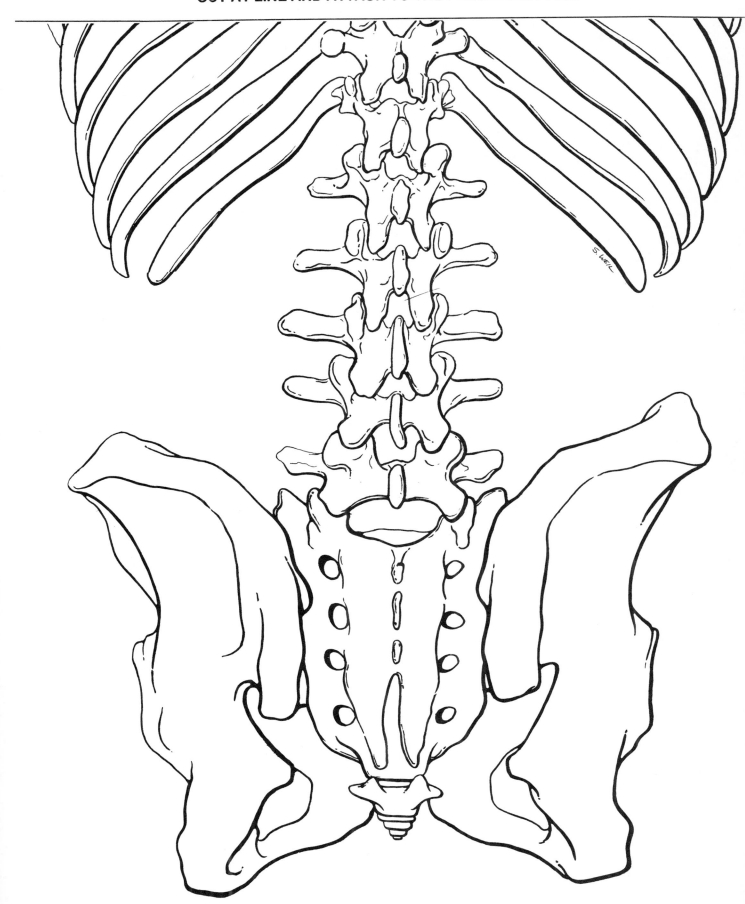

143 Back muscles I: superficial layer

RP

T8

T12

L1

L4

13

13

14

14

15

Color and label

1 Trapezius
2 Semispinalis
3 Splenius capitis
4 Splenius cervicis
5 Levator scapulae
6 Rhomboid minor
7 Rhomboid major
8 Supraspinatus

9   Deltoid
10 Infraspinatus
11 Teres minor
12 Teres major
13 Latissimus dorsi
14 External abdominal oblique
15 Thoracolumbar fascia

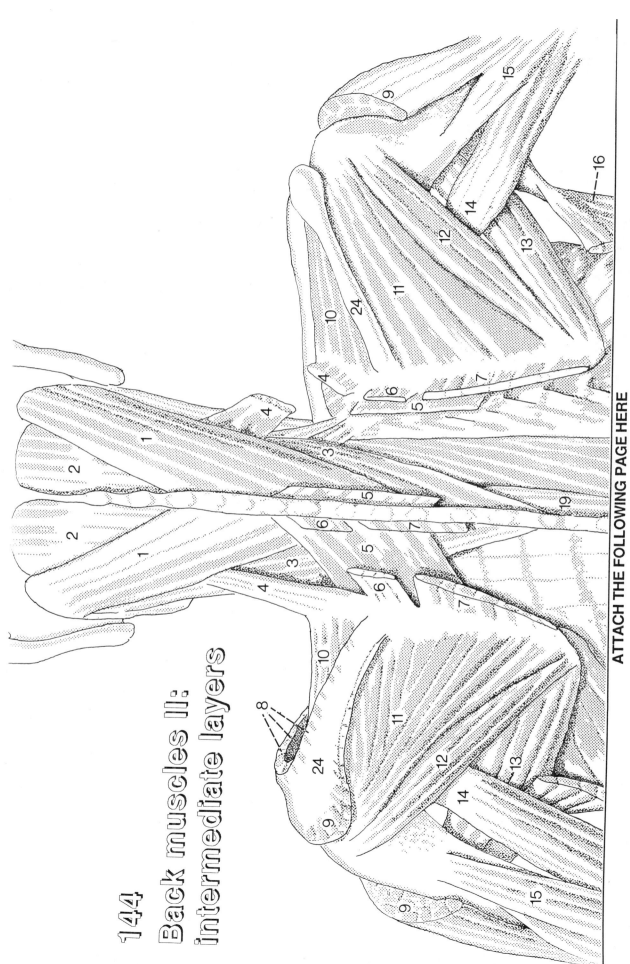

144

Back muscles II:
intermediate layers

Color and label

1 Splenius capitis
2 Semispinalis capitis
3 Splenius cervicis
4 Levator scapulae
5 Serratus posterior superior
6 Rhomboideus minor
7 Rhomboideus major
8 Trapezius
9 Deltoid
10 Supraspinatus
11 Infraspinatus
12 Teres minor
13 Teres major
14 Triceps brachii, long head
15 Triceps brachii, lateral head
16 Latissimus dorsi
17 Serratus anterior
18 Serratus posterior inferior
19 Spinalis thoracis
20 Longissimus
21 Iliocostalis
22 Latissimus dorsi and aponeurosis
23 Thoracolumbar fascia
24 Spine of scapula

RP

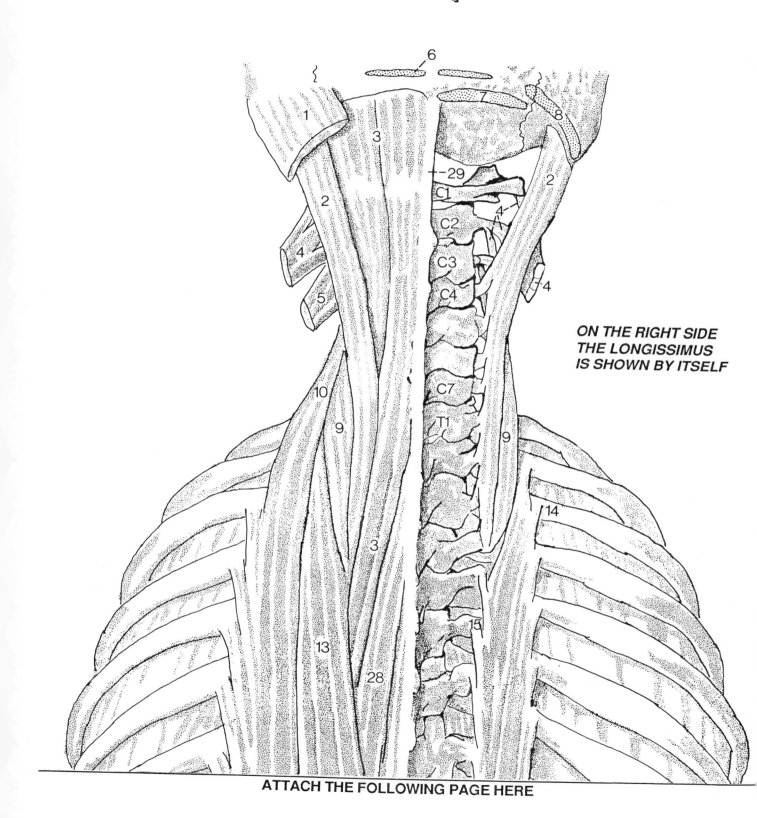

ON THE RIGHT SIDE
THE LONGISSIMUS
IS SHOWN BY ITSELF

ATTACH THE FOLLOWING PAGE HERE

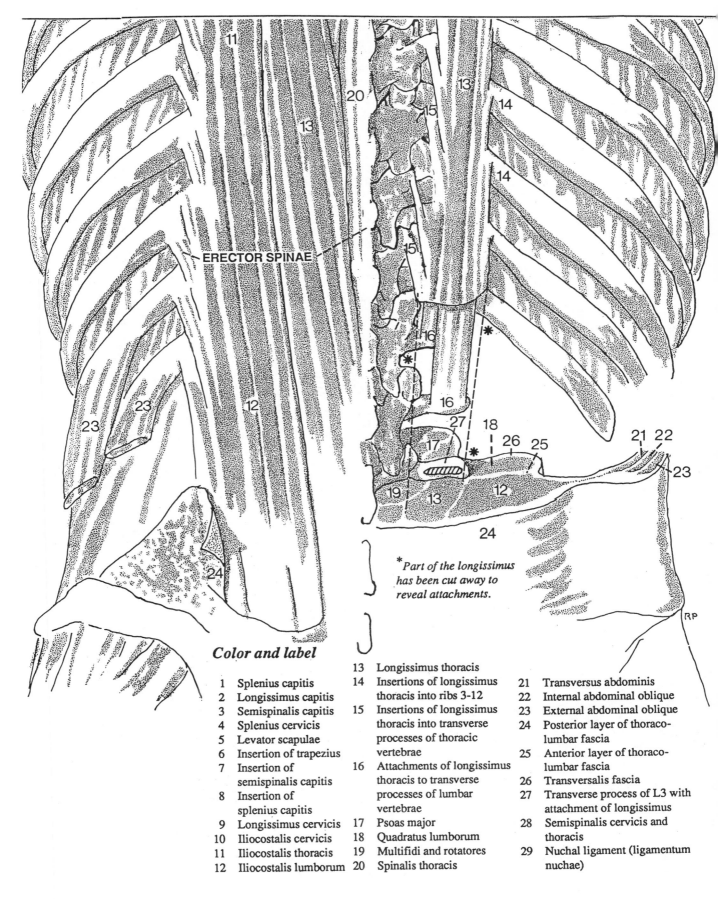

ERECTOR SPINAE

*Part of the longissimus
has been cut away to
reveal attachments.*

Color and label

1	Splenius capitis
2	Longissimus capitis
3	Semispinalis capitis
4	Splenius cervicis
5	Levator scapulae
6	Insertion of trapezius
7	Insertion of semispinalis capitis
8	Insertion of splenius capitis
9	Longissimus cervicis
10	Iliocostalis cervicis
11	Iliocostalis thoracis
12	Iliocostalis lumborum

13	Longissimus thoracis
14	Insertions of longissimus thoracis into ribs 3-12
15	Insertions of longissimus thoracis into transverse processes of thoracic vertebrae
16	Attachments of longissimus thoracis to transverse processes of lumbar vertebrae
17	Psoas major
18	Quadratus lumborum
19	Multifidi and rotatores
20	Spinalis thoracis

21	Transversus abdominis
22	Internal abdominal oblique
23	External abdominal oblique
24	Posterior layer of thoraco-lumbar fascia
25	Anterior layer of thoraco-lumbar fascia
26	Transversalis fascia
27	Transverse process of L3 with attachment of longissimus
28	Semispinalis cervicis and thoracis
29	Nuchal ligament (ligamentum nuchae)

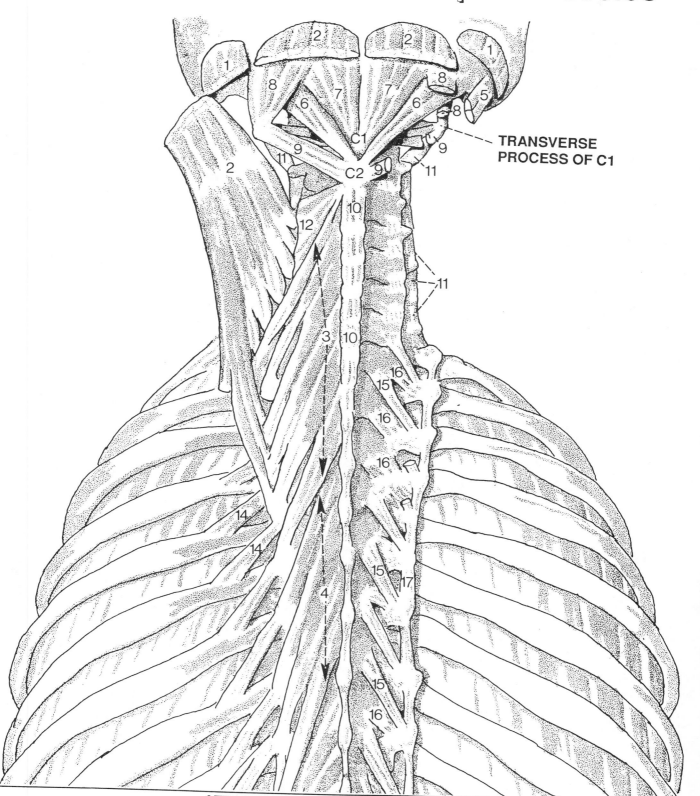

TRANSVERSE PROCESS OF C1

ATTACH THE FOLLOWING PAGE HERE

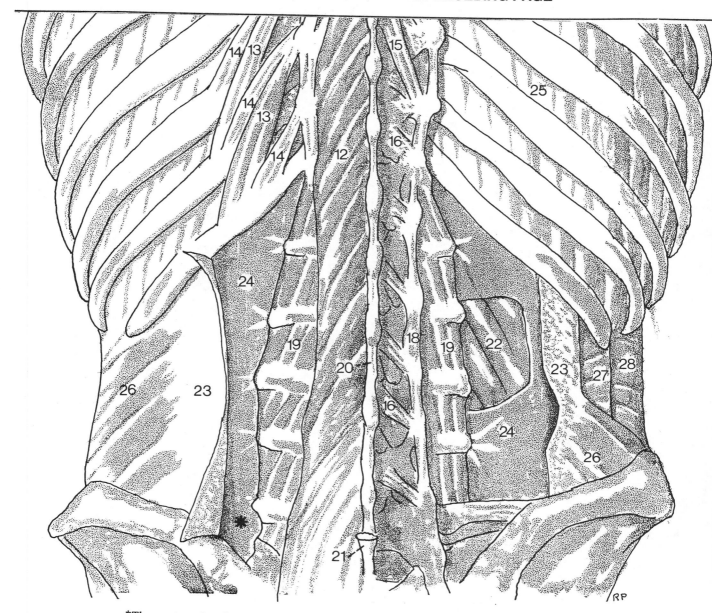

*The erector spinae lies between the anterior and posterior layers of the thoracolumbar fascia.

Color and label

1	Splenius capitis	15	Rotatores longi
2	Semispinalis capitis	16	Rotatores breves
3	Semispinalis cervicis	17	Intertransversarii thoracis
4	Semispinalis thoracis	18	Intertransversarii lumborum *(medial)*
5	Longissimus capitis	19	Intertransversarii lumborum *(lateral)*
6	Rectus capitis posterior major	20	Interspinales lumborum
7	Rectus capitis posterior minor	21	Supraspinous ligament *(cut)*
8	Obliquus capitis superior	22	Quadratus lumborum
9	Obliquus capitis inferior	23	Thoracolumbar fascia *(posterior layer, cut)*
10	Interspinales cervicis	24	Thoracolumbar fascia *(anterior layer)*
11	Intertransversarii cervicis *(posterior)*	25	External intercostal
12	Multifidus	26	External abdominal oblique
13	Levatores costarum longi	27	Internal abdominal oblique
14	Levatores costarum breves	28	Transversus abdominis

The multifidus extends from the sacrum to the axis (C2). On the left, several bundles have a common origin from the same mamillary process. The longest bundle (1) extends up to the spinous process of T12, thus reaching the 5th vertebra above. The next longest bundle (2) reaches L1 (the 4th vertebra above). Bundle 3 extends to L2 (3rd vertebra above) and bundle 4 extends to the 2nd vertebra above. This is the general pattern of the multifidus, with three or four bundles of different lengths arising from a common origin. The origins of the multifidus are the back of the sacrum (indicated by the dotted area), the mamillary processes of the lumbar vertebrae, the transverse processes of thoracic vertebrae, and the articular process of the lower four cervical vertebrae. It inserts into the spinous processes of all vertebrae up to and including the axis.

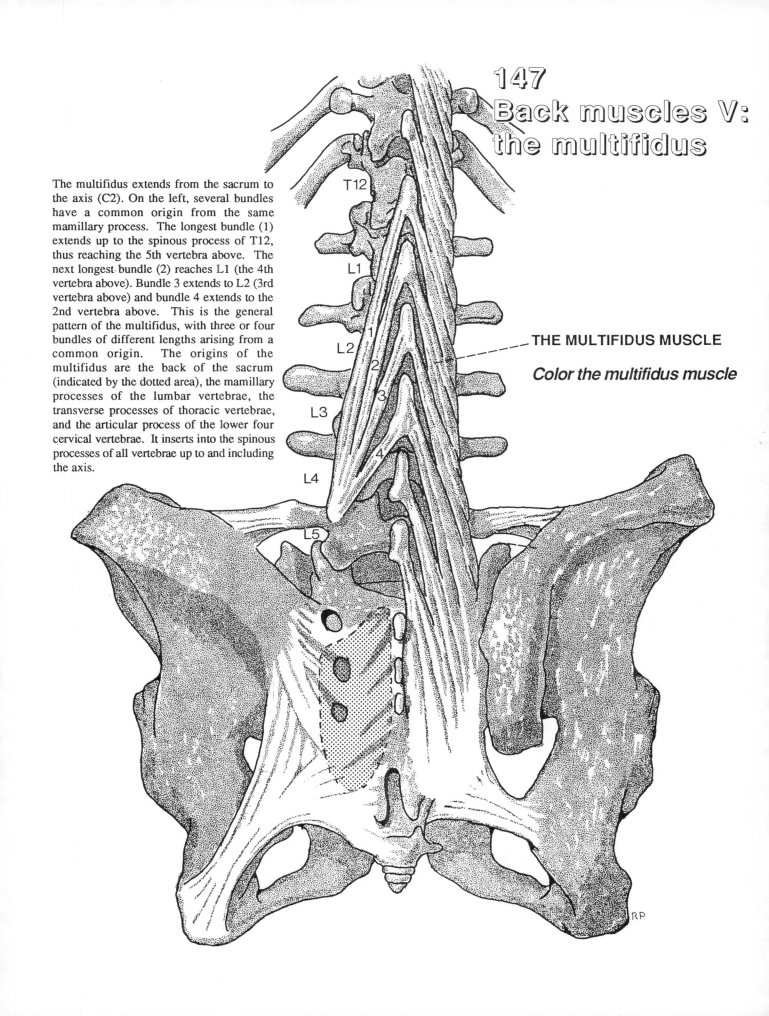

THE MULTIFIDUS MUSCLE

Color the multifidus muscle

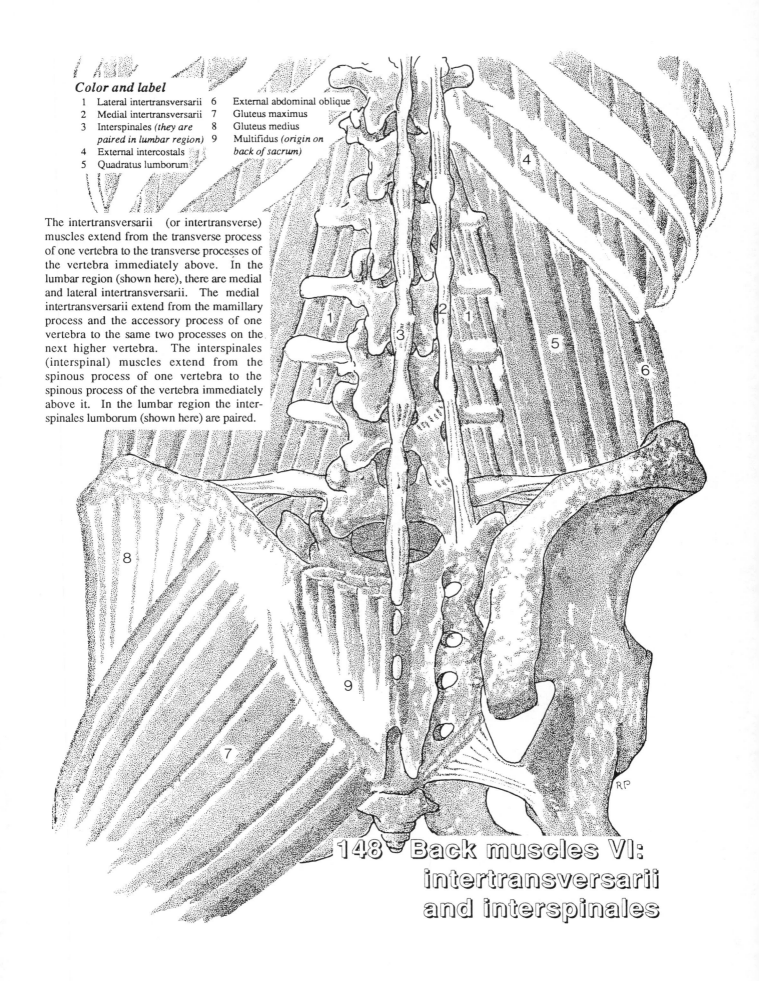

The intertransversarii (or intertransverse) muscles extend from the transverse process of one vertebra to the transverse processes of the vertebra immediately above. In the lumbar region (shown here), there are medial and lateral intertransversarii. The medial intertransversarii extend from the mamillary process and the accessory process of one vertebra to the same two processes on the next higher vertebra. The interspinales (interspinal) muscles extend from the spinous process of one vertebra to the spinous process of the vertebra immediately above it. In the lumbar region the interspinales lumborum (shown here) are paired.

148 Back muscles VI: intertransversarii and interspinales

149 Ligaments of the posterior sacrum

Color and label

1. Sacrotuberous ligament
2. Sacrospinous ligament
3. Iliolumbar ligament
4. Posterior sacroiliac ligament
5. Supraspinous ligament *(this runs from spinous process to spinous process for the entire length of the vertebral column)*
6. Joint capsule of "facet" joint between articular processes *(each of these joints has a joint capsule; only two are shown here)*
7. Spine of ischium
8. Ischial tuberosity

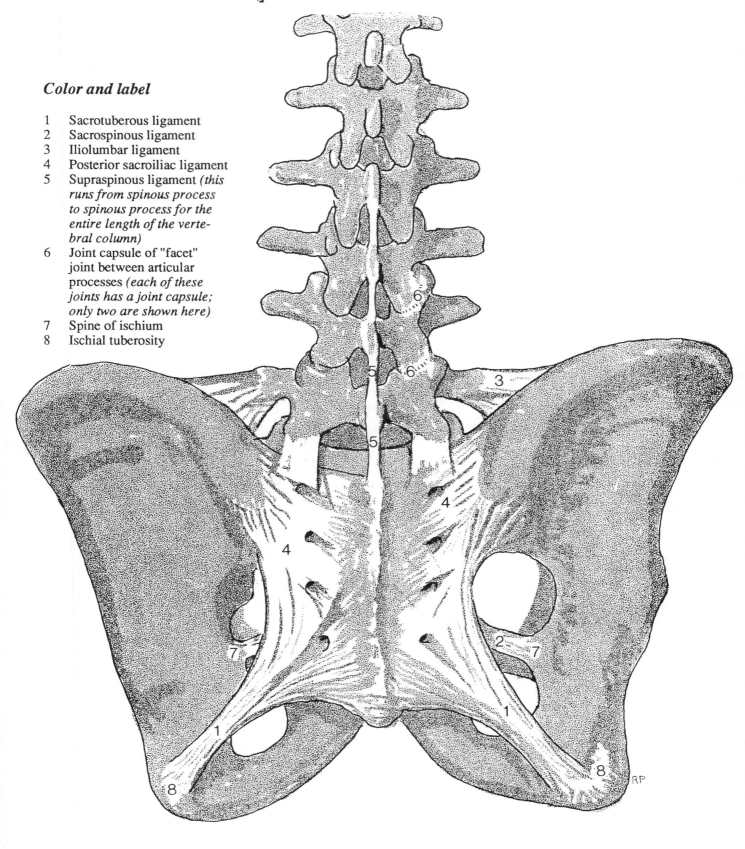

150 Lumbar vertebrae

Color and label

1	Spinous process
2	Transverse process
3	Superior articular process
4	Inferior articular process
5	Superior articular facet
6	Lamina
7	Mamillary process
8	Accessory process
9	Body
10	Posterior superior iliac spine
L1	First lumbar vertebra
L2	Second lumbar vertebra
L3	Third lumbar vertebra
L4	Fourth lumbar vertebra
L5	Fifth lumbar vertebra

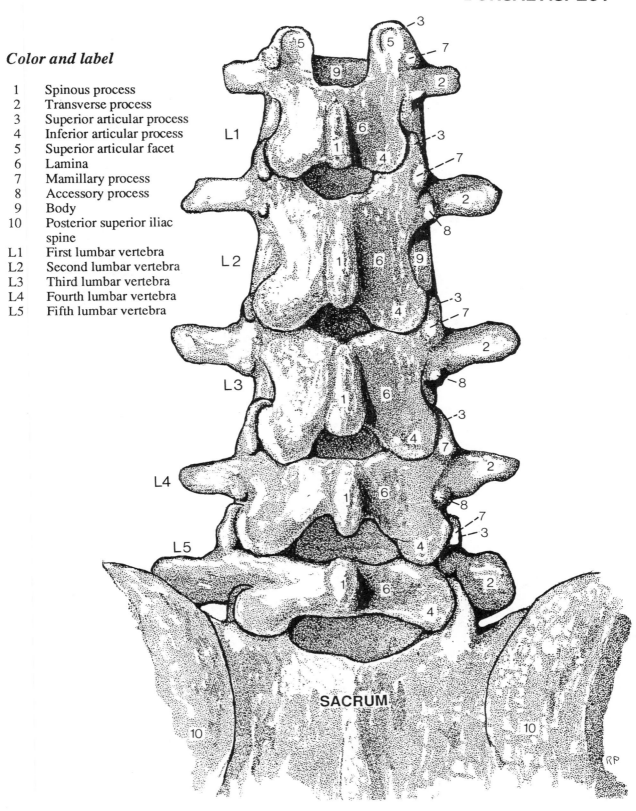

SACRUM

FIFTH LUMBAR VERTEBRA

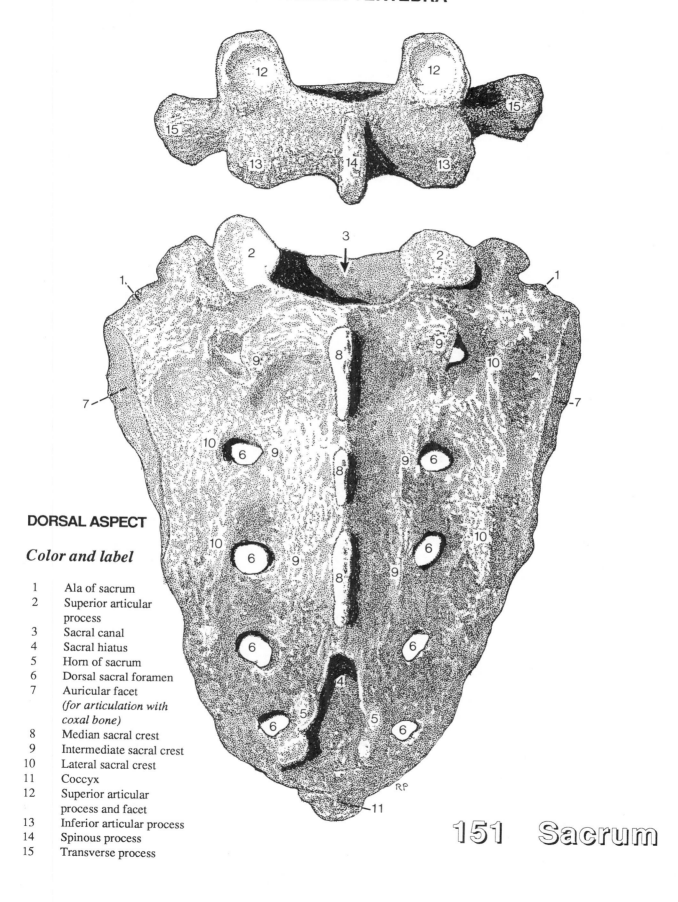

DORSAL ASPECT

Color and label

1 Ala of sacrum
2 Superior articular process
3 Sacral canal
4 Sacral hiatus
5 Horn of sacrum
6 Dorsal sacral foramen
7 Auricular facet
   (for articulation with coxal bone)
8 Median sacral crest
9 Intermediate sacral crest
10 Lateral sacral crest
11 Coccyx
12 Superior articular process and facet
13 Inferior articular process
14 Spinous process
15 Transverse process

151 Sacrum

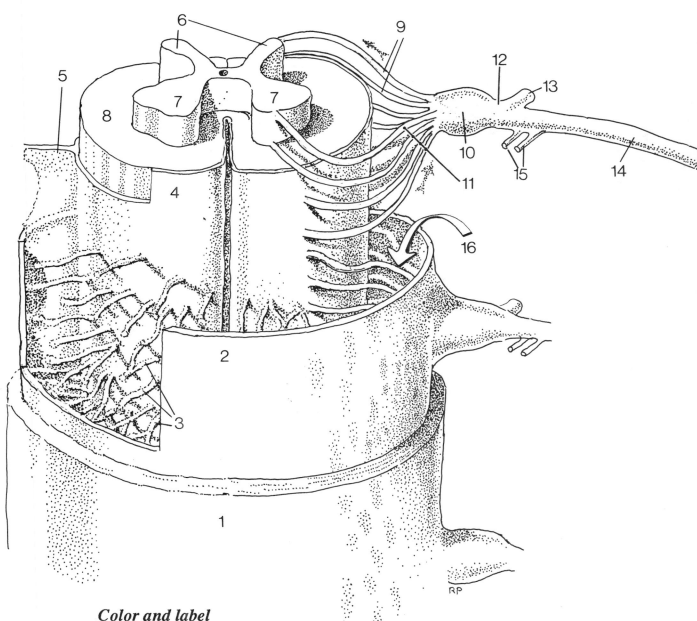

RP

Color and label

1	Dura mater	9	Dorsal root filaments
2	Arachnoid mater	10	Dorsal root ganglion
3	Arachnoid trabeculae	11	Ventral root filaments
4	Pia mater	12	Spinal nerve trunk
5	Denticulate ligament	13	Dorsal ramus
6	Dorsal horn *(of gray matter)*	14	Ventral ramus
7	Ventral horn *(of gray matter)*	15	Communicating rami
8	White matter	16	Subarachnoid space

From Poritsky R: Neuroanatomical Pathways.
Philadelphia, W.B. Saunders, 1984, with permission.

153 Functional components of spinal nerves

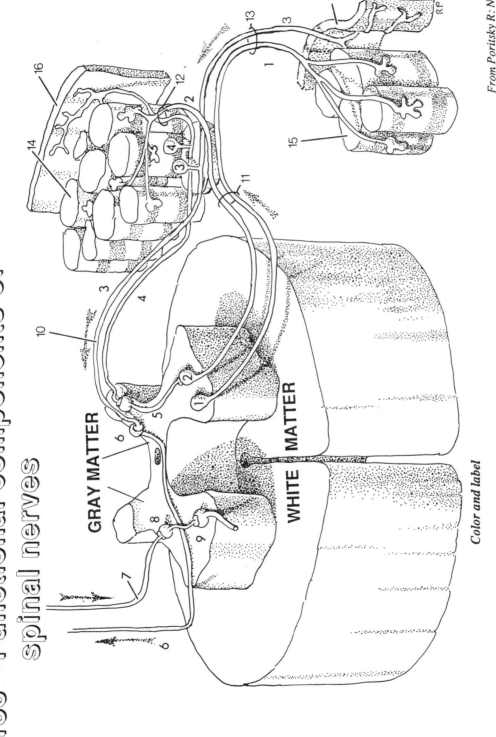

GRAY MATTER

WHITE MATTER

RP

From Poritsky R: Neuroanatomical Pathways. Philadelphia, W.B. Saunders, 1984, with permission.

Color and label

1   Motor neuron to limb muscle
2   Motor neuron to back muscle
3   Sensory neuron from skin of limb
4   Sensory neuron from skin of back
5   Interneuron connecting sensory neuron 4 with motor neuron 2
6   Second-order sensory neuron conveying information up spinal cord
7   Descending fiber bringing motor commands to interneuron (8), which
8   relays commands to motor neuron (9)

10   Dorsal root
11   Ventral root
12   Dorsal ramus
13   Ventral ramus
14   Intrinsic back muscles
15   Muscles of arm, leg, and trunk (*but not back*)
16   Skin of back
17   Skin of remainder of body

PART VI: LEG

PLATES 154-194

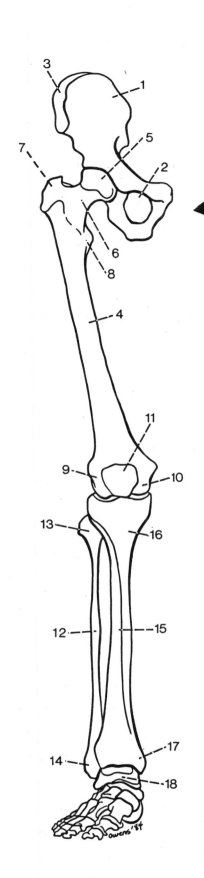

**RIGHT LEG,
ANTERIOR VIEW**

Color and label

1   Coxal bone (hip bone)
2   Obturator foramen
3   Iliac crest
4   Femur
5   Head of femur
6   Neck of femur
7   Greater trochanter
8   Lesser trochanter
9   Lateral epicondyle
10   Medial epicondyle
11   Patella
12   Fibula
13   Head of fibula
14   Lateral malleolus
15   Tibia
16   Tibial tuberosity
17   Medial malleolus
18   Talus

**RIGHT LEG,
POSTERIOR VIEW**

Color and label

1   Ischial tuberosity
2   Greater trochanter
3   Lesser trochanter
4   Intertrochanteric crest
5   Linea aspera
6   Adductor tubercle
7   Medial condyle
8   Lateral condyle
9   Tibia
10   Fibula
11   Talus
12   Calcaneus

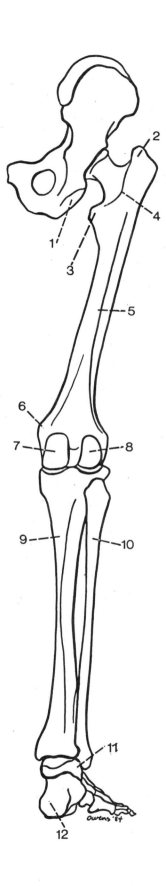

154   Hip bone and bones of leg

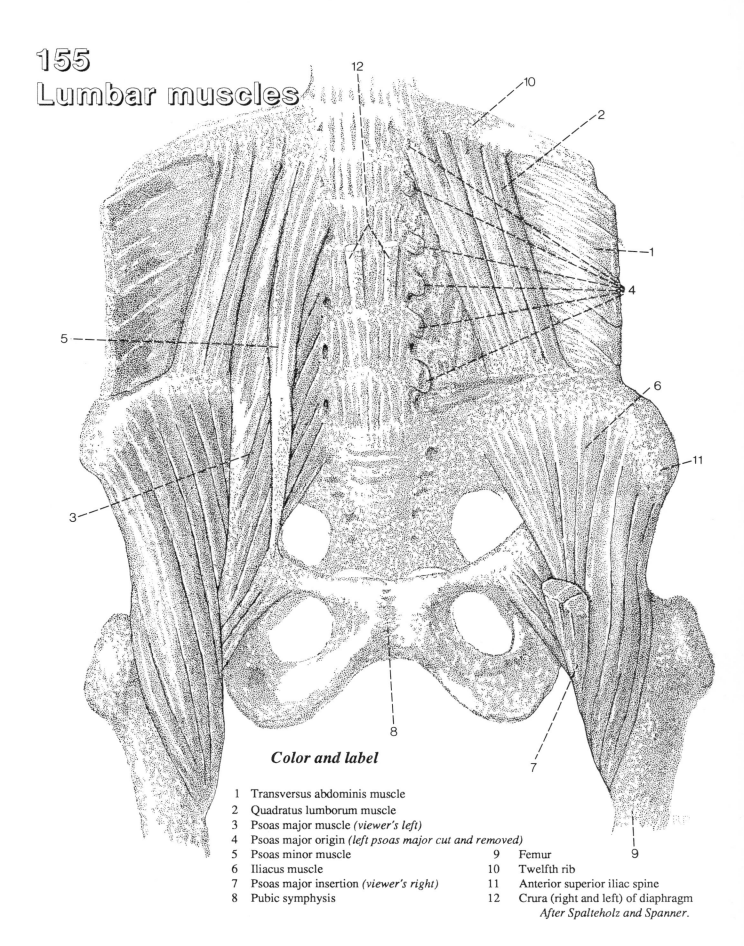

Color and label

1 Transversus abdominis muscle
2 Quadratus lumborum muscle
3 Psoas major muscle *(viewer's left)*
4 Psoas major origin *(left psoas major cut and removed)*
5 Psoas minor muscle
6 Iliacus muscle
7 Psoas major insertion *(viewer's right)*
8 Pubic symphysis

9 Femur
10 Twelfth rib
11 Anterior superior iliac spine
12 Crura (right and left) of diaphragm

After Spalteholz and Spanner.

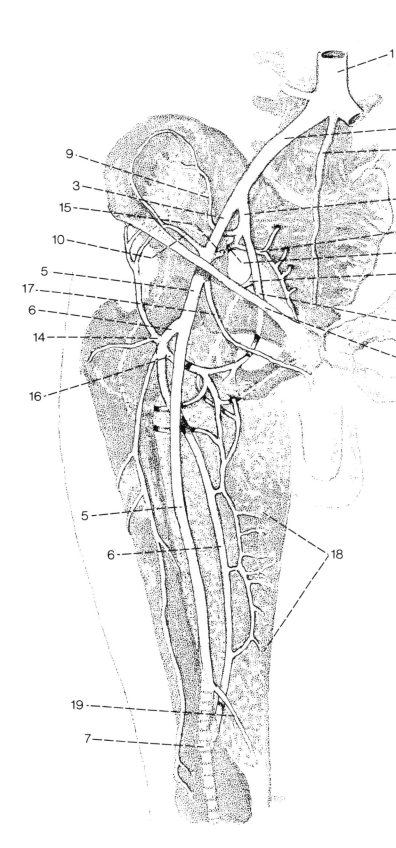

156
Arteries of anterior thigh

Collateral circulation is exaggerated

Color and label

1 Abdominal aorta
2 Common iliac artery
3 External iliac artery
4 Internal iliac artery
5 Femoral artery (the external iliac artery becomes the femoral artery below the inguinal ligament)
6 Deep femoral artery
7 Popliteal artery (the femoral artery becomes the popliteal artery below the adductor hiatus)
8 Median sacral artery
9 Iliolumbar artery
10 Deep iliac circumflex artery
11 Superior gluteal artery
12 Lateral sacral artery
13 Obturator artery
14 Lateral femoral circumflex artery
15 Inferior epigastric artery (cut)
16 Medial femoral circumflex artery
17 External pudendal artery
18 Perforating branches of deep femoral artery
19 Descending genicular artery
20 Inferior gluteal artery
21 Inguinal ligament

After Eycleshymer and Jones.

Color and label

N L1–N L5, lumbar nerves 1–5 (ventral rami)

L1–L5, lumbar vertebrae 1–5

 1 Subcostal nerve (12th intercostal nerve)
 2 Iliohypogastric nerve
 3 Ilioinguinal nerve
 4 Anterior scrotal (labial in female)
   branches of ilioinguinal nerve
 5 Genitofemoral nerve
 6 Genital branch of genitofemoral nerve
 7 Femoral branch of genitofemoral nerve
 8 Lateral femoral cutaneous nerve
 9 Obturator nerve (notice that both the
   obturator nerve and the femoral nerve
   arise from lumbar nerves L2, L3, L4)

10 Anterior branch of obturator nerve
11 Posterior branch of obturator nerve
12 Femoral nerve
13 Saphenous nerve (off femoral nerve)
14 Muscular branches of femoral nerve
   (the femoral nerve supplies all the
   muscles in the anterior compartment
   of the thigh)
15 Anterior cutaneous branches of the
   femoral nerve
16 Lumbosacral trunk
17 Ventral rami of sacral nerves S1–S5
18 Sacral plexus
19 Twelfth rib
20 Spermatic cord and testes
21 Inguinal canal

After Spalteholz and Spanner.

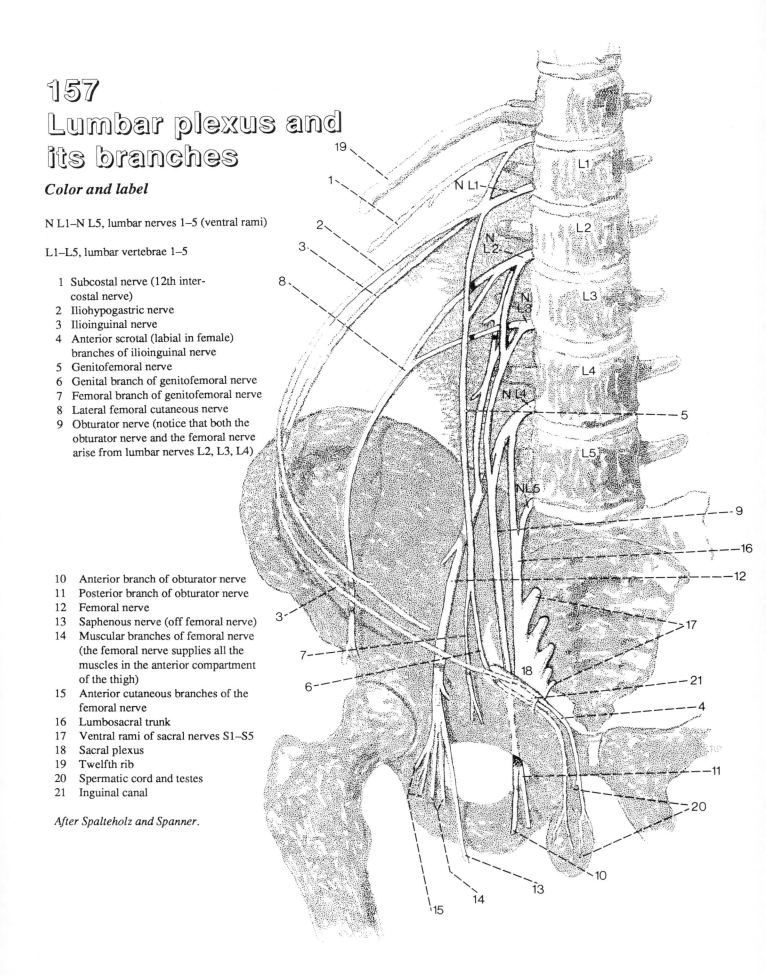

RIGHT

The shaded nerves are dorsal derivatives
of the plexus. These originally
innervated dorsal extensor muscles.

Color and label

T12, subcostal nerve (twelfth thoracic nerve, ventral ramus)
L1–L5, ventral rami of lumbar nerves 1–5
S1–S5, ventral rami of sacral nerves 1–5
Co, coccygeal nerve

1 Rami to intertransversarii muscle
2 Rami to quadratus lumborum muscle
3 Iliohypogastric nerve
4 Ilioinguinal nerve
5 Lateral cutaneous branch
6 Genitofemoral nerve
7 Femoral branch of genitofemoral nerve
8 Genital branch of genitofemoral nerve
9 Ramus to psoas minor muscle
10 Ramus to psoas major muscle
11 Femoral nerve
12 Branch to iliacus muscle (of femoral nerve)
13 Anterior cutaneous branch (of femoral nerve)
  and branch to sartorius muscle (of femoral nerve)
14 Branch to quadriceps femoris muscle (of femoral nerve)
15 Saphenous nerve (of femoral nerve)
16 Medial femoral cutaneous branch (of femoral nerve)
17 Branch to pectineus muscle (of femoral nerve)
18 Branch to pectineus and psoas major muscles
19 Accessory obturator nerve *(present in about
  10% of legs examined)*
20 Obturator nerve
21 Lumbosacral trunk
22 Superior gluteal nerve
23 Rami to piriformis muscle
24 Peroneal nerve (common peroneal nerve)
25 Inferior gluteal nerve
26 Tibial nerve *(the tibial nerve and the common
  peroneal nerve usually combine to form the
  largest nerve in the body, the sciatic nerve)*
27 Branch of tibial nerve to adductor magnus
  (posterior part), semimembranosus,
  semitendinosus, and long head of
  biceps femoris muscles
28 Branch to quadratus femoris and
  gemellus inferior muscles
29 Branch to obturator internus and
  gemellus superior muscles
30 Posterior femoral cutaneous nerves
31 Inferior cluneal nerve
32 Perineal nerve and dorsal nerve of penis (clitoris)
33 Inferior rectal nerve
34 Branch to levator ani muscle
35 Branch to coccygeus muscle
36 Anococcygeal nerves
37 Lateral femoral cutaneous nerve

After Spalteholz and Spanner (Eisler).

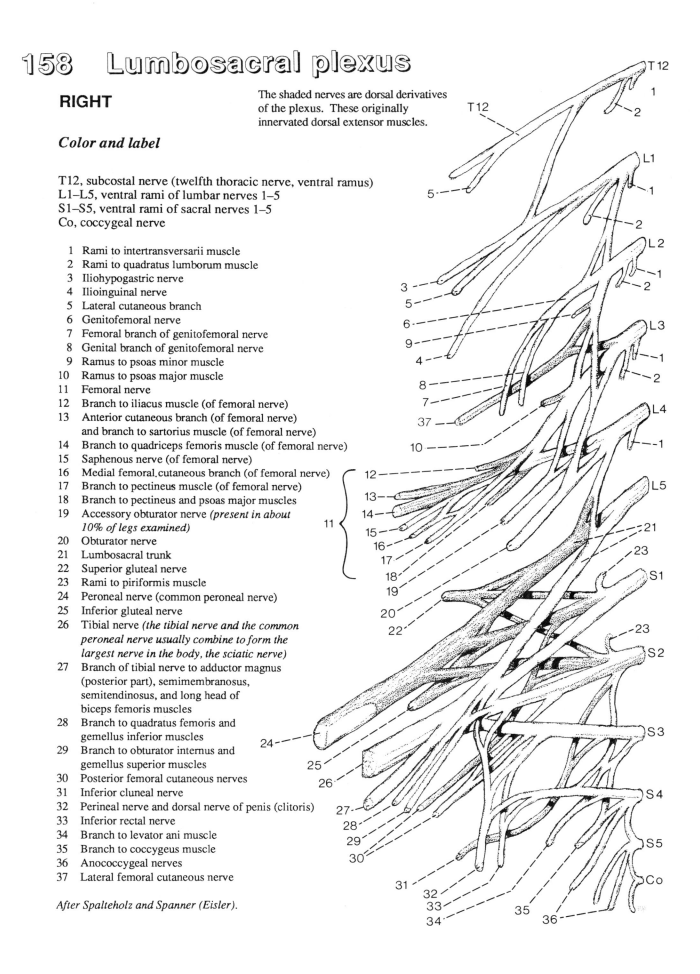

159
Motor distribution of
the femoral nerve, I

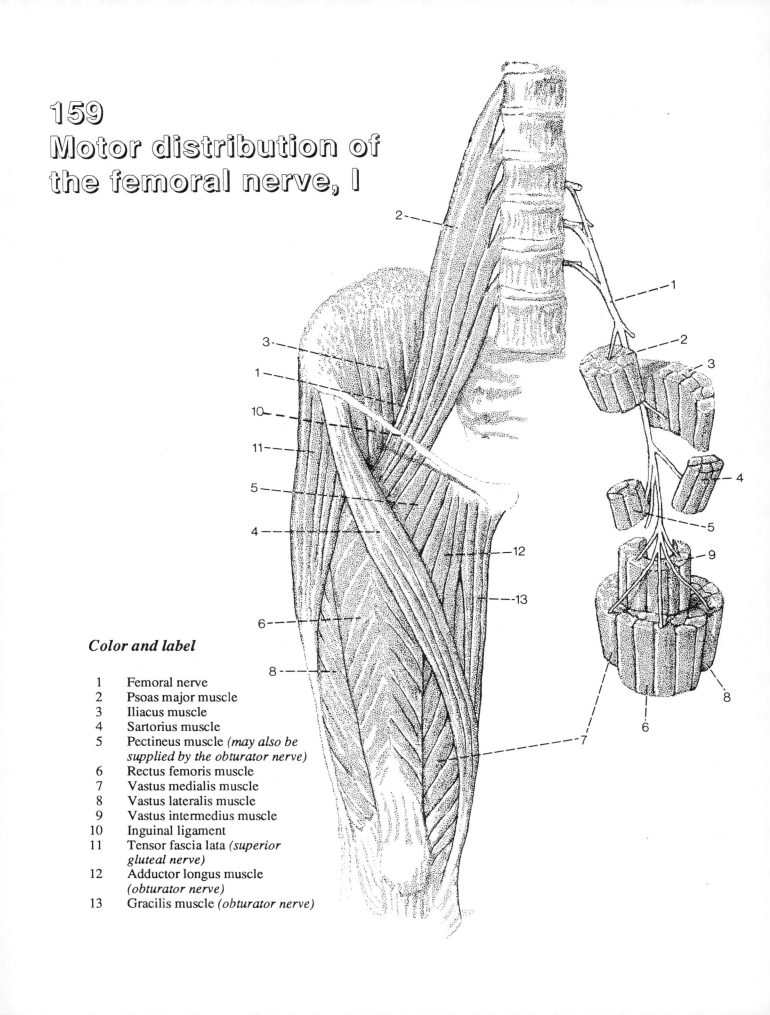

Color and label

1	Femoral nerve
2	Psoas major muscle
3	Iliacus muscle
4	Sartorius muscle
5	Pectineus muscle *(may also be supplied by the obturator nerve)*
6	Rectus femoris muscle
7	Vastus medialis muscle
8	Vastus lateralis muscle
9	Vastus intermedius muscle
10	Inguinal ligament
11	Tensor fascia lata *(superior gluteal nerve)*
12	Adductor longus muscle *(obturator nerve)*
13	Gracilis muscle *(obturator nerve)*

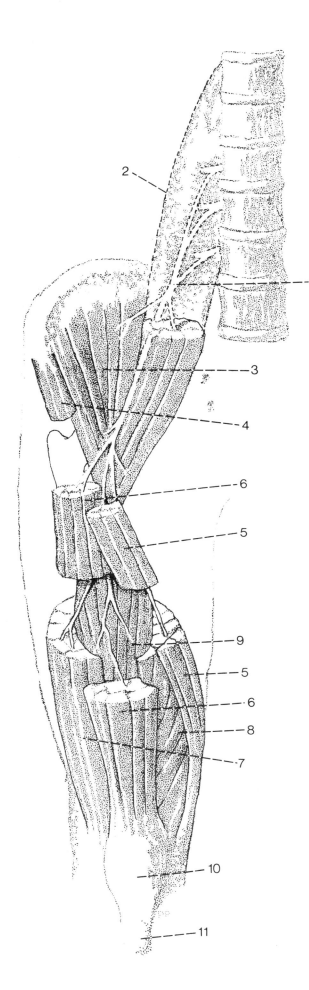

Color and label

1 Femoral nerve formed by fibers from lumbar nerves L2, L3, L4

2 Outline of psoas major muscle (*notice that the femoral nerve and other nerves of the lumbar plexus arise deep to the psoas major*)

3 Iliacus muscle (*it inserts by a tendon in common with the psoas major on the lesser trochanter, thus forming the iliopsoas muscle, which flexes the hip*)

4 Sartorius muscle (*origin on the anterior superior iliac spine*) (*cut*)

5 Sartorius muscle (*a portion*) (*sartorius means "tailor's" in Latin, in reference to the sartorius' action in flexing both hip joint and knee joint and externally rotating the leg, a position used by tailors when sewing*)

6 Rectus femoris muscle (*cut*)

7 Vastus lateralis muscle (*cut*)

8 Vastus medialis muscle (*cut*)

9 Vastus intermedius muscle (*cut*) (*the four vastus muscles and the rectus femoris form the quadriceps femoris, which means "four-headed muscle of the thigh"*)

10 Patella (*notice that the patella lies within the tendon of the quadriceps femoris; the actual insertion of the quadriceps is on the tibial tuberosity by means of the patellar ligament*)

11 Tibial tuberosity

MIDDLE OF RIGHT THIGH

Color and label

1 Femur
2 Sciatic nerve
3 Fascia lata (deep fascia of thigh)
4 Iliotibial tract (thickened fascia lata)·
5 Great saphenous vein
6 Femoral artery, vein, and saphenous nerve
   in adductor canal
7 Deep femoral artery and vein
8 Perforating vessels
9 Posterior femoral cutaneous nerve
10 Lateral femoral cutaneous nerve
11 Anterior branch of obturator nerve
12 Rectus femoris
13 Vastus lateralis
14 Vastus medialis
15 Vastus intermedius
16 Gracilis
17 Sartorius
18 Biceps femoris, long head
19 Semitendinosus
20 Semimembranosus
21 Adductor magnus
22 Adductor longus

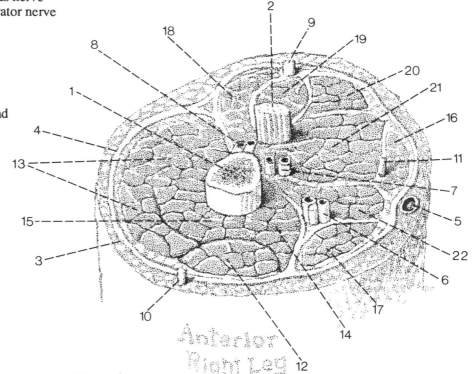

Based upon and modified from Eycleshymer and Schoemaker.

Notice that the deep fascia of the thigh, which is called the fascia lata, sends septa internally that divide the thigh into three compartments, a medial, an anterior, and a posterior compartment. The femoral nerve innervates the muscles of the anterior compartment, the obturator nerve supplies the muscles of the medial compartment, and the tibial portion of the sciatic nerve
supplies the muscles of the posterior compartment.

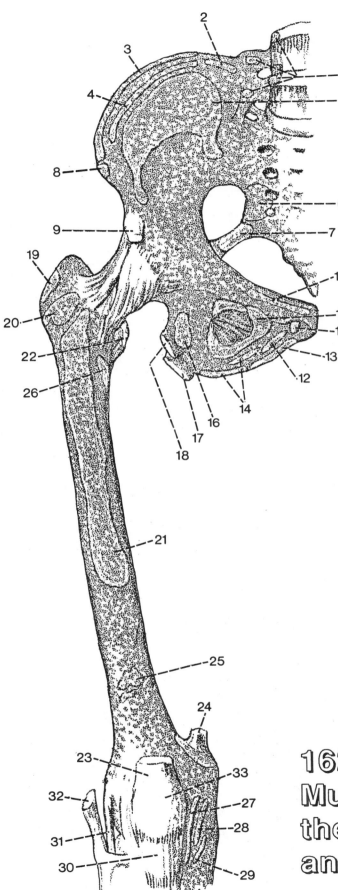

1   Psoas major (O)
2   Quadratus lumborum (O)
3   Internal abdominal oblique (O)
4   Transversus abdominis (O)
5   Iliacus (O)
6   Piriformis (O)
7   Coccygeus (O) on sacrospinous
       ligament
8   Sartorius (O)
9   Rectus femoris (O) straight head
10   Pectineus (O)
11   Adductor longus (O)
12   Adductor brevis (O)
13   Gracilis (O)
14   Adductor magnus (O)
15   Obturator externus (O)
16   Quadratus femoris (O)
17   Semimembranosus (O)
18   Biceps femoris (O)
19   Gluteus minimus (I)
20   Vastus lateralis (O)
21   Vastus intermedius (O)
22   Iliopsoas (I)
23   Quadriceps femoris (I)
24   Adductor magnus (I)
25   Articularis genu (O)
26   Vastus medialis (O)
27   Sartorius (I)
28   Gracilis (I)
29   Semitendinosus (I)
30   Patellar ligament
31   Fibular collateral ligament
32   Biceps femoris (I)
33   Patella

After Clemente.

162
Muscle attachments on the anterior pelvis and femur

*Color the origins (O) red
and the insertions (I) blue*

1   External abdominal oblique (I)
2   Gluteus medius (O)
3   Gluteus minimus (O)
4   Gluteus maximus (O) arising on posterior
    sacroiliac ligament and sacrotuberous ligament
5   Tensor fascia lata (O)
6   Piriformis (O)
7   Rectus femoris oblique head (O)
8   Gemellus superior (O)
9   Gemellus inferior (O)
10 Obturator internus (O)
11 Levator ani (pubococcygeus) (O)
12 Deep transverse perineus (in male) (O)
13 Piriformis (I)
14 Obturator internus with two gemelli (I)
15 Gluteus medius (I)
16 Gluteus minimus (I)
17 Obturator externus (I)
18 Quadratus femoris (I)
19 Iliopsoas (I)
20 Vastus medialis (O)
21 Pectineus (I)
22 Adductor brevis (I)
23 Gluteus maximus
24 Vastus lateralis (O)
25 Vastus intermedius (O)
26 Adductor longus (I)
27 Adductor magnus (I) (anterior oblique part)
28 Biceps femoris short head (O)
29 Plantaris (O)
30 Gastrocnemius (lateral and medial heads) (O)
31 Biceps femoris (I)
32 Semimembranosus (I) *(inserts by three tendons)*
33 Sartorius (I)
34 Gracilis (I)
35 Semitendinosus (I)
36 Semitendinosus (O)
37 Biceps femoris (O)
38 Adductor magnus (I) (posterior vertical part)

After Clemente.

163
Muscle attachments on
the posterior pelvis
and femur

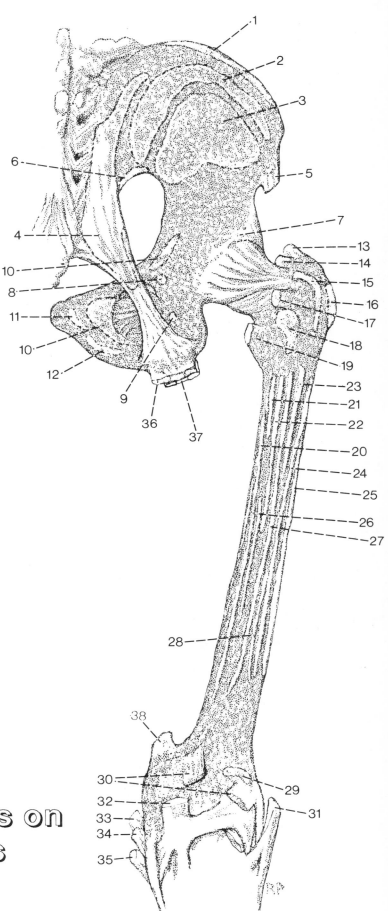

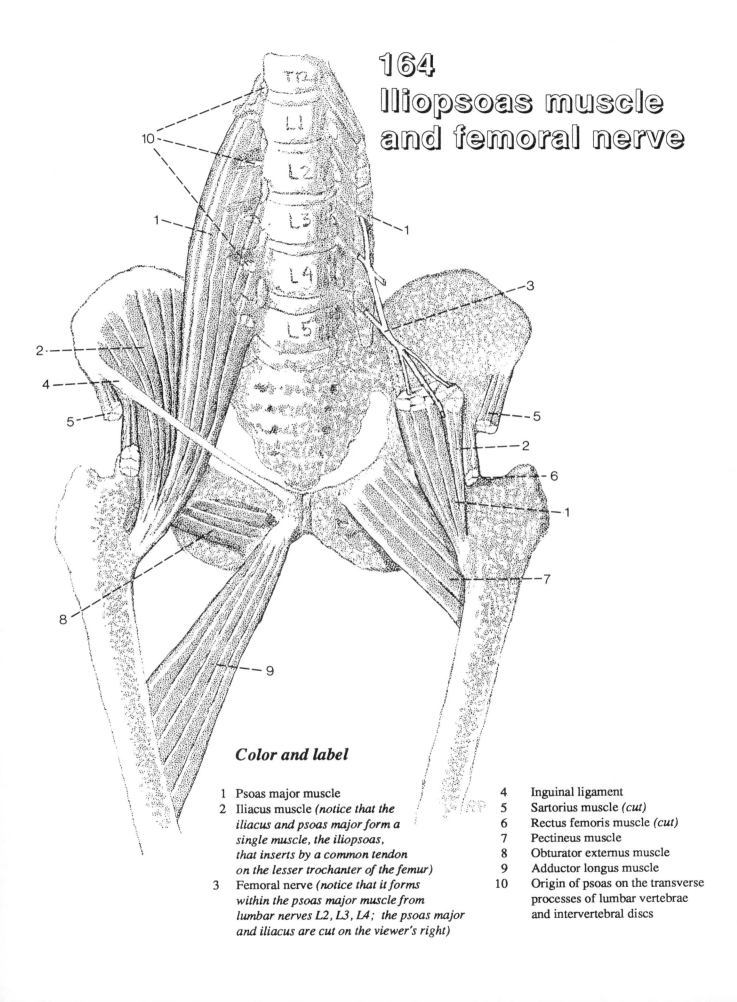

164
Iliopsoas muscle and femoral nerve

Color and label

1 Psoas major muscle
2 Iliacus muscle *(notice that the iliacus and psoas major form a single muscle, the iliopsoas, that inserts by a common tendon on the lesser trochanter of the femur)*
3 Femoral nerve *(notice that it forms within the psoas major muscle from lumbar nerves L2, L3, L4; the psoas major and iliacus are cut on the viewer's right)*

4 Inguinal ligament
5 Sartorius muscle *(cut)*
6 Rectus femoris muscle *(cut)*
7 Pectineus muscle
8 Obturator externus muscle
9 Adductor longus muscle
10 Origin of psoas on the transverse processes of lumbar vertebrae and intervertebral discs

Color and label

1 Obturator nerve *(notice that it is formed from fibers from lumbar nerves L2, L3, L4)*
2 Anterior branch of obturator nerve *(notice that it lies behind the pectineus and adductor longus, and in front of the obturator externus and adductor brevis; it supplies the adductor brevis, adductor longus, and gracilis muscles)*
3 Pectineus muscle *(cut on viewer's right)*
4 Obturator externus muscle
5 Adductor brevis and its insertion on the posterior femur *(notice that it lies posterior to and is largely covered by the pectineus and adductor longus muscles)*
6 Adductor longus and its insertion on the posterior femur *(cut on viewer's right)*
7 Adductor magnus (oblique part)
8 Adductor magnus (vertical part)
9 Gracilis muscle *(cut on viewer's right; gracilis means "slender" in Latin)*

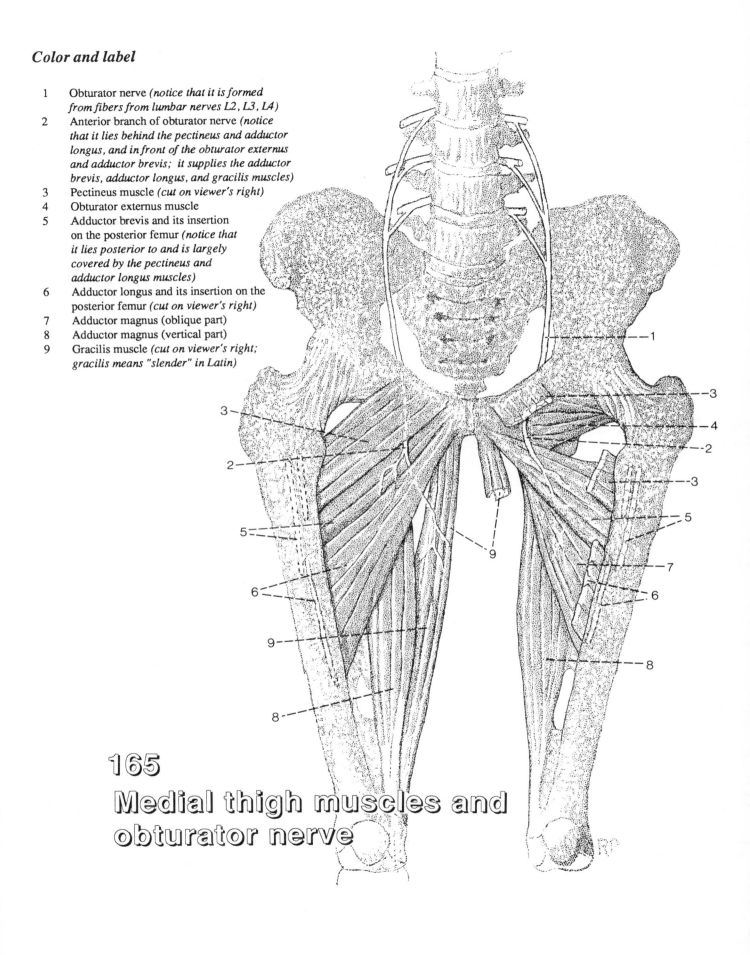

165
Medial thigh muscles and obturator nerve

Color and label

1 Obturator nerve *(notice that the obturator nerve arises within the psoas major muscle from lumbar nerves L2, L3, L4 and before passing through the obturator foramen it divides into an anterior and a posterior branch)*

2 Anterior branch of obturator nerve *(cut)*

3 Posterior branch of obturator nerve *(notice that it penetrates the obturator externus muscle, which it supplies)*

4 Adductor magnus muscle (anterior horizontal part) *(this part of the adductor magnus is sometimes a separate muscle, in which case it is called the adductor minimus)*

5 Adductor magnus (anterior oblique part) *(The anterior horizontal part and anterior oblique part of the adductor magnus are both supplied by the posterior branch of the obturator nerve)*

6 Adductor magnus (posterior vertical part) *(notice that this part arises from the ischial tuberosity, descends vertically, and forms a tendon that inserts on the adductor tubercle; this part of the adductor magnus is innervated by the tibial portion of the sciatic nerve)*

7 Femoral artery and vein passing through the adductor hiatus

8 Fibrous expansion of adductor magnus tendon

9 Pectineus muscle *(cut) (usually supplied by femoral nerve, sometimes by obturator nerve or accessory obturator nerve)*

10 Obturator externus muscle *(shown passing behind femur)*

11 Origin and outline of anterior parts of adductor magnus *(the vertical ischiotuberal part is shown by itself on the viewer's right)*

12 Accessory obturator nerve *(present 10% of the time; notice that it passes over the pubis and not through the obturator canal)*

13 Obturator* foramen

14 Insertion of adductor magnus on posterior surface of femur

15 Insertion of iliopsoas on lesser trochanter

16 Origin of pectineus

*Obturator is derived from the Latin obturo, "to stop up," and refers to the obturator foramen's being almost completely stopped up by a membrane and two muscles, which do, however, contain a small obturator canal for the passage of the obturator vessels and nerve.

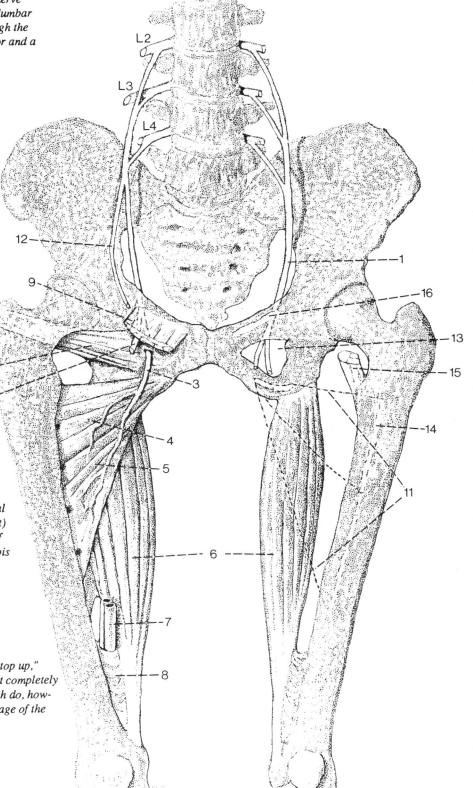

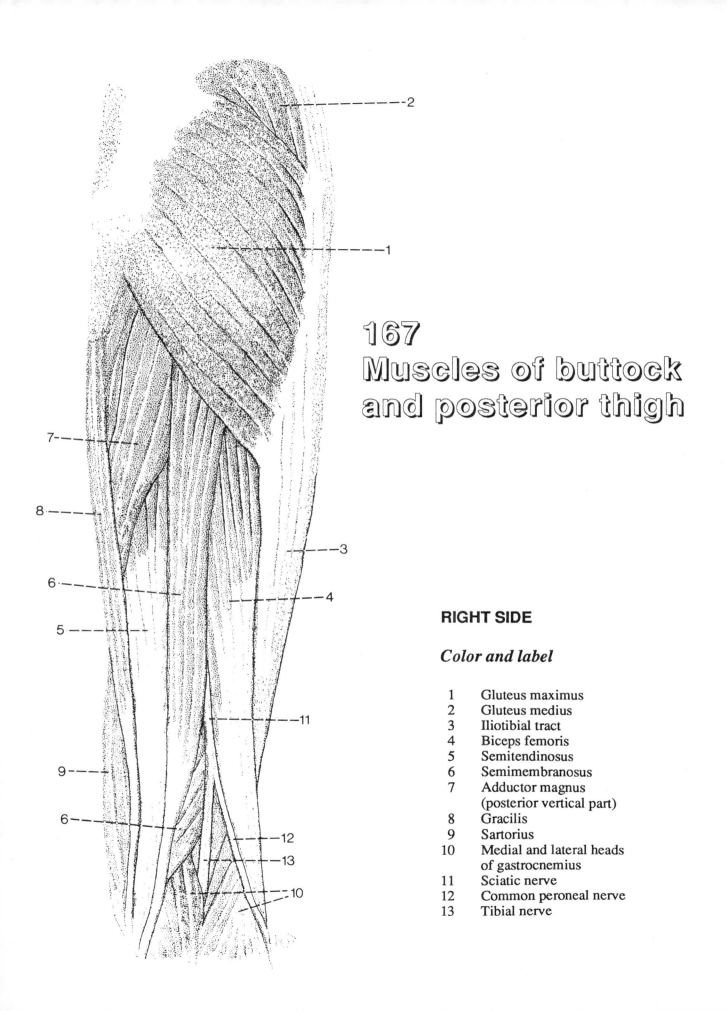

167
Muscles of buttock and posterior thigh

RIGHT SIDE

Color and label

1   Gluteus maximus
2   Gluteus medius
3   Iliotibial tract
4   Biceps femoris
5   Semitendinosus
6   Semimembranosus
7   Adductor magnus
     (posterior vertical part)
8   Gracilis
9   Sartorius
10   Medial and lateral heads
     of gastrocnemius
11   Sciatic nerve
12   Common peroneal nerve
13   Tibial nerve

168
Gluteus maximus
and iliotibial tract

RIGHT LEG, POSTERIOR VIEW

Color and label

1   Gluteus maximus
2   Origin of gluteus maximus
3   Insertion of gluteus maximus
    on iliotibial tract
4   Insertion of gluteus maximus
    on femur
5   Tensor fasciae latae muscle
6   Iliotibial tract (thickened
    portion of fascia lata)
7   Insertion of iliotibial tract on
    anterior tibia
8   Sacrotuberous ligament
9   Small section of fascia lata
    (deep fascia of thigh)

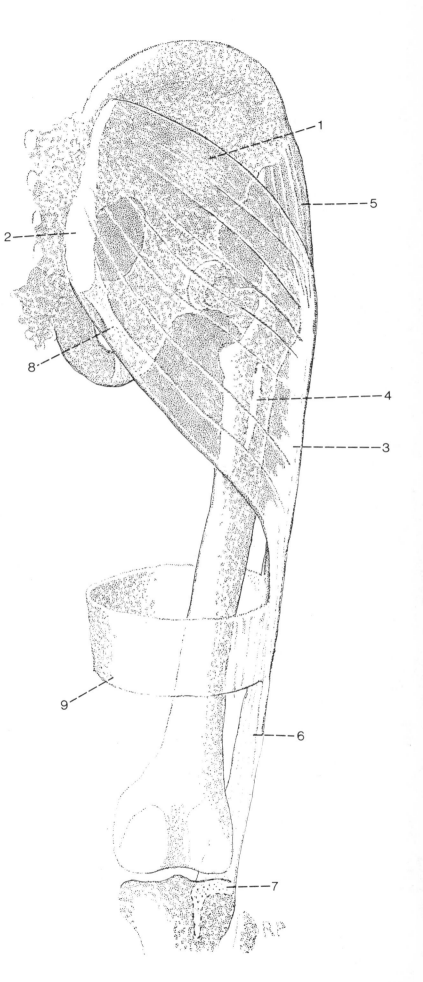

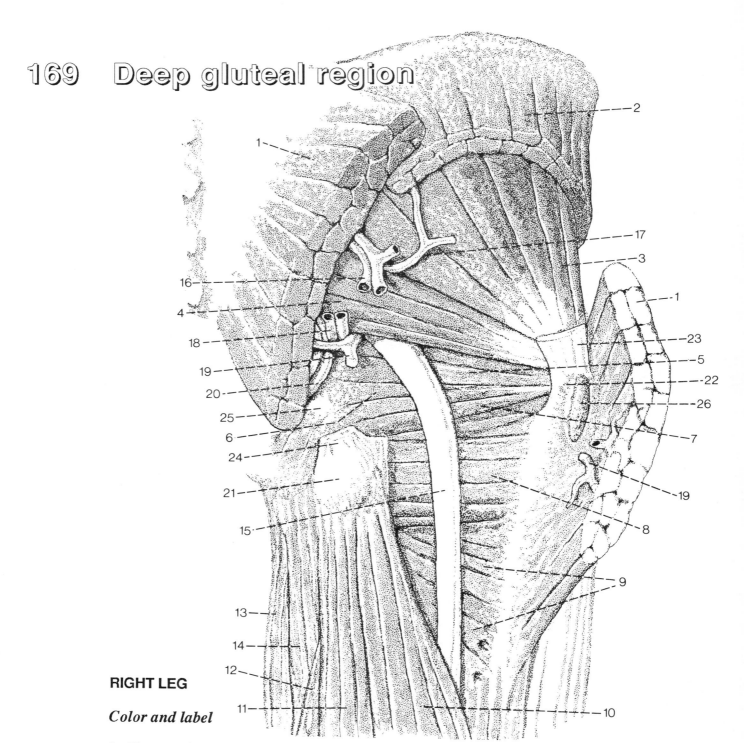

RIGHT LEG

Color and label

1. Gluteus maximus muscle *(cut)*
2. Gluteus medius muscle *(cut)*
3. Gluteus minimus muscle
4. Piriformis muscle
5. Superior gemellus muscle
6. Obturator internus muscle
7. Inferior gemellus muscle
8. Quadratus femoris muscle
9. Adductor magnus (horizontal and oblique parts)
10. Biceps femoris muscle
11. Semitendinosus muscle

12. Semimembranosus muscle
13. Gracilis muscle
14. Adductor magnus muscle (vertical part)
15. Sciatic nerve
16. Superior gluteal artery and vein
17. Superior gluteal nerve *(cut; supplies gluteus medius and gluteus minimus)*
18. Inferior gluteal artery and vein
19. Inferior gluteal nerve *(supplies gluteus maximus)*

20. Internal pudendal artery and vein *(travel with pudendal nerve not shown)*
21. Ischial tuberosity
22. Greater trochanter of femur
23. Tendon of gluteus medius
24. Sacrotuberous ligament *(cut)*
25. Bend in obturator internus muscle on lesser sciatic notch
26. Trochanteric bursa *(beneath gluteus maximus muscle)*

RIGHT LEG

Color and label

1   Gluteus maximus
     (cut and pulled aside)
2   Gluteus medius
3   Piriformis
4   Superior gemellus
5   Obturator internus
6   Inferior gemellus
7   Quadratus femoris
8   Biceps femoris
     (long head)
9   Semitendinosus
10   Semimembranosus
11   Biceps femoris
     (short head)
12   Iliotibial tract
13   Adductor magnus
     (horizontal part)
14   Adductor magnus
     (oblique part)
15   Adductor magnus
     (vertical part)
16   Gastrocnemius medial
     and lateral heads

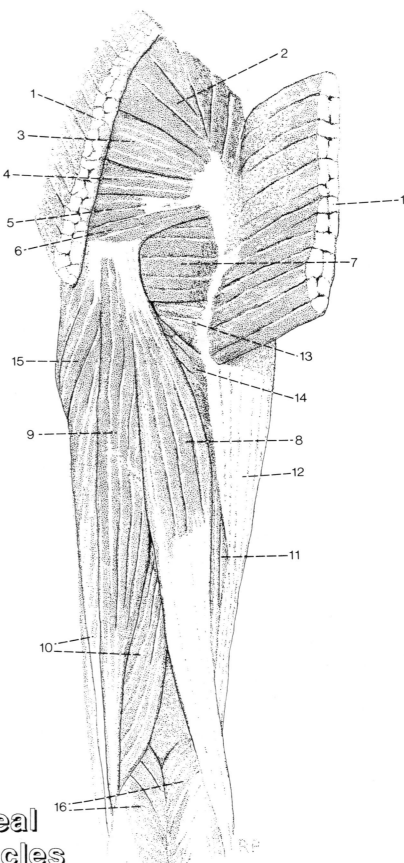

170
Posterior gluteal
and thigh muscles

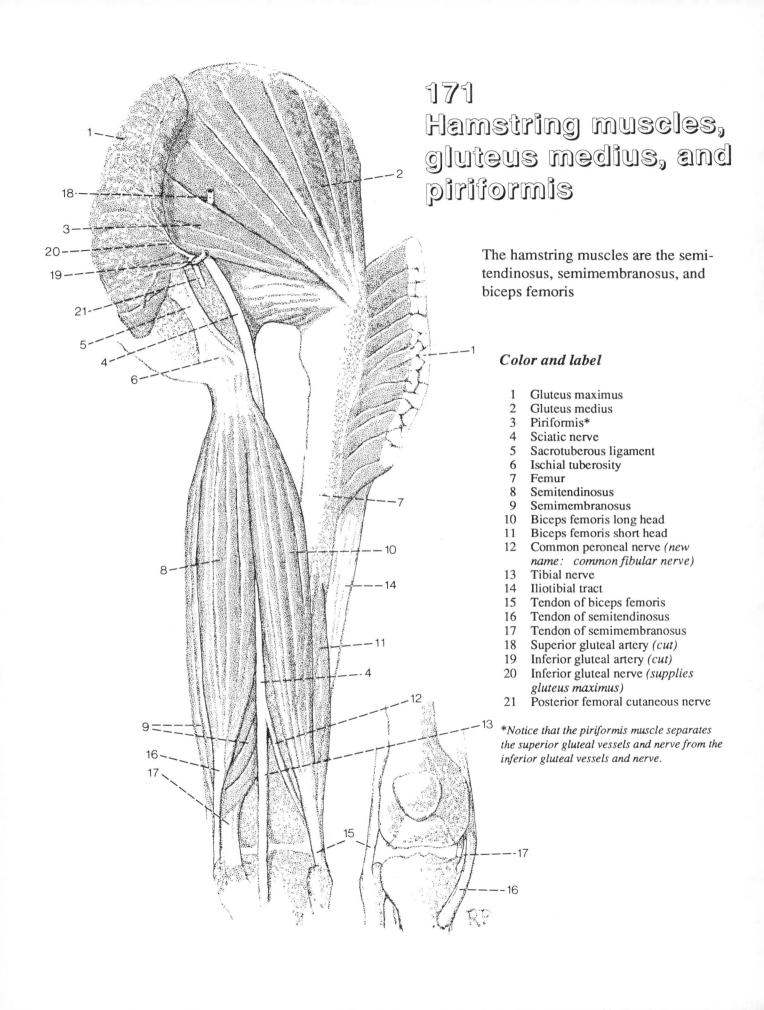

171
Hamstring muscles, gluteus medius, and piriformis

The hamstring muscles are the semitendinosus, semimembranosus, and biceps femoris

Color and label

1 Gluteus maximus
2 Gluteus medius
3 Piriformis*
4 Sciatic nerve
5 Sacrotuberous ligament
6 Ischial tuberosity
7 Femur
8 Semitendinosus
9 Semimembranosus
10 Biceps femoris long head
11 Biceps femoris short head
12 Common peroneal nerve *(new name: common fibular nerve)*
13 Tibial nerve
14 Iliotibial tract
15 Tendon of biceps femoris
16 Tendon of semitendinosus
17 Tendon of semimembranosus
18 Superior gluteal artery *(cut)*
19 Inferior gluteal artery *(cut)*
20 Inferior gluteal nerve *(supplies gluteus maximus)*
21 Posterior femoral cutaneous nerve

Notice that the piriformis muscle separates the superior gluteal vessels and nerve from the inferior gluteal vessels and nerve.

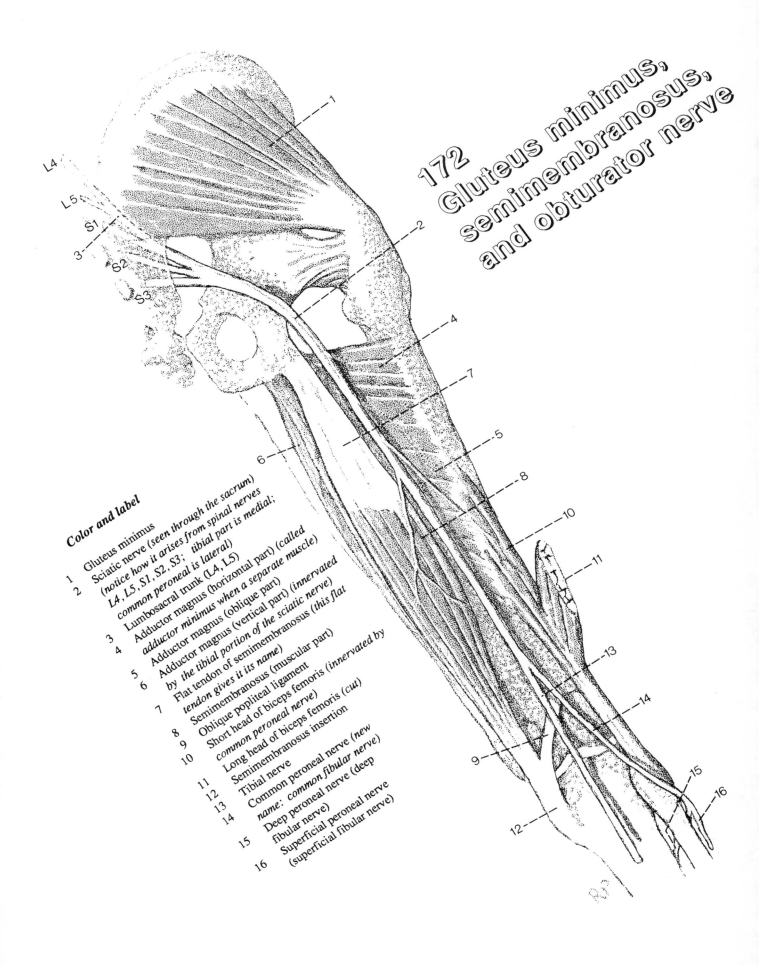

L4

L5

S1

3

S2

S3

1

2

4

7

6

5

8

10

11

13

14

9

15

16

12

Color and label

1　Gluteus minimus

2　Sciatic nerve (seen through the sacrum)
(notice how it arises from spinal nerves
L4, L5, S1, S2, S3; tibial part is medial;
common peroneal is lateral)

3　Lumbosacral trunk (L4, L5)

4　Adductor minimus when a separate muscle)
adductor magnus (horizontal part) (called

5　Adductor magnus (oblique part) (innervated
by the tibial portion of the sciatic nerve)

6　Adductor magnus (vertical part) (innervated
by the tibial portion of the sciatic nerve)

7　Flat tendon of semimembranosus (this flat
tendon gives it its name)

8　Semimembranosus (muscular part)

9　Oblique popliteal ligament

10　Short head of biceps femoris (innervated by
common peroneal nerve) (cut)

11　Long head of biceps femoris

12　Semimembranosus insertion

13　Tibial nerve

14　Common peroneal nerve (new
name: common fibular nerve)

15　Deep peroneal nerve (deep
fibular nerve)

16　Superficial peroneal nerve
(superficial fibular nerve)

173 Gastrocnemius

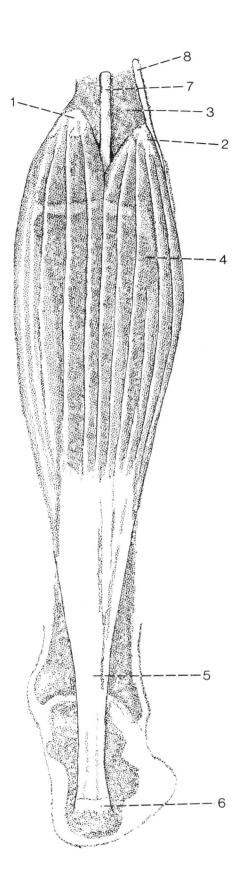

Color and label

1 Gastrocnemius (origin of medial head)
2 Gastrocnemius (origin of lateral head)
3 Femur
4 Gastrocnemius
5 Tendo calcaneus (Achilles tendon)
6 Insertion of gastrocnemius and soleus
   (triceps surae) on calcaneus
7 Tibial nerve
8 Common peroneal nerve (common
   fibular nerve)

RIGHT LEG

Color and label

1 Femur
2 Adductor tubercle and insertion of vertical part of adductor magnus
3 Lateral tibial condyle
4 Medial tibial condyle
5 Patella
6 Head of fibula
7 Lateral malleolus
8 Tibia
9 Tibial tuberosity
10 Medial malleolus
11 Talus

Color the origins (O) RED and the insertions (I) BLUE

12 Biceps femoris (I)
13 Peroneus longus (fibularis longus) (O)
14 Peroneus brevis (fibularis brevis) (O)
15 Extensor digitorum longus (O)
16 Extensor hallucis longus (O)
17 Tibialis posterior (O)
18 Iliotibial tract (I)
19 Tibialis anterior (O)
20 Quadriceps femoris (patellar "ligament") (I)
21 Sartorius (I)
22 Gracilis (I)
23 Semitendinosus (I)

*In anatomy the lower leg (from knee to ankle) is the leg, and the upper leg (from hip to knee) is the thigh.

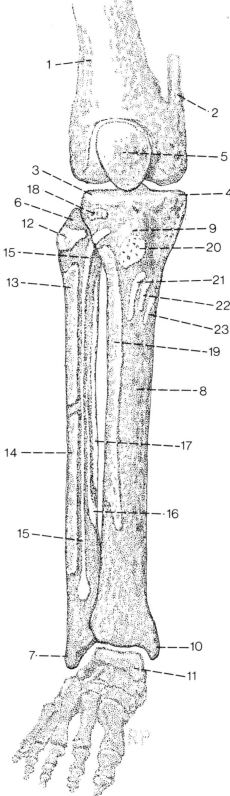

RIGHT LEG

*Label and color the origins (O) red
and the insertions (I) blue*

1   Medial and lateral femoral condyles
2   Tendon of vertical part of adductor
    magnus (I)
3   Gastrocnemius (medial head) (O)
4   Gastrocnemius (lateral head) (O)
5   Intercondylar eminence
6   Medial tibial condyle

7   Lateral tibial condyle
8   Tibia
9   Fibula
10 Lateral malleolus
11 Medial malleolus
12 Head of fibula
13 Talus
14 Calcaneus
15 Semimembranosus (I)
16 Tibial collateral ligament
17 Popliteus (O)
18 Soleus (O)
19 Flexor digitorum longus (O)
20 Tibialis posterior (O)
21 Flexor hallucis longus (O)
22 Peroneus brevis (fibularis brevis) (O)
23 Biceps femoris (I)
24 Fibular collateral ligament
25 Popliteus (I)
26 Groove for tendon of flexor hallucis longus
27 Insertion of tendo calcaneus
    (gastrocnemius and soleus) (I)
28 Plantaris (O)

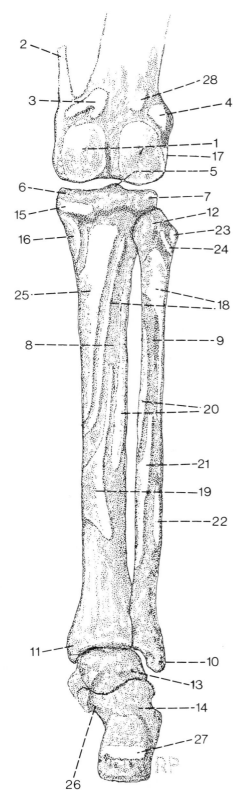

176
Soleus,
gastrocnemius,
and plantaris

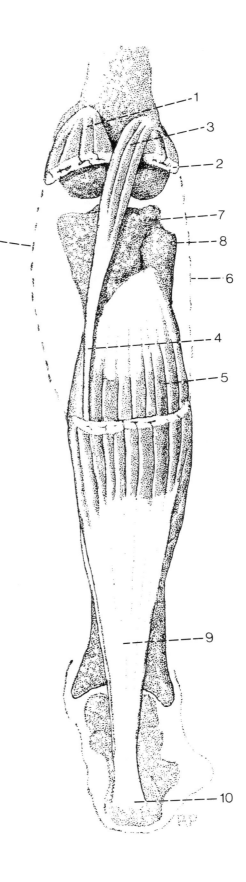

RIGHT LEG, POSTERIOR VIEW

Color and label

1   Medial head of gastrocnemius *(cut)*
2   Lateral head of gastrocnemius *(cut)*
3   Plantaris *(this muscle is small and almost insignificant in the human)*
4   Tendon of plantaris *(long and thin and easily mistaken for a nerve; it may combine with the tendo calcaneus or insert separately on the tubercle of the calcaneus)*
5   Soleus *(it, along with the two heads of the gastrocnemius, inserts by the tendo calcaneus on the tubercle of the calcaneus; the term triceps surae [Latin for "three heads of the calf"] refers to the two heads of the gastrocnemius and the soleus)*
6   Outline of the gastrocnemius
7   Tibia
8   Fibula
9   Tendo calcaneus
10   Insertion of tendo calcaneus

**POSTERIOR VIEW OF RIGHT LEG;
FOOT IS PLANTARFLEXED**

Color and label

1 Origin of flexor hallucis longus on fibula
2 Flexor hallucis muscle
3 Tendon of flexor hallucis longus
4 Medial and lateral sesamoid bones *(in tendons of flexor hallucis brevis [not shown])*
5 Insertion of flexor hallucis longus tendon
   on distal phalanx of big toe (hallux)
6 Origin of flexor digitorum longus on tibia
7 Tubercle of calcaneus
8 Sustentaculum tali with groove for tendon
   of flexor hallucis longus

MEDIAL VIEW OF RIGHT LEG

Color and label

1 Flexor hallucis longus muscle
2 Tendon of flexor hallucis longus
3 Talus
4 Sustentaculum tali
5 Medial sesamoid bone
6 Tibia
7 Medial malleolus
8 Calcaneus

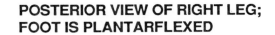

177 Flexor hallucis longus

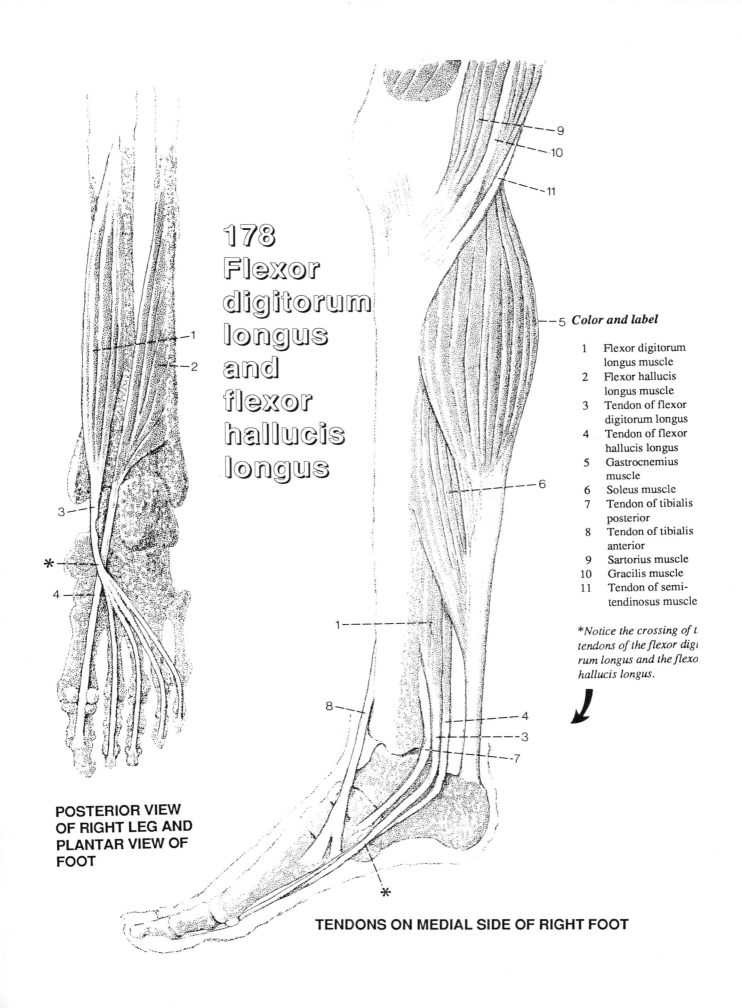

178
Flexor digitorum longus and flexor hallucis longus

Color and label

1 Flexor digitorum longus muscle
2 Flexor hallucis longus muscle
3 Tendon of flexor digitorum longus
4 Tendon of flexor hallucis longus
5 Gastrocnemius muscle
6 Soleus muscle
7 Tendon of tibialis posterior
8 Tendon of tibialis anterior
9 Sartorius muscle
10 Gracilis muscle
11 Tendon of semi-tendinosus muscle

*Notice the crossing of t_ tendons of the flexor dig_ rum longus and the flexo_ hallucis longus.

POSTERIOR VIEW OF RIGHT LEG AND PLANTAR VIEW OF FOOT

TENDONS ON MEDIAL SIDE OF RIGHT FOOT

PLANTAR (INFERIOR) ASPECT OF THE RIGHT FOOT

Color and label

1   Calcaneus (heel bone)
2   Tuber calcanei
3   Lateral process of tuber calcanei
4   Medial process of tuber calcanei
5   Sustentaculum tali
6   Groove for tendon of flexor hallucis
    longus muscle
7   Head of the talus (caput tali)
8   Cuboid bone
9   Tuberosity of cuboid bone
10 Navicular bone
11 Tuberosity of navicular bone
12 Medial cuneiform bone
13 Intermediate cuneiform bone
14 Lateral cuneiform bone
15 Tuberosity of first metatarsal bone
16 Groove for tendon of peroneus
    longus muscle
17 Tuberosity of fifth metatarsal bone
18 Proximal phalanx of big toe (hallux)
19 Distal phalanx of big toe

179   Bones of foot, inferior aspect

RIGHT FOOT

Color and label

1   Calcaneus
2   Talus
3   Navicular bone
4   Medial cuneiform bone
5   Intermediate cuneiform bone
6   First metatarsal bone
7   Proximal phalanx of big toe (hallux)
8   Distal phalanx of big toe
9   Sesamoid bones (in tendons of flexor hallucis brevis)
10   Medial malleolus (tibia)
11   Medial malleolar surface of talar trochlea
12   Tuberosity of calcaneus
13   Sustentaculum tali (of calcaneus)
14   Medial process of calcaneal tuberosity

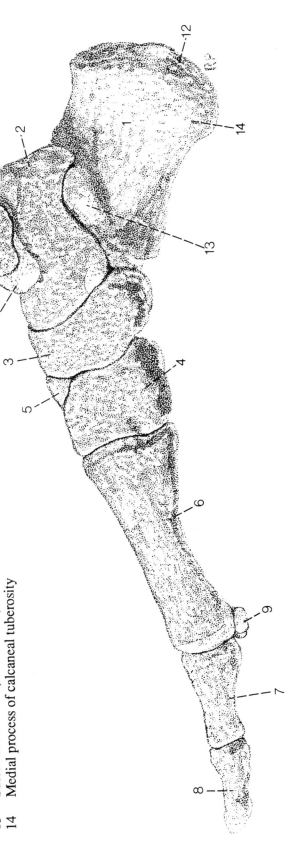

RIGHT FOOT

*Color the origins (O) RED
and the insertions (I) BLUE*

1 Flexor digitorum brevis (O)
2 Abductor hallucis (O)
3 Abductor digiti minimi (O)
4 Quadratus plántae (O)
5 Tibialis posterior (I)
6 Tibialis anterior (I)
7 Peroneus longus (I)
8 Flexor hallucis brevis (O)
9 Flexor hallucis brevis (I)
10 Adductor hallucis oblique head (O)
11 Adductor hallucis transverse
     head (O)
12 Adductor hallucis (I) (with flexor
     hallucis brevis)
13 Abductor hallucis (I) (with flexor
     hallucis brevis)
14 Flexor digiti minimi (O)
15 Flexor digiti minimi (I)
16 Flexor hallucis longus (I)
17 Plantar interosseous (O)
18 Plantar interosseous (I)
19 Flexor digitorum brevis (I)
20 Flexor digitorum longus (I)
21 Sesamoid bones in tendon of
     flexor hallucis brevis
22 Abductor digiti minimi (I)
23 Dorsal interosseous (O)

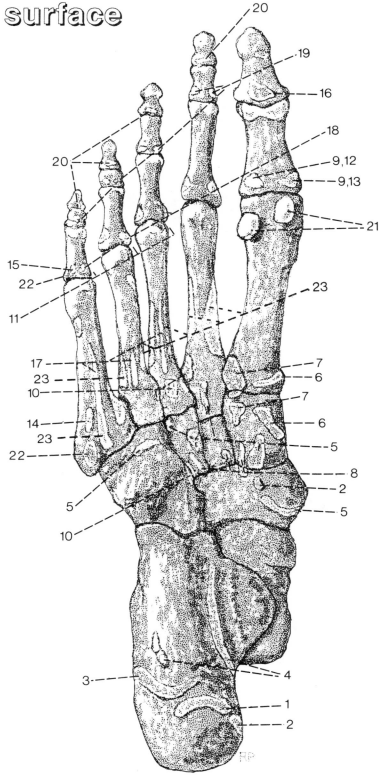

RIGHT LEG

Color and label

1	Popliteus	6	Tendon of flexor hallucis longus
2	Tibialis posterior	7	Peroneus longus (lateral compartment)
3	Flexor digitorum longus	8	Peroneus brevis (lateral compartment)
4	Flexor hallucis longus	9	Tendon of peroneus longus
5	Tendon of flexor digitorum longus	10	Medial malleolus

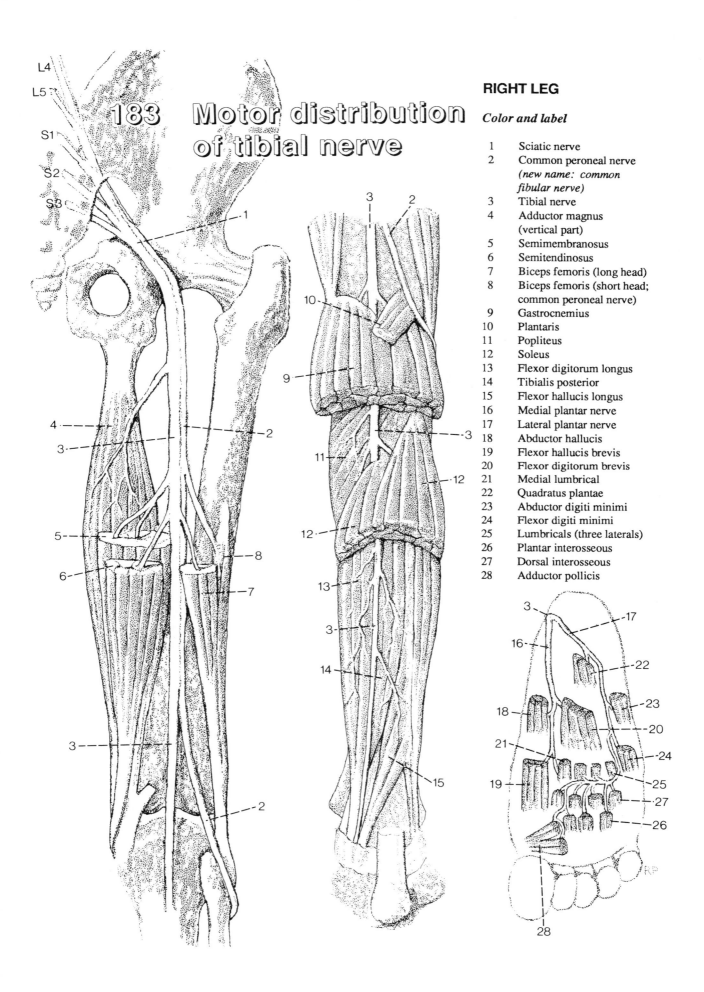

L4
L5
S1
S2
S3

RIGHT LEG

Color and label

1   Sciatic nerve
2   Common peroneal nerve
    (*new name: common
    fibular nerve*)
3   Tibial nerve
4   Adductor magnus
    (vertical part)
5   Semimembranosus
6   Semitendinosus
7   Biceps femoris (long head)
8   Biceps femoris (short head;
    common peroneal nerve)
9   Gastrocnemius
10 Plantaris
11 Popliteus
12 Soleus
13 Flexor digitorum longus
14 Tibialis posterior
15 Flexor hallucis longus
16 Medial plantar nerve
17 Lateral plantar nerve
18 Abductor hallucis
19 Flexor hallucis brevis
20 Flexor digitorum brevis
21 Medial lumbrical
22 Quadratus plantae
23 Abductor digiti minimi
24 Flexor digiti minimi
25 Lumbricals (three laterals)
26 Plantar interosseous
27 Dorsal interosseous
28 Adductor pollicis

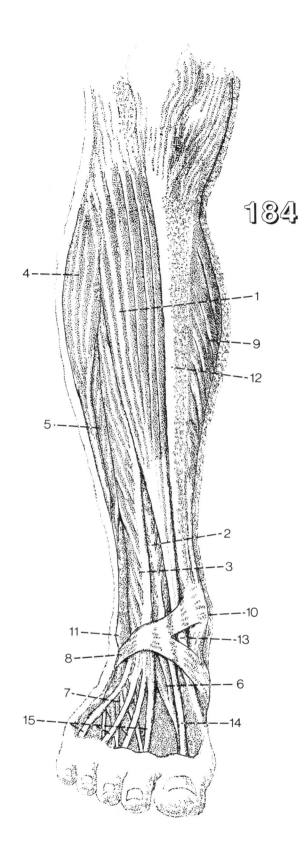

184 Muscles of anterior leg

ANTERIOR ASPECT OF RIGHT LEG

Color and label

1	Tibialis anterior
2	Extensor hallucis longus
3	Extensor digitorum longus
4	Peroneus longus (fibularis longus)
5	Peroneus brevis (fibularis brevis)
6	Extensor hallucis brevis
7	Extensor digitorum brevis
8	Inferior extensor retinaculum
9	Gastrocnemius
10	Medial malleolus
11	Lateral malleolus
12	Tibia
13	Tendon of tibialis anterior
14	Tendon of extensor hallucis longus
15	Tendons of extensor digitorum longus

After Clemente.

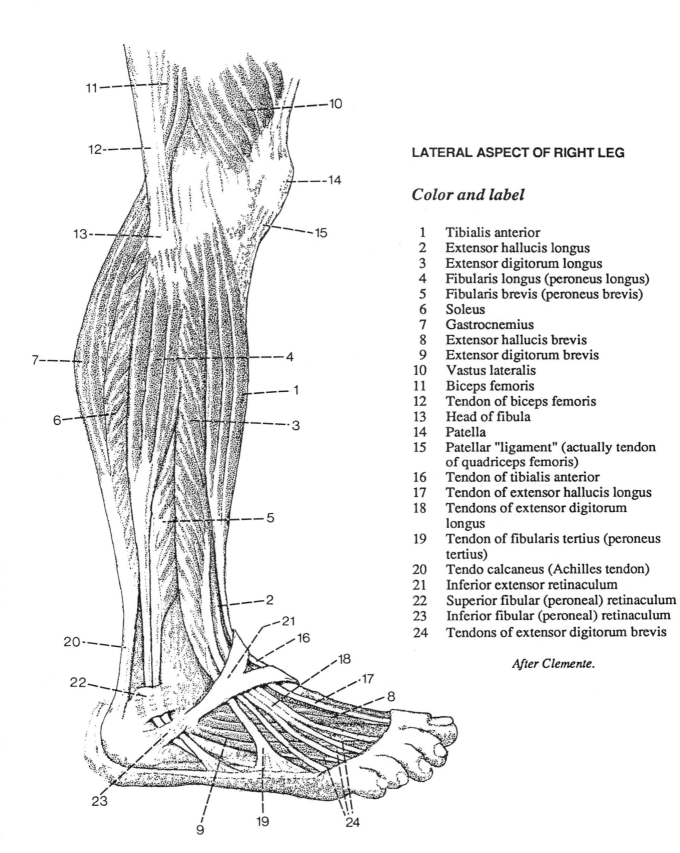

LATERAL ASPECT OF RIGHT LEG

Color and label

1 Tibialis anterior
2 Extensor hallucis longus
3 Extensor digitorum longus
4 Fibularis longus (peroneus longus)
5 Fibularis brevis (peroneus brevis)
6 Soleus
7 Gastrocnemius
8 Extensor hallucis brevis
9 Extensor digitorum brevis
10 Vastus lateralis
11 Biceps femoris
12 Tendon of biceps femoris
13 Head of fibula
14 Patella
15 Patellar "ligament" (actually tendon of quadriceps femoris)
16 Tendon of tibialis anterior
17 Tendon of extensor hallucis longus
18 Tendons of extensor digitorum longus
19 Tendon of fibularis tertius (peroneus tertius)
20 Tendo calcaneus (Achilles tendon)
21 Inferior extensor retinaculum
22 Superior fibular (peroneal) retinaculum
23 Inferior fibular (peroneal) retinaculum
24 Tendons of extensor digitorum brevis

After Clemente.

185   Muscles of lateral leg

RIGHT LEG, ANTERIOR ASPECT

Color and label

1   Common fibular (peroneal) nerve
2   Deep fibular (peroneal) nerve
3   Superficial fibular (peroneal) nerve
4   Tibialis anterior muscle *(cut)*
5   Tendon of tibialis anterior muscle *(cut)*
6   Extensor digitorum longus muscle *(cut)*
7   Tendon of extensor digitorum longus
8   Extensor hallucis longus muscle
9   Tendon of extensor hallucis longus
10 Extensor hallucis brevis
11 Extensor digitorum brevis
12 Lateral malleolus
13 Peroneus (fibularis) longus *(cut)*
14 Peroneus (fibularis) brevis
15 Tendon of fibularis longus

Notice that the superficial fibular nerve supplies the two fibular (peroneal) muscles that lie in the lateral compartment. The deep fibular nerve supplies the muscles in the anterior compartment.

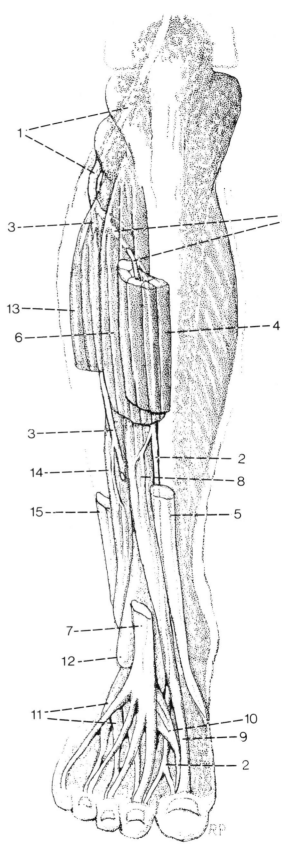

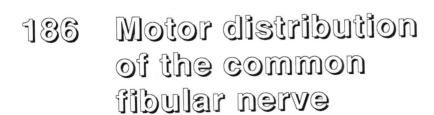

186 Motor distribution of the common fibular nerve

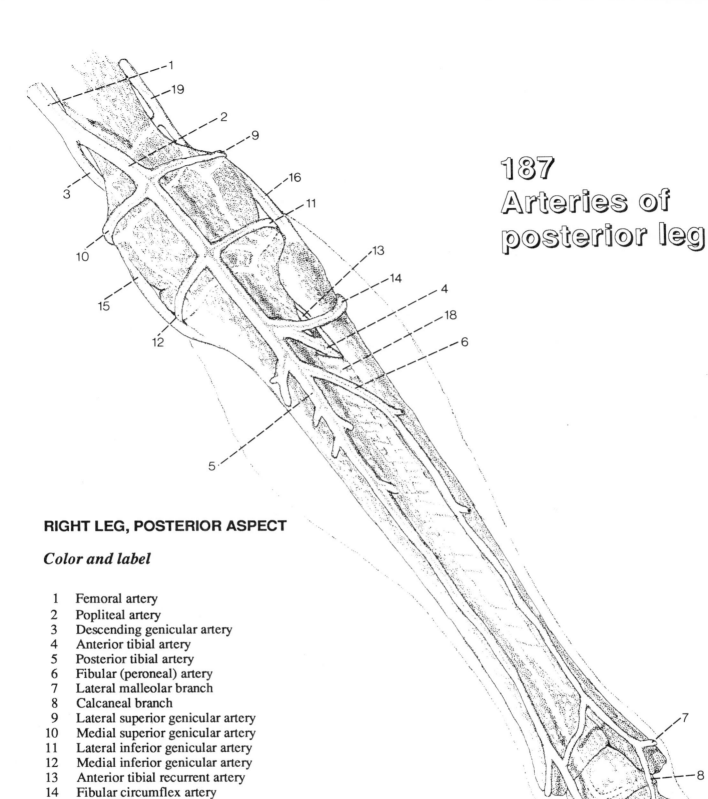

RIGHT LEG, POSTERIOR ASPECT

Color and label

1 Femoral artery
2 Popliteal artery
3 Descending genicular artery
4 Anterior tibial artery
5 Posterior tibial artery
6 Fibular (peroneal) artery
7 Lateral malleolar branch
8 Calcaneal branch
9 Lateral superior genicular artery
10 Medial superior genicular artery
11 Lateral inferior genicular artery
12 Medial inferior genicular artery
13 Anterior tibial recurrent artery
14 Fibular circumflex artery
15 Tibial collateral ligament
16 Fibular collateral ligament
17 Dorsalis pedis artery
18 Interosseous membrane
19 Descending branch of lateral
    femoral circumflex artery

After Hollinshead.

188
Foot: anterior–superior aspect

LEFT FOOT

Color and label

1   Tibia
2   Fibula
3   Inteosseous membrane
4   Inferior extensor retinaculum
5   Medial malleolus
6   Lateral malleolus
7   Tibialis anterior muscle and tendon
8   Tendon of extensor hallucis longus
9   Extensor digitorum longus muscle
10 Tendons of extensor digitorum longus
11 Extensor hallucis brevis
12 Extensor digitorum brevis
13 Deep peroneal (fibular) nerve
14 Anterior tibial artery
15 Abductor hallucis muscle
16 Peroneus (fibularis) brevis muscle
17 Peroneus (fibularis) longus muscle
    and tendon
18 Tibial nerve and posterior tibial
    artery and vein
19 Superficial fibular (peroneal) nerve,
    divided
20 Medial dorsal cutaneous branch of
    superficial fibular nerve
21 Intermediate dorsal cutaneous branch of
    superficial fibular nerve
22 Lateral dorsal cutaneous nerve
    (continuation of sural nerve)
23 Dorsal pedal digital nerves
24 Deep peroneal (fibular) nerve
    (cutaneous branches)
25 Dorsalis pedis artery (continuation of
    anterior tibial artery)
26 Dorsal digital nerves
27 First dorsal metatarsal artery
28 Lateral tarsal artery
29 Tendo calcaneus (Achilles tendon)
30 Soleus muscle
31 Tibialis posterior muscle
32 Flexor digitorum longus muscle
33 Flexor hallucis longus muscle

Based on and slightly modified from a Somso model.

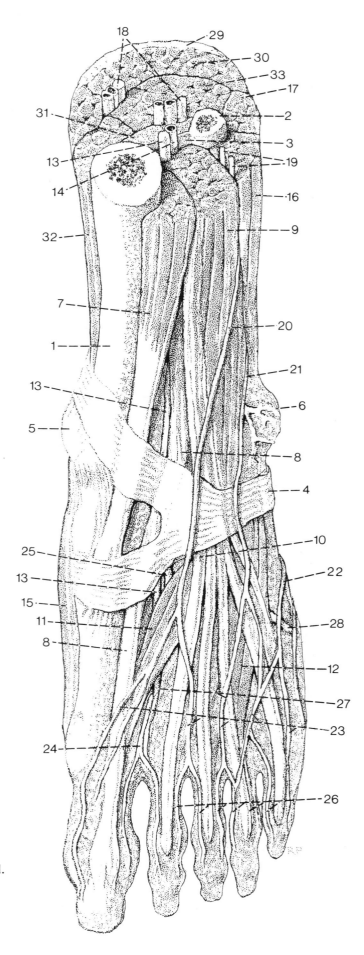

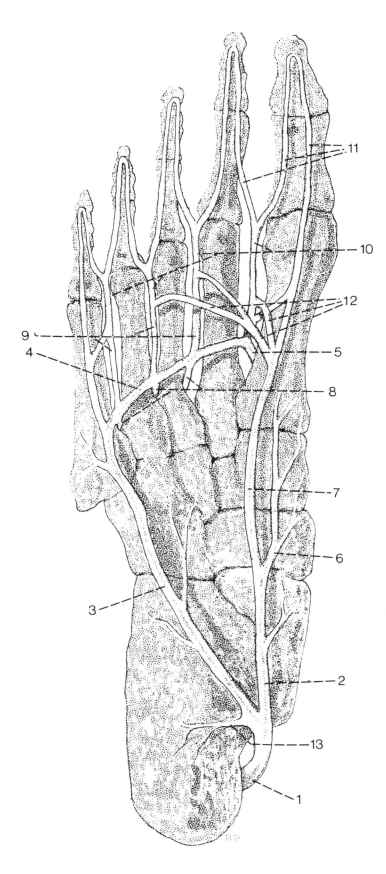

RIGHT FOOT, PLANTAR (INFERIOR) ASPECT

Color and label

1 Posterior tibial artery
2 Medial plantar artery
3 Lateral plantar artery
4 Deep plantar arch
5 Deep plantar artery (from dorsalis pedis artery)
6 Deep branch of medial plantar artery
7 Superficial branch of medial plantar artery
8 Perforating branches of plantar arch
9 Plantar metatarsal arteries
10 Common plantar digital arteries
11 Proper plantar digital arteries
12 Communicating branches
13 Calcaneal branch

After Hollinshead.

189 Plantar arteries

190 Knee: ligaments and menisci

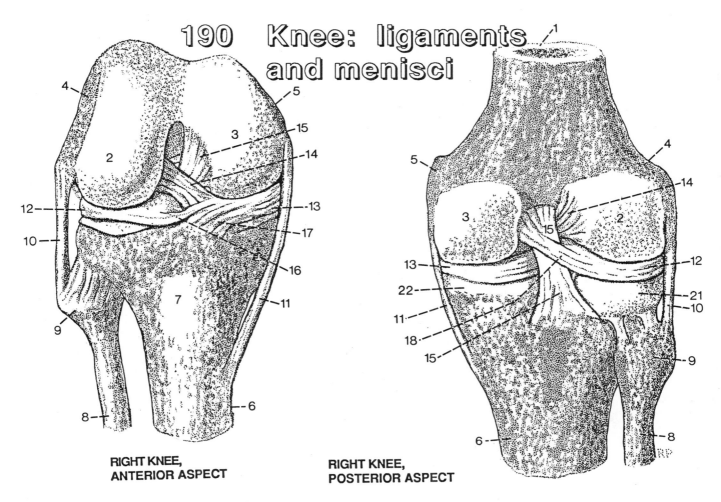

RIGHT KNEE, ANTERIOR ASPECT

RIGHT KNEE, POSTERIOR ASPECT

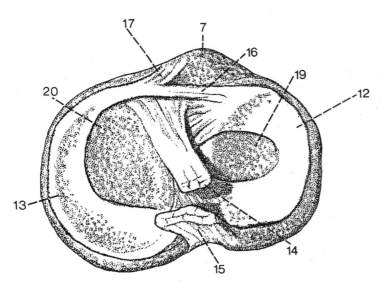

RIGHT TIBIA, SUPERIOR SURFACE

Menisci and ligaments in the positions they occupy in extension of the knee

After Spalteholz and Spanner.

Color and label

1 Femur
2 Lateral condyle of femur
3 Medial condyle of femur
4 Lateral epicondyle of femur
5 Medial epicondyle of femur
6 Tibia
7 Tibial tuberosity
8 Fibula
9 Head of fibula
10 Fibular collateral ligament
11 Tibial collateral ligament
12 Lateral meniscus
13 Medial meniscus
14 Anterior cruciate ligament
15 Posterior cruciate ligament
16 Transverse ligament of the knee
17 Anterior insertion of medial meniscus
18 Posterior meniscofemoral ligament
19 Superior articular surface of lateral tibial condyle
20 Superior articular surface of medial tibial condyle
21 Lateral tibial condyle
22 Medial tibial condyle

191
First layer* of plantar muscles

AND RELATED STRUCTURES OF LEFT FOOT

Color and label

1 Abductor hallucis*
2 Flexor digitorum brevis*
3 Abductor digiti minimi*
4 Tendon of flexor hallucis longus
5 Medial plantar nerve *(this nerve innervates four plantar muscles: flexor digitorum brevis, abductor hallucis, flexor hallucis brevis, medial lumbrical; it corresponds to the median nerve in the hand)*
6 Common plantar digital nerves
7 Proper plantar digital nerves *(branches of medial plantar nerve)*
8 Lateral plantar nerve *(this nerve innervates the remaining 12 plantar muscles, including the quadratus plantae; it corresponds to the ulnar nerve in the hand)*
9 Deep plantar arch
10 Superficial branch of lateral plantar nerve
11 Proper digital nerves *(branches of the lateral plantar nerve)*

Based on a Somso model.

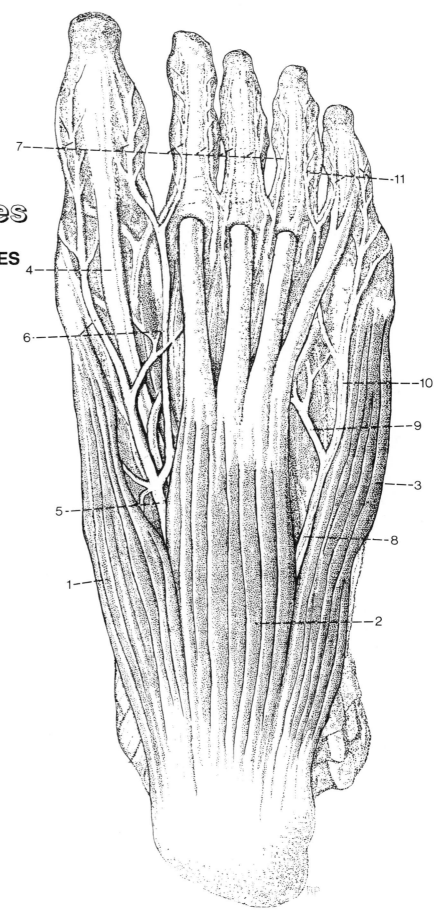

AND RELATED STRUCTURES OF LEFT FOOT

Color and label

1 Quadratus plantae* *(notice its insertion on tendon of flexor digitorum longus)*
2 Lumbrical muscles*
3 Tendon of flexor digitorum longus muscle*
4 Posterior tibial artery
5 Lateral plantar artery
6 Medial plantar artery
7 Deep plantar arch
8 Superficial branch of lateral plantar artery
9 Deep branch of medial plantar artery
10 Superficial branch of medial plantar artery
11 Plantar metatarsal arteries
12 Proper plantar digital arteries
13 Tibial nerve
14 Lateral plantar nerve
15 Medial plantar nerve
16 Common plantar digital neves
17 Proper plantar digital nerves
18 Calcaneal tuberosity
19 Flexor hallucis brevis muscle
20 Flexor digiti minimi muscle
21 Tendon of flexor hallucis longus muscle
22 Abductor hallucis muscle *(cut)*
23 Abductor digiti muscle *(cut)*
24 Tendons of flexor digitorum brevis *(cut)*
25 Tendon of peroneus longus (fibularis longus)
26 Tendon of peroneus brevis (fibularis brevis)
27 Deep branch of lateral plantar nerve
28 Superficial branches of lateral plantar nerve

Based on and modified from a Somso model.

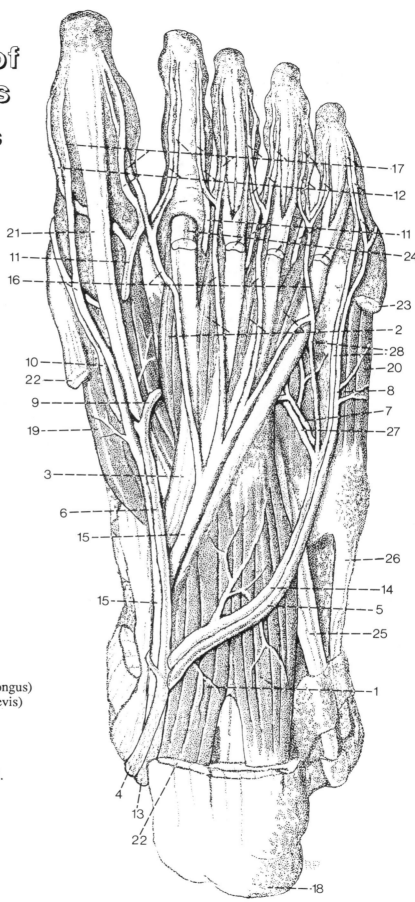

193
Third layer* of plantar muscles

AND RELATED STRUCTURES OF LEFT FOOT

Color and label

1 Flexor hallucis brevis*
2 Adductor hallucis* oblique head
3 Adductor hallucis* transverse head
4 Flexor digiti minimi*
5 Quadratus plantae *(cut)*
6 Tendon of flexor hallucis longus
7 Abductor hallucis *(cut)*
8 Abductor digiti minimi *(cut)*
9 Tendon of peroneus longus
10 Tendon of peroneus brevis
11 Superior fibular retinaculum
12 Inferior fibular retinaculum
13 Tendon of tibialis posterior
14 Posterior tibial artery
15 Medial plantar artery *(cut)*
16 Lateral plantar artery *(cut)*
17 Medial plantar nerve *(cut)*
18 Lateral plantar nerve *(cut)*
19 Tendon of flexor digitorum longus *(cut)*
20 Flexor retinaculum *(cut)*
21 Long plantar ligament
22 Interosseous muscles

Based on a Somso model.

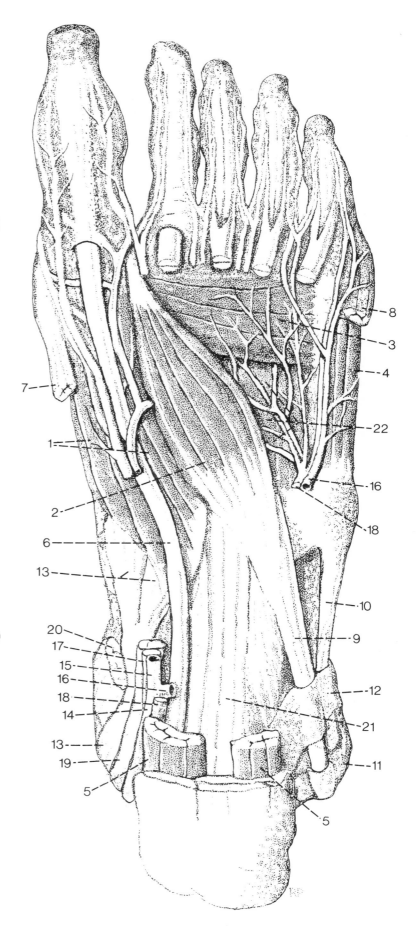

194
Fourth layer* of plantar muscles

AND RELATED STRUCTURES OF LEFT FOOT

Color and label

1 Plantar interosseous muscles*
  (*planta, Latin, sole*)
2 Dorsal interosseous muscles* *(the
  dorsum of the foot is the superior
  surface)*
3 Lateral plantar artery
4 Deep plantar arch
5 Plantar metatarsal arteries
6 Common digital plantar arteries
7 Proper digital arteries
8 Medial plantar artery
9 Deep branch of medial plantar artery
10 Superficial branch of medial plantar
   artery
11 Lateral plantar nerve
12 Deep branch of lateral plantar nerve
13 Superficial branch of lateral plantar
   nerve
14 Tendon of fibularis (peroneus)
   longus
15 Tendon of tibialis posterior
16 Posterior tibial artery
17 Medial plantar nerve
18 Superficial branch of lateral plantar artery

Modified from a Somso model.

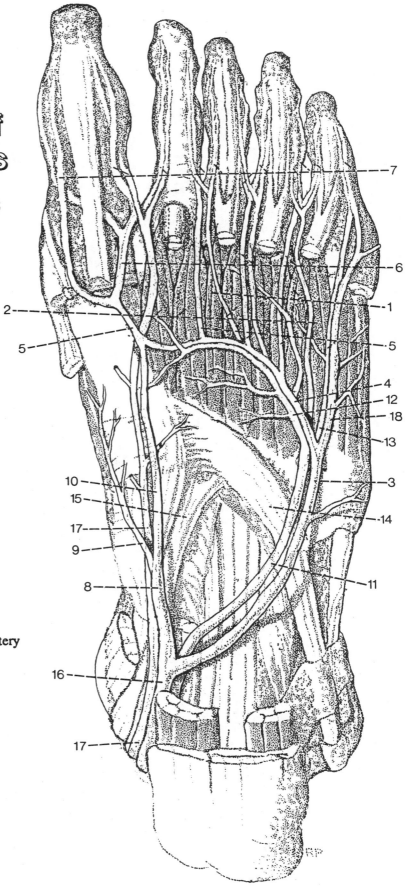

PART VII: HEAD AND NECK
PLATES 195-263

195 MUSCLES OF FACIAL EXPRESSION

(See opposite page)

Color and label

1   Galea aponeurotica (*cut edge*) (epicranial aponeurosis)
2   Frontal belly of occipitofrontalis
3   Temporoparietalis *(highly variable)*
4   Orbicularis oculi
   4A Orbital part
   4B Palpebral part
   4C Lacrimal part
   4D Origin of orbital
   part on orbit
5   Medial palpebral ligament
6   Superior tarsus of eyelid
7   Inferior tarsus of eyelid
8   Orbital septum
9   Tendon of levator palpebrae
10 Corrugator supercilii
11 Procerus
12 Auricularis anterior
13 Zygomaticus major
14 Zygomaticus minor
15 Levator labii superioris (*English: raiser of the superior lip*)
16 Levator labii superioris alaeque nasi
17 Levator anguli oris
18 Masseter
19 Parotid duct
20 Risorius
21 Nasalis
   21A Transverse part
   21B Alar part
22 Depressor septi
23 Orbicularis oris
   23A Marginal part
   23B Labial part
24 Depressor anguli oris (*depressor of the mouth angle*)
25 Depressor labii inferioris
26 Mentalis
27 Buccinator (trumpeter)
28 Platysma
29 Outline of the masseter

All of these muscles except the masseter are innervated by the facial nerve.

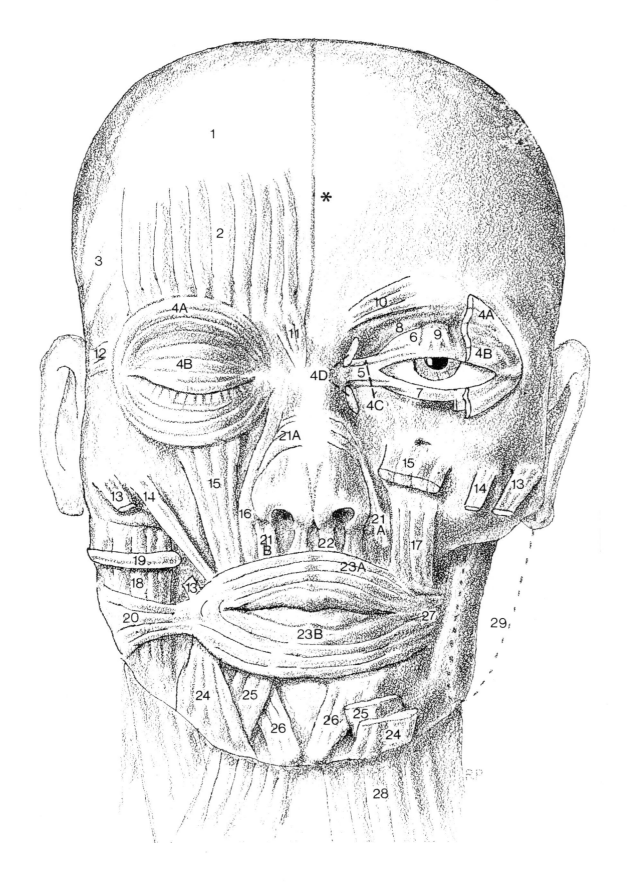

195 MUSCLES OF FACIAL EXPRESSION

SUPERFICIAL STRUCTURES ON THE LATERAL HEAD

(See opposite page)

Color and label

1 Parotid gland
2 Parotid duct
3 Temporal branches of facial nerve (VII)
4 Zygomatic branches of facial nerve (VII)
5 Buccal branches of facial nerve (VII)
6 Marginal mandibular branch of facial nerve (VII)
7 Cervical branch of facial nerve (VII)
8 Transverse facial artery
9 Facial artery and vein
10 Superficial temporal artery and vein
11 Auriculotemporal nerve
   (branch of mandibular nerve V₃)

12 External jugular vein
13 Great auricular nerve
14 Transverse cervical nerve(s)
15 Supraclavicular nerves
16 Lesser occipital nerve
17 Accessory parotid gland
18 Buccal fat pad
19 Accessory nerve (XI)
20 Angular artery and vein
21 Masseter muscle
22 Orbicularis oculi
23 Zygomaticus major
24 Zygomaticus minor
25 Platysma
26 Sternocleidomastoid
27 Trapezius
28 Occipital artery
29 Greater occipital nerve

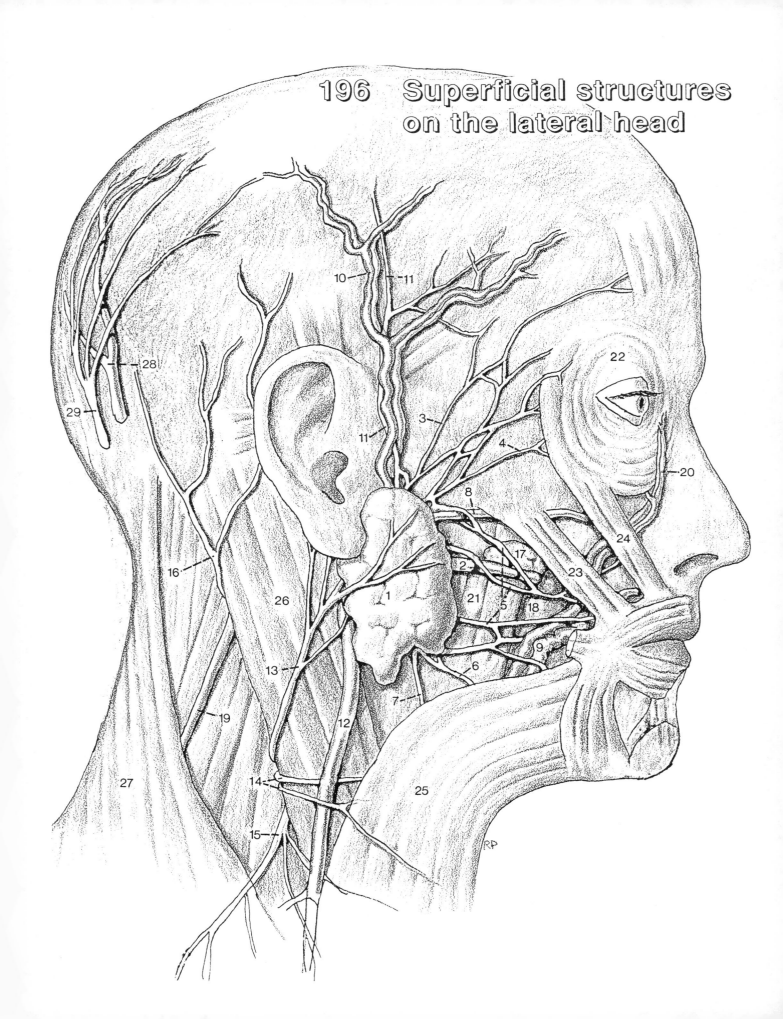

197 Bones of the skull, anterior aspect

Color and label these bones

1 Frontal bone
  1A Squamous part
  1B Orbital part
2 Sphenoid bone
  2A Greater wing orbital surface
  2B Lesser wing
  2C Greater wing temporal surface
3 Zygomatic bone
  3A Lateral surface
  3B Frontal process
  3C Orbital surface
4 Maxillary bone (maxilla)
  4A Body
  4B Nasal process
  4C Orbital surface
5 Mandible
  5A Mental protuberance
  5B Body
  5C Ramus
6 Nasal bone
7 Temporal bone
  7A Squamous part
  7B Mastoid process
  7C Zygomatic process
8 Inferior nasal concha
9 Lacrimal bone
10 Parietal bone
11 Vomer
12 Ethmoid bone
  12A Perpendicular plate
  12B Middle nasal concha

Label these foramina

13 Optic canal
14 Superior orbital fissure
15 Inferior orbital fissure
16 Infraorbital groove
17 Supraorbital foramen
  (sometimes notch)
18 Infraorbital foramen
19 Mental foramen

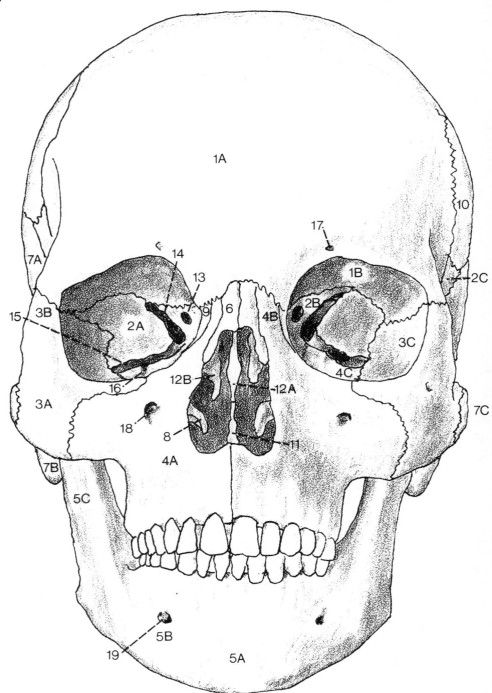

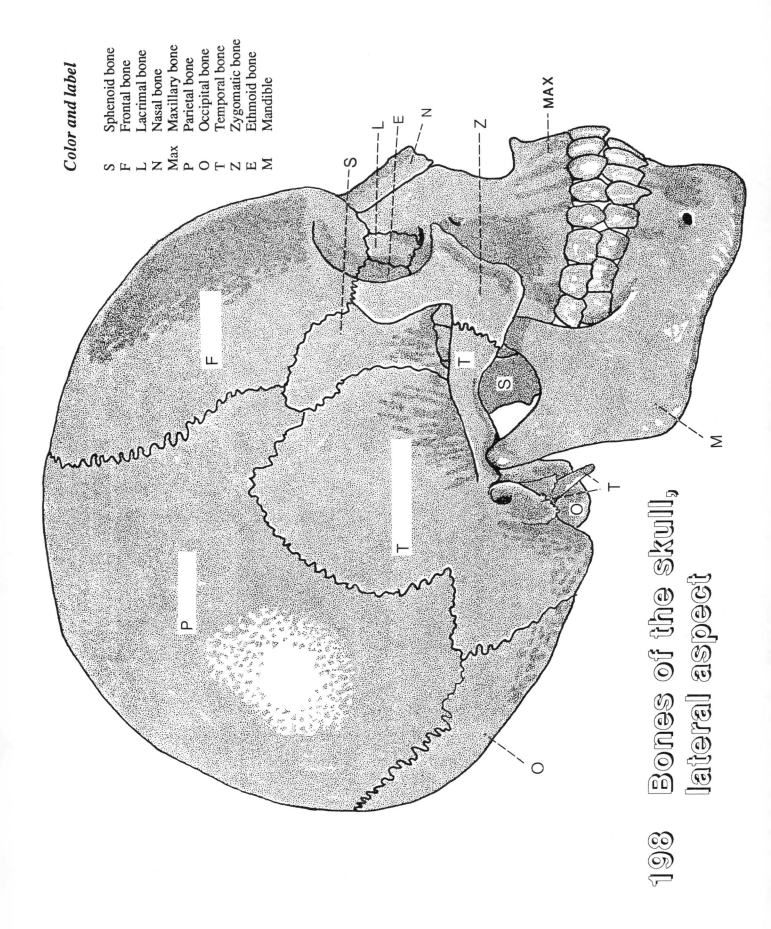

198   Bones of the skull, lateral aspect

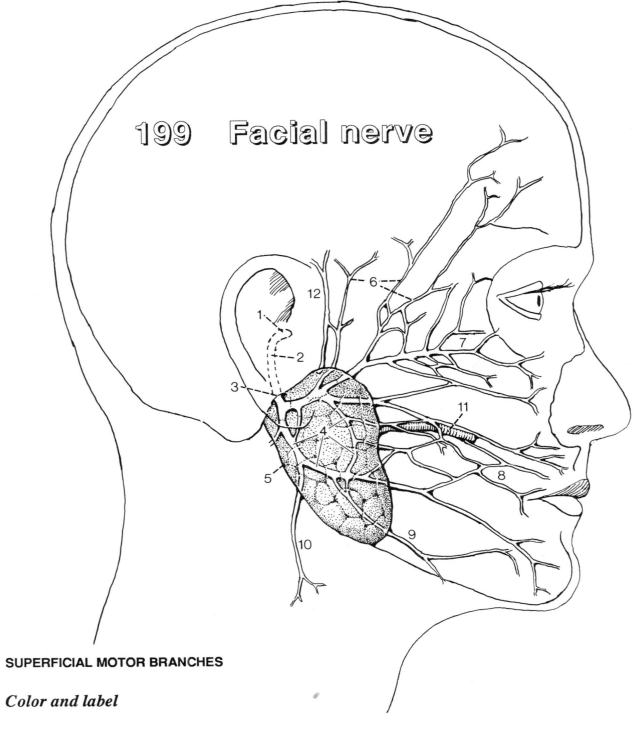

199　Facial nerve

SUPERFICIAL MOTOR BRANCHES

Color and label

1　Geniculate ganglion *(within temporal bone)*
2　Facial nerve within bony facial canal
3　Stylomastoid foramen
4　Facial nerve within parotid gland
5　Parotid gland
6　Temporal branches of facial nerve
7　Zygomatic branches of facial nerve

8　Buccal branches of facial nerve
9　Mandibular branch of facial nerve
10　Cervical branch of facial nerve
11　Parotid duct
12　Auriculotemporal nerve *(a branch of the mandibular nerve)*

The interconnecting rami form the parotid plexus. Earlier anatomists likened the parotid plexus to the webbed foot of a goose and called it pes anserinus (Latin, goose's foot).

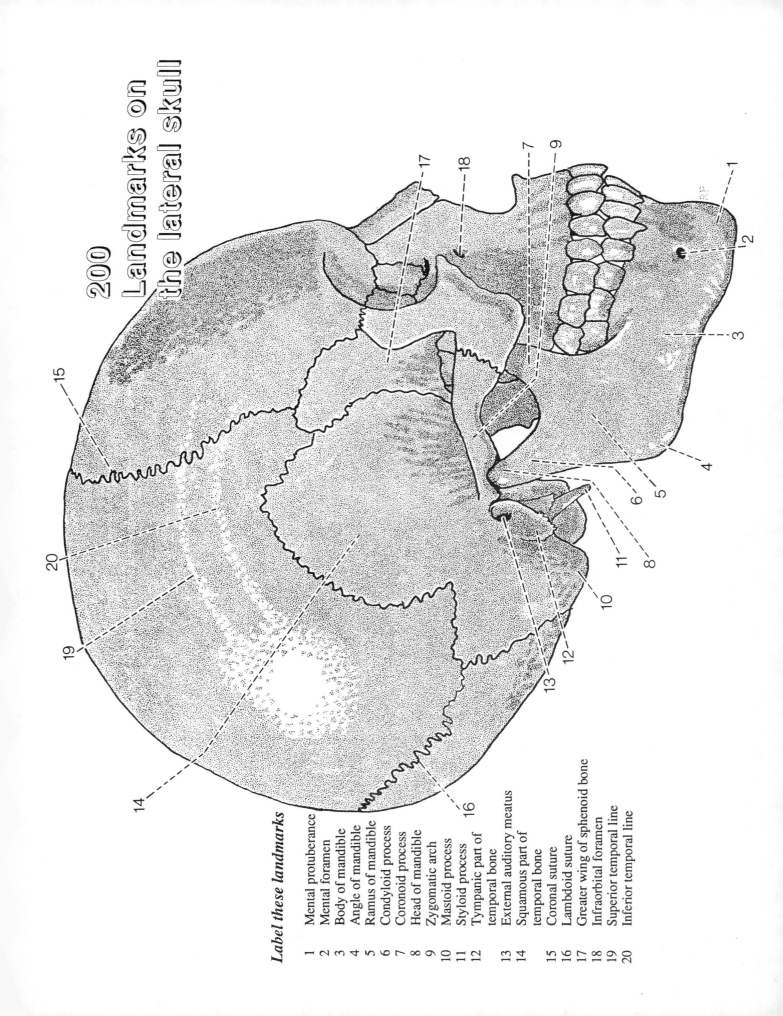

Label these landmarks

1 Mental protuberance
2 Mental foramen
3 Body of mandible
4 Angle of mandible
5 Ramus of mandible
6 Condyloid process
7 Coronoid process
8 Head of mandible
9 Zygomatic arch
10 Mastoid process
11 Styloid process
12 Tympanic part of temporal bone
13 External auditory meatus
14 Squamous part of temporal bone
15 Coronal suture
16 Lambdoid suture
17 Greater wing of sphenoid bone
18 Infraorbital foramen
19 Superior temporal line
20 Inferior temporal line

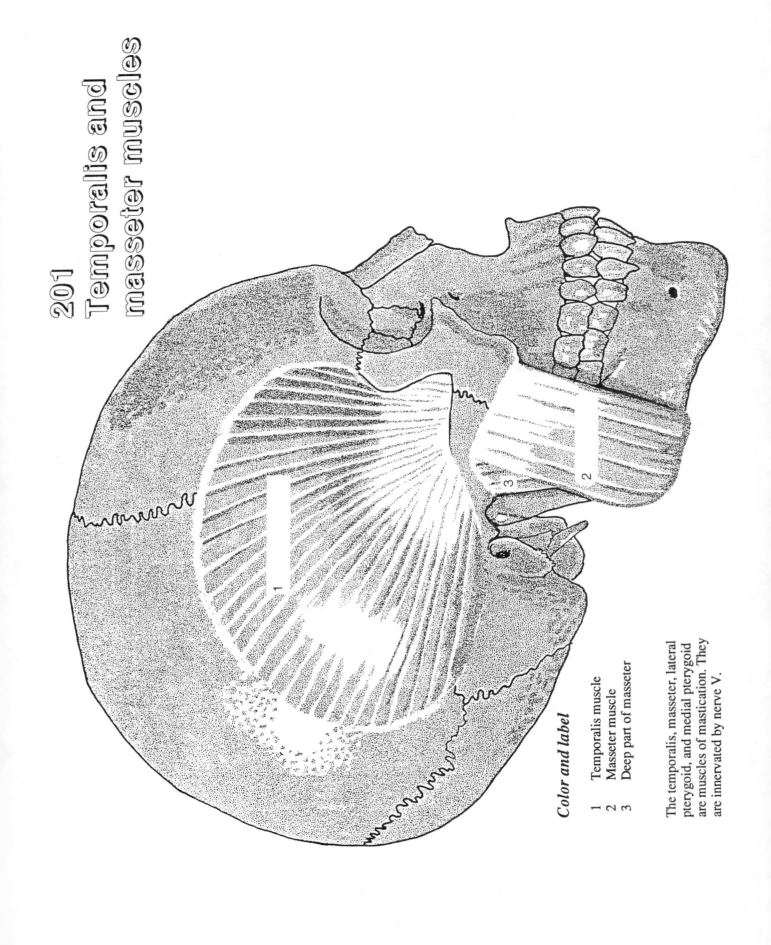

Color and label

1 Temporalis muscle
2 Masseter muscle
3 Deep part of masseter

The temporalis, masseter, lateral pterygoid, and medial pterygoid are muscles of mastication. They are innervated by nerve V.

Color and label

1 Temporalis muscle
2 Insertion of temporalis
   on coronoid process of mandible
3 Zygomatic arch (*cut*)
4 Insertion of masseter on ramus
   and angle of mandible

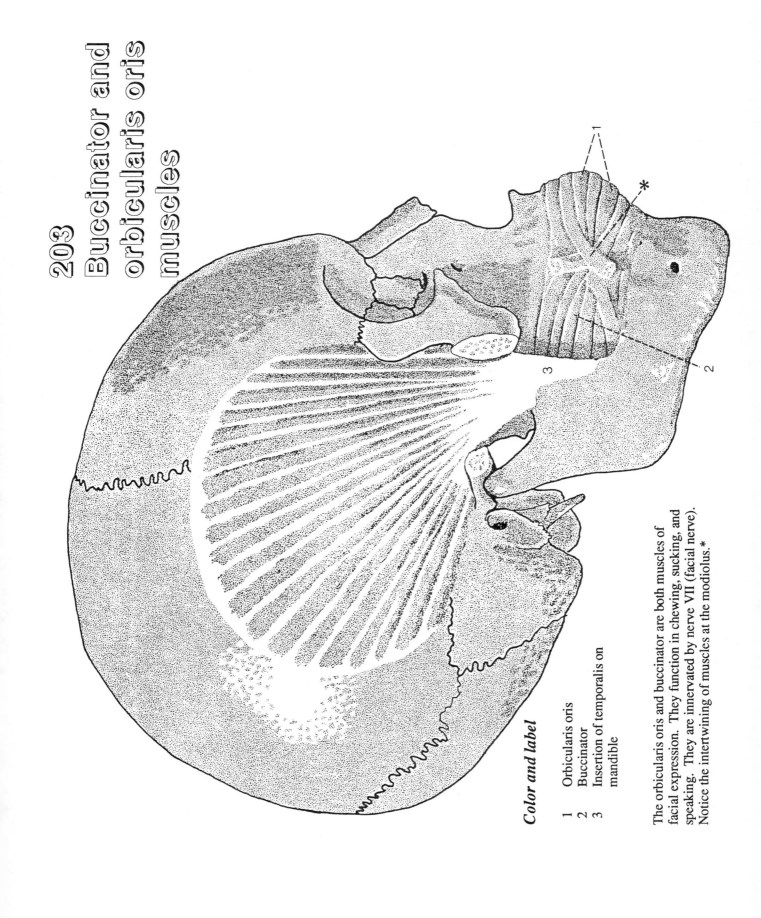

Color and label

1   Orbicularis oris
2   Buccinator
3   Insertion of temporalis on
      mandible

The orbicularis oris and buccinator are both muscles of
facial expression. They function in chewing, sucking, and
speaking. They are innervated by nerve VII (facial nerve).
Notice the intertwining of muscles at the modiolus.*

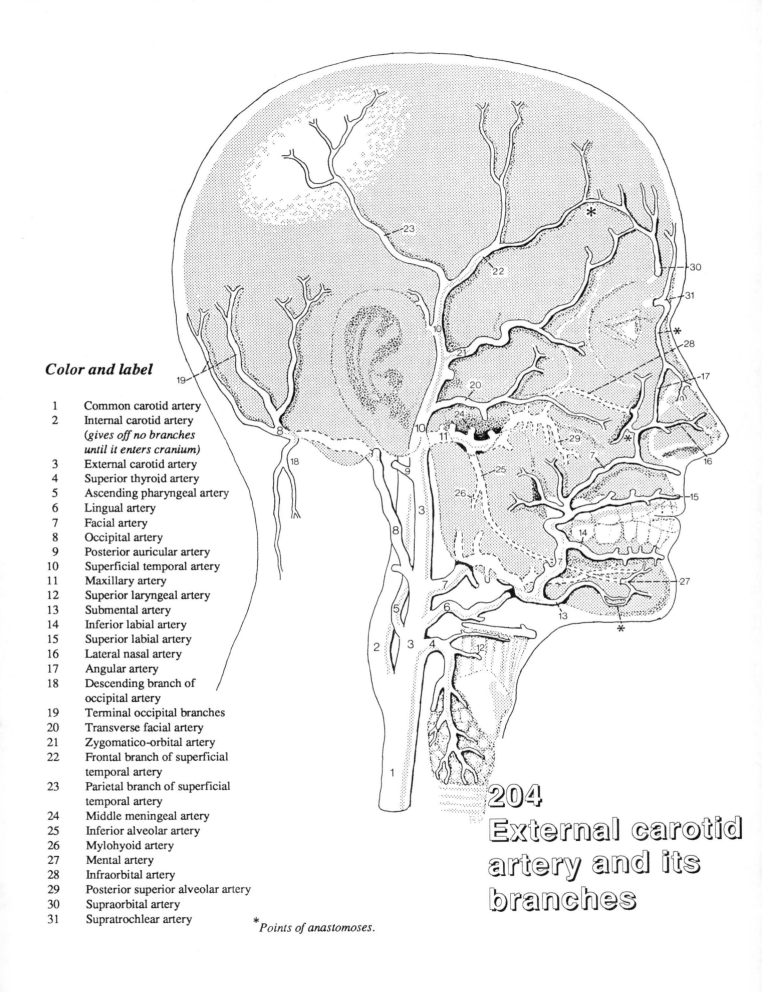

Color and label

1	Common carotid artery
2	Internal carotid artery *(gives off no branches until it enters cranium)*
3	External carotid artery
4	Superior thyroid artery
5	Ascending pharyngeal artery
6	Lingual artery
7	Facial artery
8	Occipital artery
9	Posterior auricular artery
10	Superficial temporal artery
11	Maxillary artery
12	Superior laryngeal artery
13	Submental artery
14	Inferior labial artery
15	Superior labial artery
16	Lateral nasal artery
17	Angular artery
18	Descending branch of occipital artery
19	Terminal occipital branches
20	Transverse facial artery
21	Zygomatico-orbital artery
22	Frontal branch of superficial temporal artery
23	Parietal branch of superficial temporal artery
24	Middle meningeal artery
25	Inferior alveolar artery
26	Mylohyoid artery
27	Mental artery
28	Infraorbital artery
29	Posterior superior alveolar artery
30	Supraorbital artery
31	Supratrochlear artery

*Points of anastomoses.

204
External carotid artery and its branches

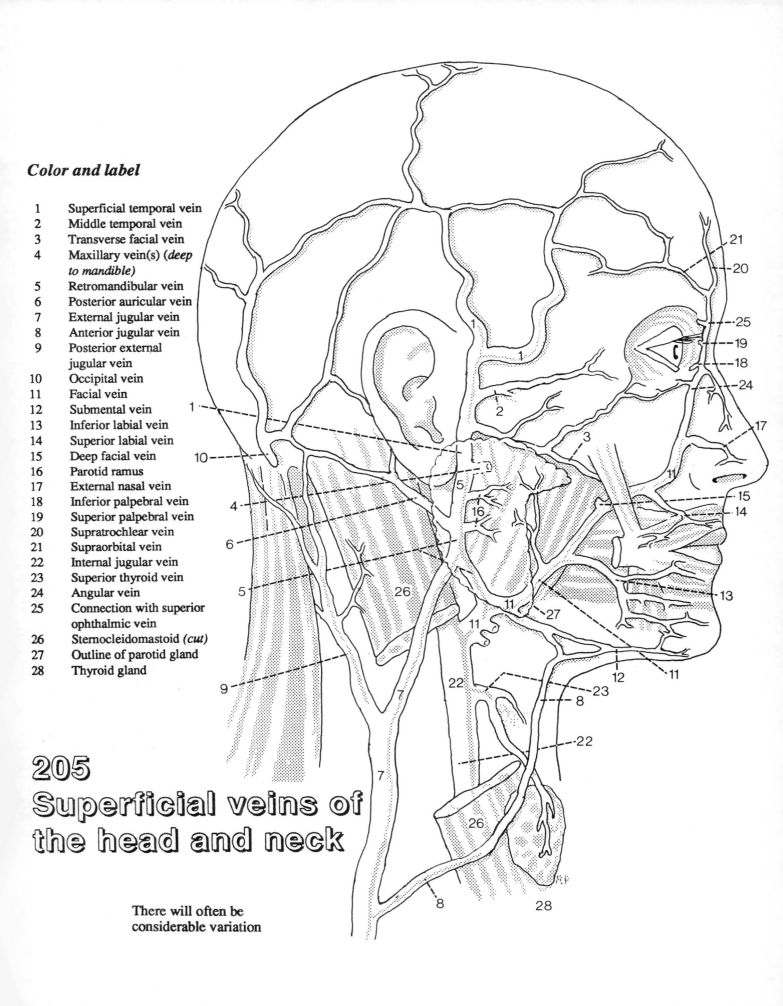

Color and label

1	Superficial temporal vein
2	Middle temporal vein
3	Transverse facial vein
4	Maxillary vein(s) *(deep to mandible)*
5	Retromandibular vein
6	Posterior auricular vein
7	External jugular vein
8	Anterior jugular vein
9	Posterior external jugular vein
10	Occipital vein
11	Facial vein
12	Submental vein
13	Inferior labial vein
14	Superior labial vein
15	Deep facial vein
16	Parotid ramus
17	External nasal vein
18	Inferior palpebral vein
19	Superior palpebral vein
20	Supratrochlear vein
21	Supraorbital vein
22	Internal jugular vein
23	Superior thyroid vein
24	Angular vein
25	Connection with superior ophthalmic vein
26	Sternocleidomastoid *(cut)*
27	Outline of parotid gland
28	Thyroid gland

205
Superficial veins of
the head and neck

There will often be
considerable variation

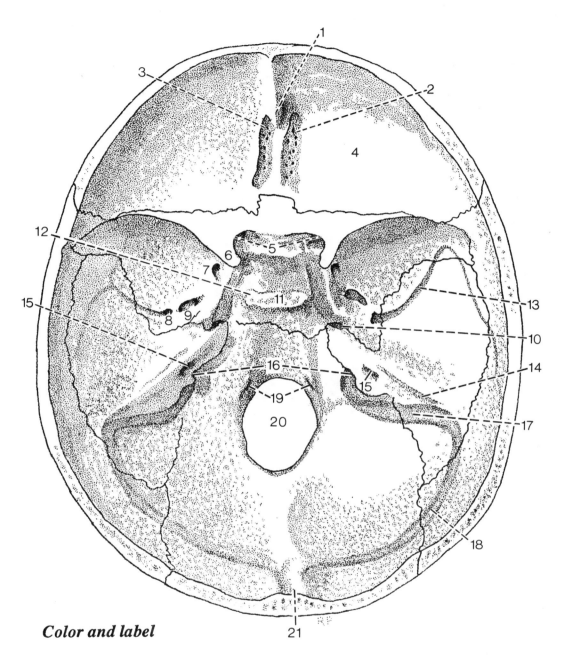

Color and label

1	Crista galli
2	Cribriform plate of ethmoid bone
3	Foramina for olfactory nerve fibers
4	Orbital part of frontal bone
5	Optic canal
6	Anterior clinoid process
7	Foramen rotundum
8	Foramen spinosum
9	Foramen ovale
10	Foramen lacerum
11	Dorsum sellae
12	Posterior clinoid process
13	Groove for middle meningeal artery
14	Groove for superior petrosal sinus
15	Internal auditory meatus
16	Jugular foramen
17	Sulcus for sigmoid sinus
18	Sulcus for transverse sinus
19	Hypoglossal canal
20	Foramen magnum
21	Sulcus for superior sagittal sinus

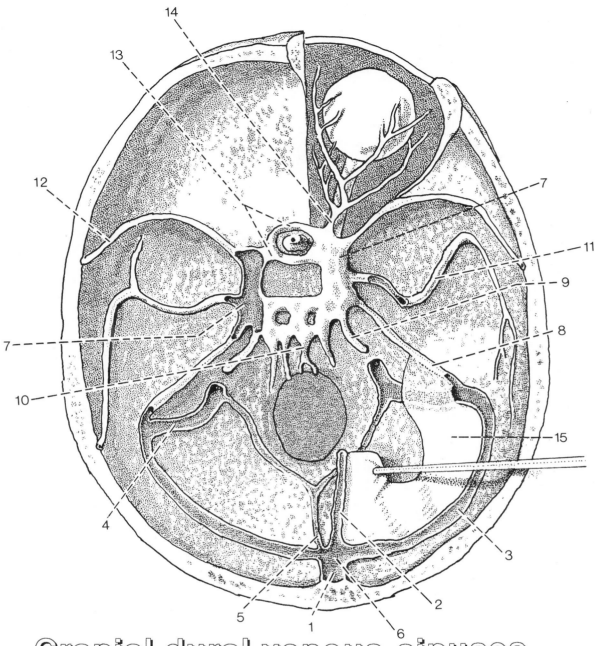

207 Cranial dural venous sinuses

BENEATH THE BRAIN

Color and label

1 Superior sagittal sinus
  (*cut open*)
2 Straight sinus (*cut open*)
3 Right transverse sinus
  (*cut open*)
4 Sigmoid sinus (*cut open*)
5 Occipital sinus
6 Confluence of sinuses
7 Cavernous sinus (*cut open on left*)

8 Superior petrosal sinus
9 Inferior petrosal sinus
10 Basilar venous plexus
11 Middle meningeal vein
12 Sphenoparietal sinus
13 Anterior and posterior inter-
  cavernous sinuses
14 Superior ophthalmic vein
15 Tentorium cerebelli (*cut*)

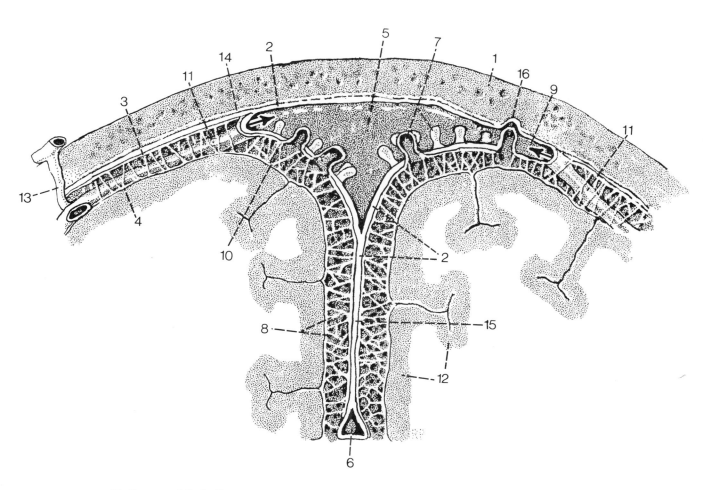

Color and label

1   Bone of skull
2   Dura mater *(Latin, tough mother)*
3   Arachnoid mater *(Greek, spider-web-like)*
4   Pia mater *(Latin, tender, faithful mother)*
5   Superior sagittal sinus *(this is a large vein formed by walls of dura mater)*
6   Inferior sagittal sinus
7   Arachnoid granulations *(these allow the cerebrospinal fluid in the subarachnoid space to enter the superior sagittal sinus and mix with its venous blood)*
8   Arachnoid trabeculae *(these form a meshwork of small fibers that crisscross the subarachnoid space)*
9   Lateral lacunae *(these are outpouchings of the superior sagittal sinus)*
10   Subarachnoid space containing cerebrospinal fluid
11   Superior cerebral vein emptying into the superior sagittal sinus
12   Cerebral cortex
13   Emissary vein *(these pass completely through the skull)*
14   Periosteum *(in most areas the dura mater and periosteum are fused together)*
15   Falx cerebri *(falx, Latin, scythe)*
16   Pits on inner surface of skull caused by arachnoid granulations

209
Dura mater
(etymological
cartoon)

Latin,
tough mother

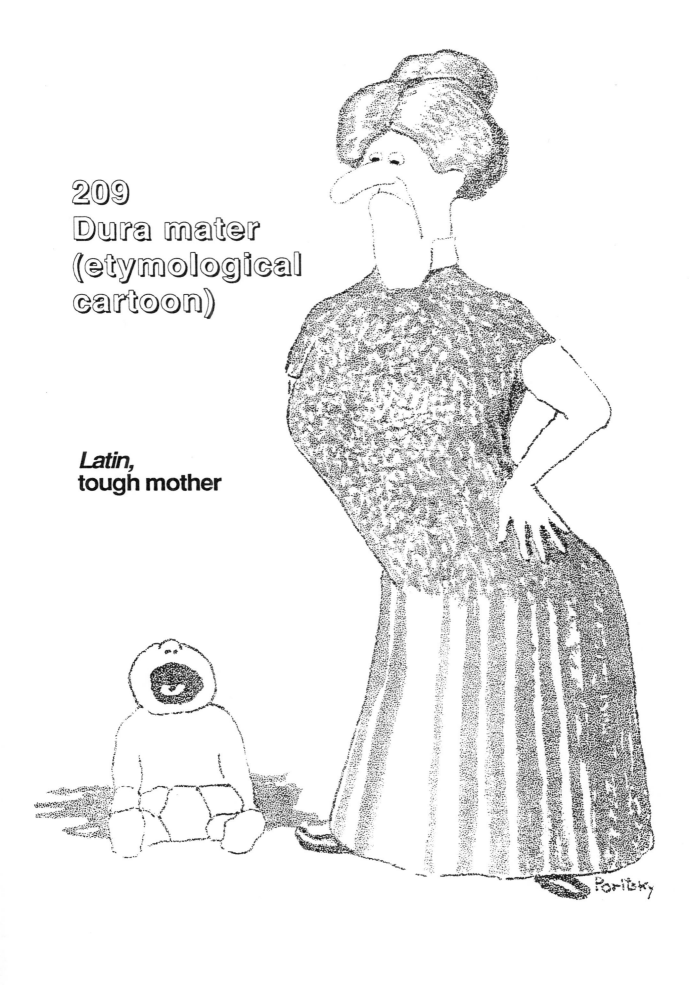

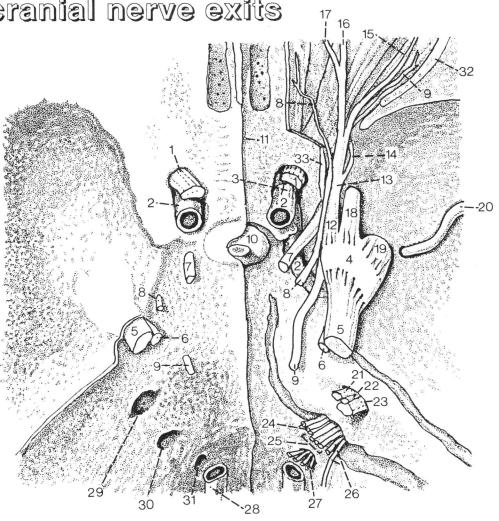

Color and label

1	Optic nerve (N II)	18	Maxillary nerve
2	Internal carotid artery	19	Mandibular nerve
3	Ophthalmic artery	20	Middle meningeal artery
4	Trigeminal ganglion	21	Facial nerve motor root (N VII)
5	Sensory root of trigeminal nerve	22	Nervus intermedius (N VII)
6	Motor root of trigeminal nerve	23	Vestibulocochlear nerve (N VIII)
7	Oculomotor nerve (N III)	24	Glossopharyngeal nerve (N IX)
8	Trochlear nerve (N IV)	25	Vagus nerve (N X)
9	Abducent nerve (N VI)	26	Accessory nerve (N XI)
10	Pituitary gland (hypophysis)	27	Hypoglossal nerve (N XII)
11	Cut edge of dura mater	28	Vertebral artery
12	Ophthalmic nerve	29	Internal auditory meatus
13	Frontal nerve	30	Jugular foramen
14	Nasociliary nerve	31	Hypoglossal canal
15	Lacrimal nerve	32	Roof of orbit removed
16	Supraorbital nerve	33	Roof of superior orbital fissure removed
17	Supratrochlear nerve		

211 Facial nerve and its branches

LATERAL VIEW OF FACIAL NERVE WITH INTERNAL AUDITORY MEATUS AND CANAL EXPOSED, CAROTID CANAL OPENED, AND GREATER WING OF SPHENOID REMOVED

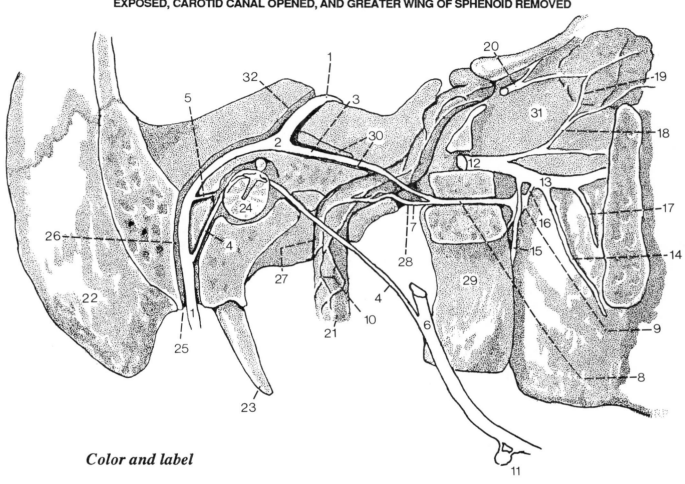

Color and label

1	Facial nerve	17	Middle superior alveolar nerve
2	Geniculate ganglion	18	Zygomatic nerve
3	Greater petrosal nerve	19	Communicating branch to lacrimal nerve
4	Chorda tympani		
5	Nerve to stapedius muscle	20	Lacrimal nerve
6	Lingual nerve *(cut; part of mandibular nerve)*	21	Internal carotid artery
		22	Mastoid process
7	Deep petrosal nerve	23	Styloid process
8	Nerve of pterygoid canal	24	Eardrum and malleus
9	Pterygopalatine ganglion	25	Stylomastoid foramen
10	Internal carotid plexus *(sympathetic)*	26	Facial canal
		27	Carotid canal
11	Submandibular ganglion	28	Foramen lacerum
12	Maxillary nerve (cut)	29	Medial pterygoid plate
13	Infraorbital nerve	30	Canal and groove for greater petrosal nerve
14	Posterior superior alveolar nerve		
		31	Orbit
15	Palatine nerves	32	Internal auditory meatus *(roof removed)*
16	Pterygopalatine nerves		

Functional components of the facial nerve

(See opposite page)

Color and label these nerve fibers and brainstem nuclei

1	Motor neuron to muscles of facial expression *(also stapedius, stylohyoid, posterior belly of digastric)*
2	Facial motor nucleus
3	Parasympathetic neuron *(preganglionic)* ending in submandibular ganglion
4	Parasympathetic neuron *(preganglionic)* ending in pterygopalatine ganglion
5	Superior salivatory nucleus
6	Cell body of taste neuron carrying taste from the tongue via chorda tympani nerve
7	Cell body of taste neuron carrying taste from the palate via greater petrosal nerve
8	Neuron of nucleus from solitary tract *(second-order; receives taste sensation from tongue)*
9	Neuron in nucleus of solitary tract *(second-order; receives taste sensation from palate)*
10	Nucleus of solitary tract
11	Parasympathetic neuron *(postganglionic)* to lacrimal gland
12	Parasympathetic neuron *(postganglionic)* to nasal glands
13	Pterygopalatine ganglion
14	Parasympathetic neuron *(postganglionic)* to submandibular gland
15	Parasympathetic neuron *(postganglionic)* to sublingual gland
16	Sympathetic neuron *(preganglionic)* in spinal cord
17	Sympathetic neurons *(postganglionic)*
18	Superior cervical ganglion
19	Internal carotid plexus
20	Geniculate ganglion
21	Greater petrosal nerve
22	Deep petrosal nerve
23	Nerve of pterygoid canal
24	Nerve to stapedius
25	Chorda tympani
26	Facial canal
27	Stylomastoid foramen
28	Maxillary nerve in foramen rotundum
29	Lacrimal nerve
30	Zygomatic nerve
31	Zygomaticotemporal nerve
32	Communicating branch between zygomaticotemporal and lacrimal nerves
33	Facial nerve (VII) exiting stylomastoid foramen
34	Genu of facial nerve

Functional components of the facial nerve

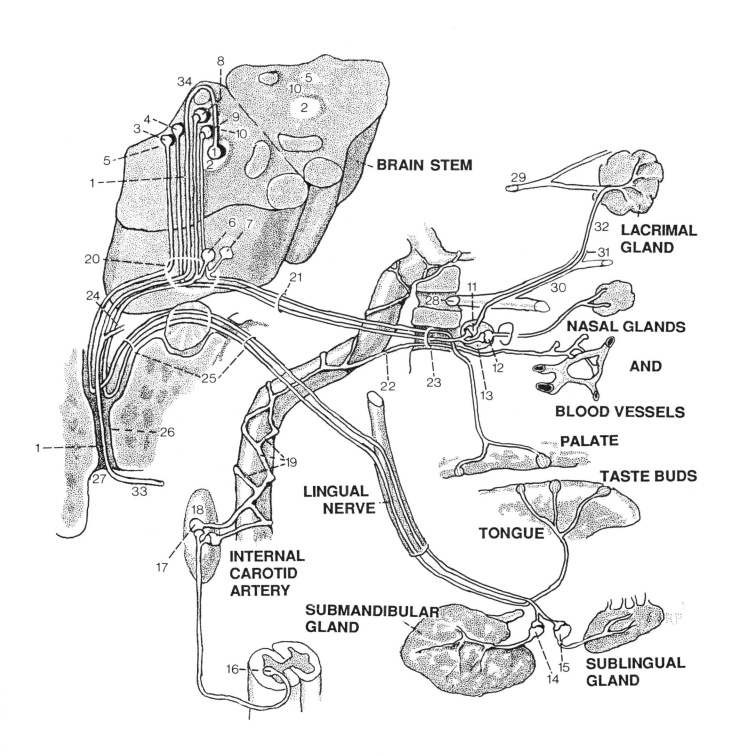

BRAIN STEM

LACRIMAL GLAND

NASAL GLANDS

AND

BLOOD VESSELS

PALATE

TASTE BUDS

TONGUE

LINGUAL NERVE

INTERNAL CAROTID ARTERY

SUBMANDIBULAR GLAND

SUBLINGUAL GLAND

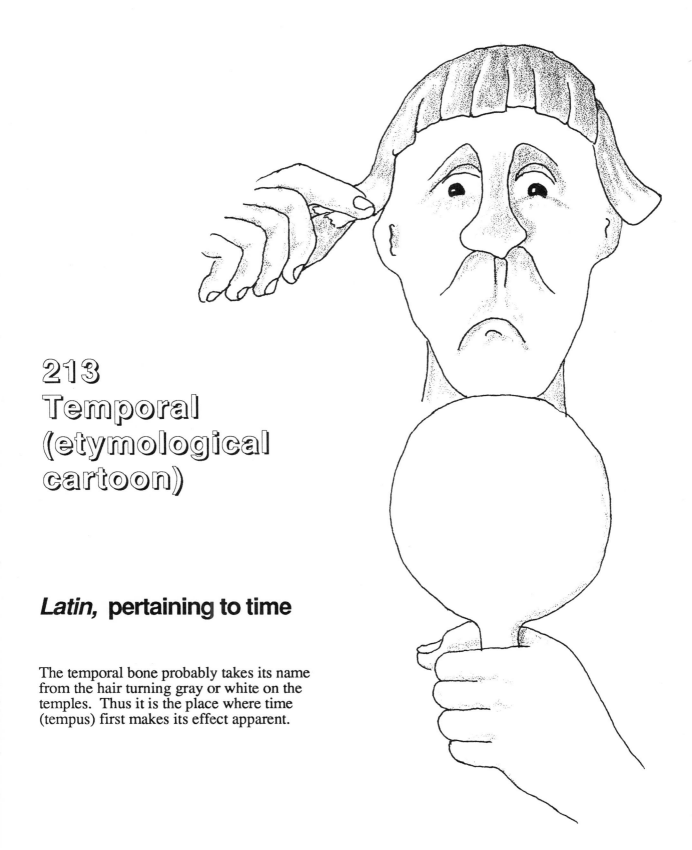

213
Temporal
(etymological
cartoon)

Latin, pertaining to time

The temporal bone probably takes its name
from the hair turning gray or white on the
temples. Thus it is the place where time
(tempus) first makes its effect apparent.

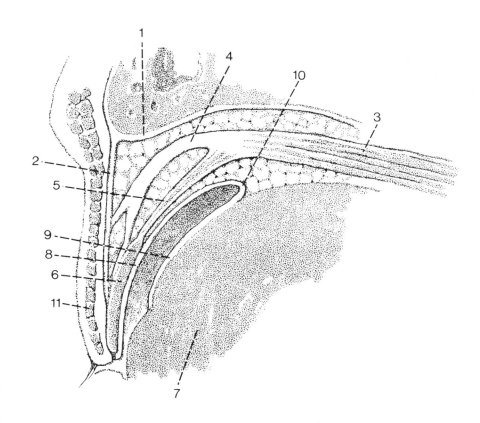

THE UPPER EYELID

Color and label

1   Periorbita (*periosteum of the orbit*)
2   Orbital septum (*dense connective tissue sheet continuous with the periorbita*)
3   Levator palpebrae muscle
4   Levator aponeurosis
5   Superior tarsal muscle (*a smooth muscle supplied by sympathetic fibers*)
6   Tarsus (*a dense curved plate of cartilage-like connective tissue*)
7   Eyeball
8   Palpebral (eyelid) conjunctiva (*a mucous membrane*)
9   Bulbar (eyeball) conjunctiva
10   Superior conjunctival fornix (*Latin, arch*)
11   Orbicularis oculi

After Hollinshead.

214   The eyelid and eye in orbit

RIGHT EYE AND ORBIT

Color and label

1   Superior tarsus
2   Inferior tarsus
3   Tendon of levator palpebrae superioris (*cut*)
4   Orbital septum (*cut*)
5   Lacrimal gland (*orbital and palpebral parts*)
6   Lateral palpebral ligament
7   Medial palpebral ligament (*cut*)
8   Superior lacrimal canaliculus
9   Inferior lacrimal canaliculus
10   Lacrimal sac
11   Nasolacrimal duct
12   Maxillary bone (*cut*)

After Wolf-Heidegger.

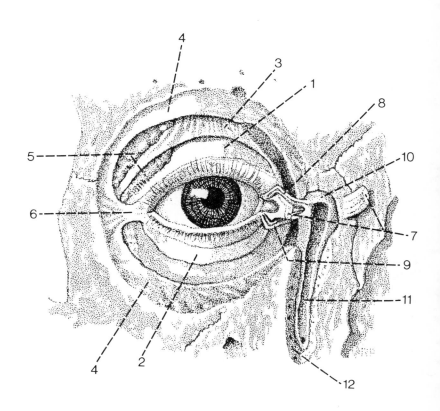

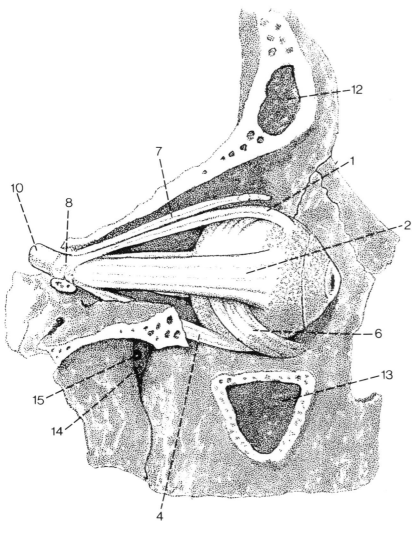

215
Extraocular muscles

**LATERAL VIEW OF RIGHT EYE (ABOVE)
WITH LATERAL WALL REMOVED**

**SUPERIOR VIEW OF RIGHT EYE (BELOW)
WITH ROOF OF ORBIT REMOVED**

Color and label

1	Superior rectus muscle
2	Lateral rectus muscle
3	Medial rectus muscle
4	Inferior rectus muscle
5	Superior oblique muscle
6	Inferior oblique muscle
7	Levator palpebrae muscle *(cut)*
8	Anulus tendineus communis
9	Trochlea
10	Optic nerve
11	Conjunctiva (tunica conjunctiva) *(cut edge)*
12	Frontal sinus
13	Maxillary sinus
14	Pterygopalatine fossa
15	Sphenopalatine foramen

After Wolf-Heidegger.

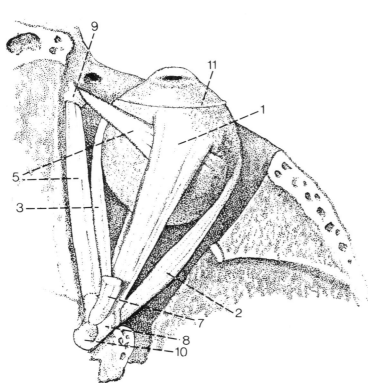

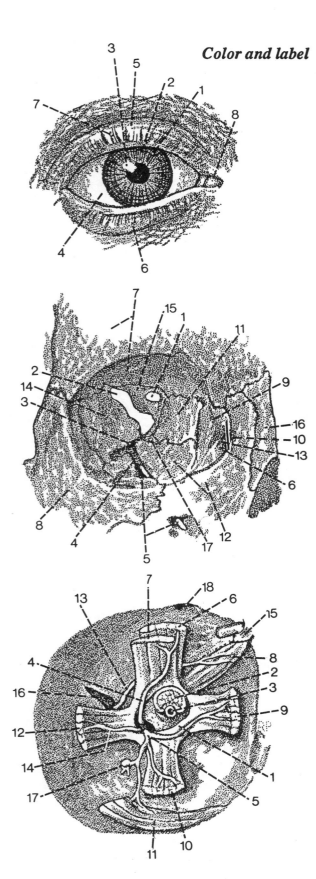

Color and label

RIGHT EYE
1 Pupil *(aperture for light in iris)*
2 Iris *(pigmented, blue, brown or green; radial dilator muscles enlarge pupil; circular constrictor muscles decrease pupil)*
3 Reflection on cornea *(the cornea's greater curvature reflects light; the cornea is transparent)*
4 Bulbar conjunctiva overlying sclera *(sclera is white fibrous coat of eye)*
5 Upper lid (palpebra superior)
6 Lower lid (palpebra inferior)
7 Cilia (eyelashes) *(notice origin on anterior lid margins)*
8 Lacrimal caruncle

RIGHT ORBIT (ANTERIOR AND SLIGHTLY LATERAL VIEW)
1 Optic canal
2 Superior orbital fissure
3 Inferior orbital fissure
4 Infraorbital groove
5 Infraorbital canal and foramen
6 Fossa for lacrimal sac
7 Frontal bone
8 Zygomatic bone
9 Lacrimal bone
10 Probe in nasolacrimal duct
11 Orbital plate of ethmoid bone
12 Maxilla (maxillary bone)
13 Posterior lacrimal crest
14 Greater wing of sphenoid bone
15 Lesser wing of sphenoid bone
16 Nasal bone
17 Palatine bone

COMMON TENDINOUS RING (ANULUS TENDINEUS COMMUNIS)
1 Common tendinous ring *(notice that it encircles both the optic canal with the optic nerve and the ophthalmic artery plus part of the superior orbital fissure with the abducent and oculomotor nerves)*
2 Optic nerve emerging from optic canal
3 Ophthalmic artery
4 Superior ramus of oculomotor nerve *(notice that it innervates the superior rectus and levator palpebrae)*
5 Inferior ramus of oculomotor nerve *(notice that it innervates the medial rectus and inferior oblique muscles plus a communicating ramus to the ciliary ganglion)*
6 Levator palpebrae
7 Superior rectus
8 Superior oblique
9 Medial rectus
10 Inferior rectus
11 Inferior oblique
12 Lateral rectus
13 Trochlear nerve
14 Abducent nerve
15 Trochlea *(Latin, pulley)*
16 Superior orbital fissure
17 Ciliary ganglion *(contains postganglionic parasympathetic nerve cell body that causes constriction of the pupil and accommodates for near vision)*
18 Supraorbital notch

216 Eye and orbit

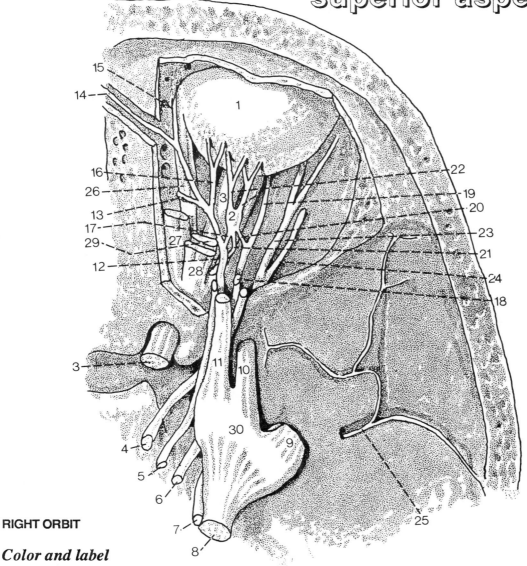

RIGHT ORBIT

Color and label

 1 Eyeball
 2 Ciliary ganglion (parasympathetic)
 3 Optic nerve
 4 Oculomotor nerve (III)
 5 Trochlear nerve (IV)
 6 Abducent nerve
 7 Motor root (portio minor) of
    trigeminal nerve (V)
 8 Sensory root (portio major) of
    trigeminal nerve (V)
 9 Mandibular nerve
10 Maxillary nerve
11 Ophthalmic nerve *(cut)*
12 Nasociliary nerve *(branch of
    ophthalmic)*
13 Posterior ethmoidal nerve
14 Anterior ethmoidal nerve

15 Infratrochlear nerve
16 Long ciliary nerves
17 Communicating ramus of nasociliary
    nerve with ciliary ganglion
18 Oculomotor nerve superior ramus *(cut)*
19 Oculomotor nerve inferior ramus
20 Oculomotor root of ciliary ganglion
21 Sympathetic branch to ciliary ganglion
22 Short ciliary nerves
23 Zygomatic nerve
24 Infraorbital nerve
25 Meningeal ramus of mandibular nerve
26 Medial rectus muscle
27 Superior oblique muscle *(cut)*
28 Levator palpebrae superioris *(cut)*
29 Superior rectus muscle *(cut)*
30 Trigeminal ganglion

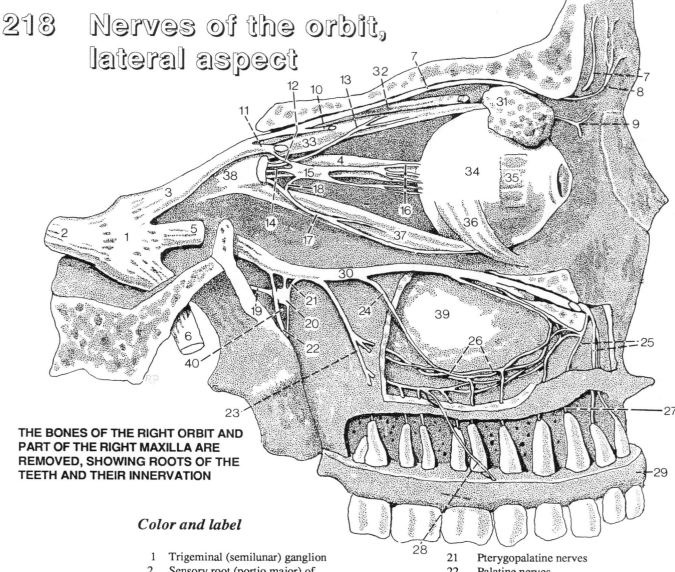

THE BONES OF THE RIGHT ORBIT AND
PART OF THE RIGHT MAXILLA ARE
REMOVED, SHOWING ROOTS OF THE
TEETH AND THEIR INNERVATION

Color and label

1	Trigeminal (semilunar) ganglion		21	Pterygopalatine nerves
2	Sensory root (portio major) of		22	Palatine nerves
	trigeminal nerve		23	Posterior superior alveolar branches
3	Ophthalmic nerve (V_1)		24	Middle superior alveolar branches
4	Optic nerve		25	Anterior superior alveolar branches
5	Maxillary nerve (V_2)		26	Superior dental plexus
6	Mandibular nerve (V_3)		27	Superior dental branches
7	Supraorbital nerve		28	Gingival branch
8	Supraorbital nerve (medial ramus)		29	Gingiva
9	Supratrochlear nerve		30	Infraorbital nerve
10	Lacrimal nerve *(cut)*		31	Lacrimal gland
11	Nasociliary nerve *(cut)*		32	Levator palpebrae superioris
12	Ramus from nasociliary nerve to			muscle *(cut)*
	ciliary ganglion		33	Superior rectus muscle
13	Superior ramus of oculomotor nerve		34	Eyeball
14	Sympathetic ramus to ciliary ganglion		35	Lateral rectus muscle *(cut)*
15	Ciliary ganglion		36	Inferior oblique muscle
16	Short ciliary nerves		37	Inferior rectus muscle
17	Inferior ramus of oculomotor nerve		38	Common tendinous ring (anulus
18	Oculomotor root to ciliary ganglion			tendineus communis)
19	Nerve of pterygoid canal		39	Mucous membrane of maxillary sinus
20	Pterygopalatine ganglion		40	Pterygopalatine fossa

After Spalteholz and Spanner.

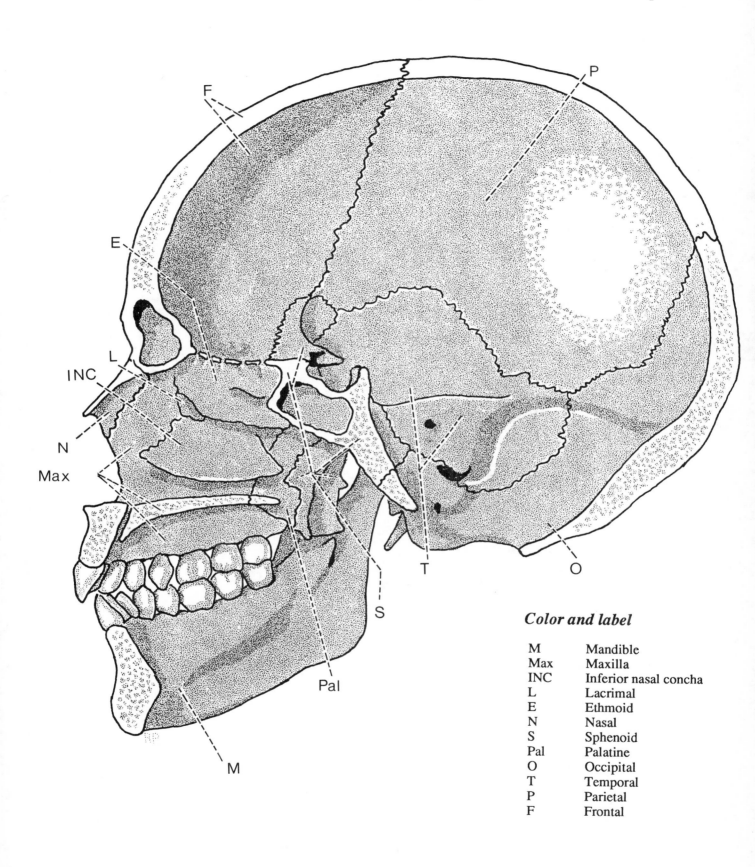

Color and label

M	Mandible
Max	Maxilla
INC	Inferior nasal concha
L	Lacrimal
E	Ethmoid
N	Nasal
S	Sphenoid
Pal	Palatine
O	Occipital
T	Temporal
P	Parietal
F	Frontal

(See opposite page)

Label

1   Cribriform plate *(ethmoid)*
2   Superior nasal concha (or turbinate) *(ethmoid)*
3   Middle nasal concha *(ethmoid)*
4   Inferior nasal concha *(a separate bone)*
5   Medial pterygoid plate *(sphenoid)*
6   Lateral pterygoid plate *(sphenoid)*
7   Hamulus
8   Lingula *(mandible)*
9   Mandibular foramen
10 Mylohyoid line
11 Mental spine (genial tubercle)
12 Palatine process of maxilla
13 Incisive canal
14 Horizontal plate of palatine
15 Lesser wing of sphenoid
16 Optic canal
17 Anterior clinoid process
18 Hypophyseal fossa
19 Greater wing of sphenoid
20 Internal acoustic (auditory) meatus
21 Jugular foramen
22 Hypoglossal canal
23 Groove for transverse sinus
24 Groove for sigmoid sinus
25 Styloid process
26 Occipital condyle
27 Foramen magnum
28 Lambdoid suture
29 Coronal suture
30 Frontal sinus
31 Sphenoid sinus
32 Sphenopalatine foramen
33 Opening of sphenoidal sinus

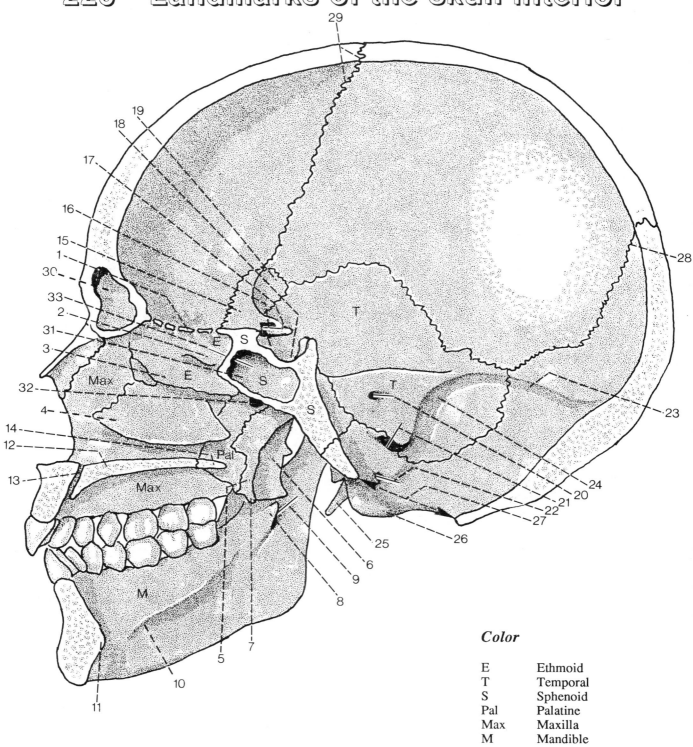

Color

E	Ethmoid
T	Temporal
S	Sphenoid
Pal	Palatine
Max	Maxilla
M	Mandible

221 Medial and lateral pterygoid muscles

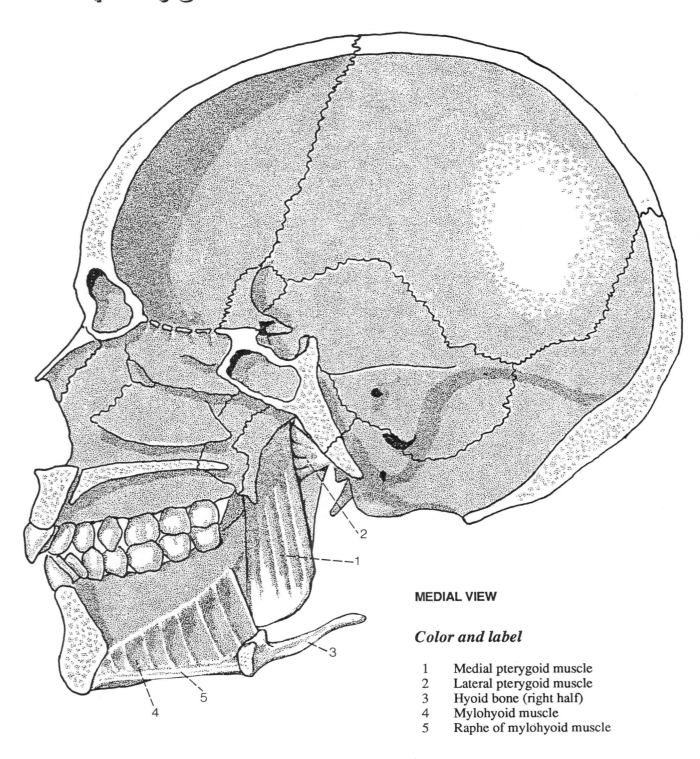

MEDIAL VIEW

Color and label

1 Medial pterygoid muscle
2 Lateral pterygoid muscle
3 Hyoid bone (right half)
4 Mylohyoid muscle
5 Raphe of mylohyoid muscle

Color and label

1 Superior sagittal sinus
2 Lateral venous lacunae
3 Superior cerebral veins
4 Inferior sagittal sinus
5 Straight sinus
6 Great cerebral vein (cut)
7 Transverse sinus
8 Sigmoid sinus
9 Internal jugular vein
10 Confluence of sinuses
11 Occipital sinus
12 Cavernous sinus
13 Superior petrosal sinus
14 Inferior petrosal sinus
15 Emissary veins
16 Superior ophthalmic vein
   (doubled)
17 Inferior ophthalmic vein
18 Supraorbital vein
19 Supratrochlear vein
20 Angular vein
21 External nasal veins
22 Superior labial vein
23 Inferior labial vein
24 Pterygoid plexus
25 Deep facial vein
26 Inferior alveolar vein
27 Maxillary vein
28 Superficial temporal vein
29 Posterior auricular vein
30 Retromandibular vein
31 External jugular vein
32 Occipital vein
33 Posterior external jugular vein
34 Submental vein
35 Lingual vein
36 Superior thyroid vein
37 Anterior jugular vein
38 Middle thyroid vein
39 Inferior thyroid veins
40 Transverse cervical vein
41 Suprascapular vein
42 Right lymphatic (thoracic) duct
43 Falx cerebri
44 Tentorium cerebelli (cut)
45 Evaginations of venous walls by
   underlying arachnoid granulations
46 Subclavian vein
47 Right brachiocephalic vein
48 Left brachiocephalic vein
49 Superior vena cava
50 Facial vein
51 Jugular foramen

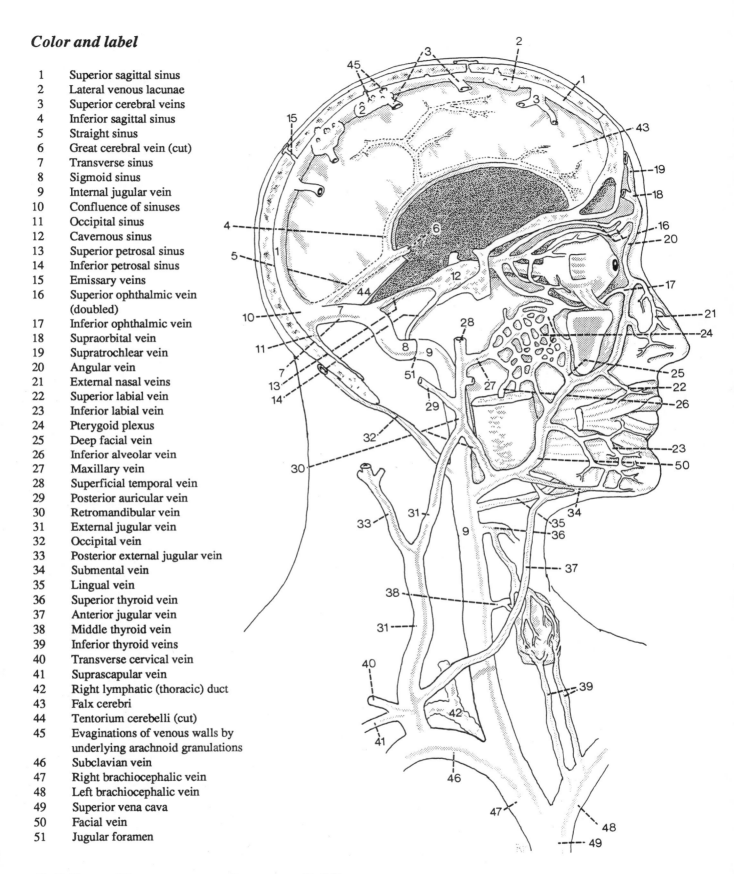

222 Deep veins of the head and neck

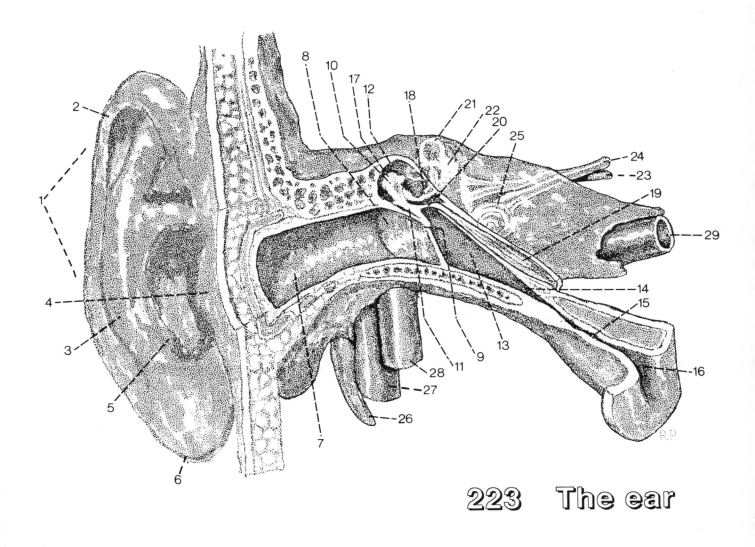

223   The ear

ANTEROLATERAL ASPECT OF RIGHT EAR

Color and label

1	Auricle (pinna)	17	Incus
2	Helix	18	Stapes
3	Antihelix	19	Tensor tympani muscle
4	Tragus	20	Tendon of tensor tympani inserting on malleus
5	Antitragus	21	Superior semicircular canal *(within petrous part of temporal bone)*
6	Lobule of auricle		
7	External auditory meatus	22	Vestibule
8	Tympanic membrane	23	Vestibular nerve (of N VIII)
9	Umbo of tympanic membrane	24	Cochlear nerve (of N VIII)
10	Head of malleus	25	Cochlea
11	Handle of malleus	26	Styloid process
12	Epitympanic recess	27	Internal jugular vein
13	Middle ear (tympanic cavity)	28	Internal carotid artery *(entering carotid canal)*
14	Auditory tube bony part		
15	Auditory tube cartilaginous part	29	Internal carotid artery *(emerging from carotid canal)*
16	Pharyngeal opening of auditory tube in nasal pharynx		

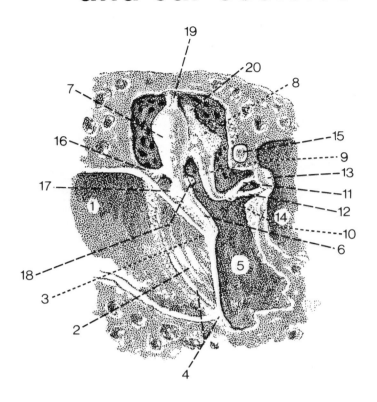

RIGHT EAR, ANTERIOR VIEW

Color and label

1   External auditory meatus
2   Tympanic membrane (eardrum)
3   Umbo *(deepest point of tympanic membrane)*
4   Fibrocartilaginous ring
5   Typanic cavity (middle ear; auris media)
6   Handle of malleus
7   Head of malleus
8   Body of incus
9   Long leg of incus
10 Head of stapes
11 Anterior leg of stapes
12 Posterior leg of stapes
13 Base of stapes covering vestibular window
    (fenestra vestibuli; *formerly oval window)*
14 Perilymph of inner ear
15 Facial nerve in its canal
16 Lateral mallear ligament
17 Lateral mallear process
18 Anterior mallear process *(cut)*
19 Superior mallear ligament
20 Superior incudial ligament

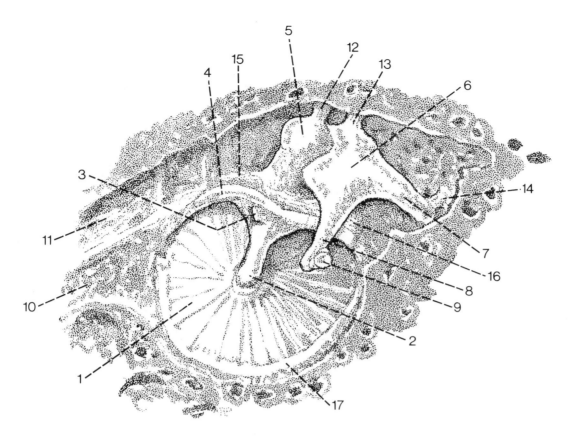

225 Tympanic membrane and ear ossicles

**RIGHT TYMPANIC MEMBRANE
FROM INSIDE MIDDLE EAR**

Color and label

1 Tympanic membrane (eardrum)
2 Handle of malleus
3 Insertion of tensor tympani muscle on malleus
4 Chorda tympani *(a branch of N VII)*
5 Head of malleus
6 Body of incus
7 Short leg of incus
8 Long leg of incus
9 Lenticular process of incus
10 Auditory tube (eustachian tube)
11 Canal for tensor tympani muscle
12 Superior mallear ligament
13 Superior incudial ligament
14 Posterior incudial ligament
15 Anterior mallear fold
16 Posterior mallear fold
17 Fibrocartilaginous ring of tympanic membrane

After Spalteholz and Spanner.

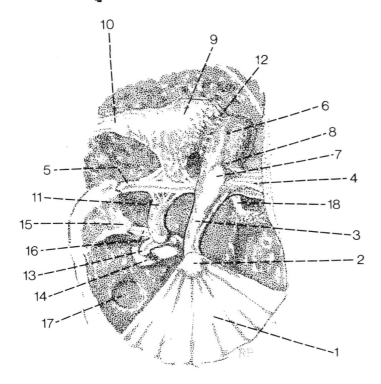

**RIGHT MIDDLE EAR WITH EARDRUM
PARTIALLY REMOVED, LATERAL VIEW**

Color and label

1	Right tympanic membrane (eardrum) *(one quarter intact; three quarters removed)*
2	Umbo *(center attachment to tip of handle of malleus; also deep point of tympanic membrane)*
3	Handle of malleus (manubrium mallei)
4	Anterior mallear process and ligament
5	Chorda tympani nerve *(a branch of nerve VII carrying taste and parasympathetic fibers)*
6	Head of malleus
7	Lateral mallear process
8	Neck of malleus
9	Body of incus
10	Short leg of incus
11	Long leg of incus
12	Incudomallear joint
13	Stapes posterior crus (leg)
14	Base of stapes on fenestra vestibuli
15	Pyramidal eminence containing stapedius muscle
16	Tendon of stapedius muscle
17	Fenestra cochleae
18	Tendon of tensor tympani muscle

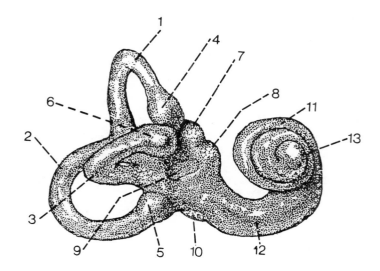

**RIGHT BONY LABYRINTH
(FROM A CAST)**

Color and label

1	Anterior semicircular canal
2	Posterior semicircular canal
3	Lateral semicircular canal
4	Anterior bony ampulla
5	Posterior bony ampulla
6	Lateral bony ampulla
7	Elliptical recess
8	Spherical recess
9	Fenestra vestibuli *(former name: oval window)*
10	Fenestra cochleae *(former name: round window)*
11	Cochlea
12	Base of cochlea
13	Cupula of cochlea

Based on Spalteholz and Spanner.

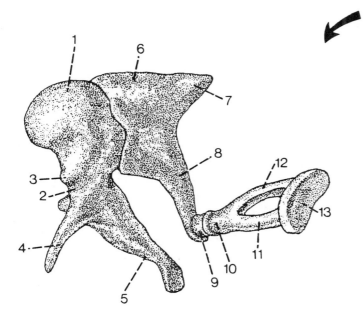

Color and label

1   Head of malleus
2   Neck of malleus
3   Lateral mallear process
4   Anterior mallear process
5   Handle of malleus
6   Body of incus
7   Short process of incus
8   Long process of incus
9   Lenticular process of incus
10   Head of stapes
11   Anterior crus (leg)
12   Posterior crus
13   Base of stapes

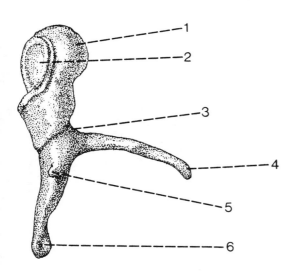

**RIGHT MALLEUS,
LATERAL VIEW**

Color and label

1   Head of malleus
2   Articular surface
3   Neck of malleus
4   Anterior (long) process
      of malleus
5   Lateral process of malleus
6   Handle of malleus

After Wolf-Heidegger.

**RIGHT MALLEUS,
POSTERIOR VIEW**

228   Ear ossicles,
detail, I

229 Ear ossicles, detail, II

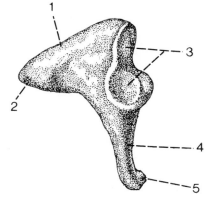

**RIGHT INCUS,
LATERAL VIEW**

Color and label

1 Body of incus
2 Short process
3 Articulating facet
4 Long process
5 Lenticular process

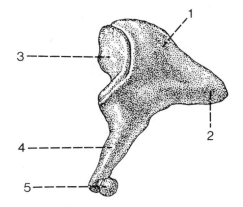

**RIGHT INCUS,
MEDIAL VIEW**

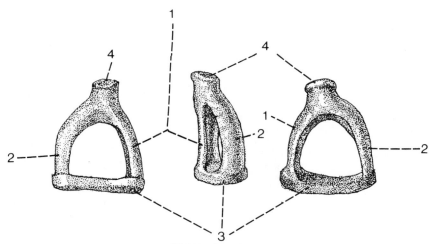

**RIGHT STAPES
INFERIOR, POSTERIOR,
AND SUPERIOR VIEWS**

Color and label

1 Anterior crus (leg)
2 Posterior crus
3 Base of stapes
4 Head of stapes

After Wolf-Heidegger.

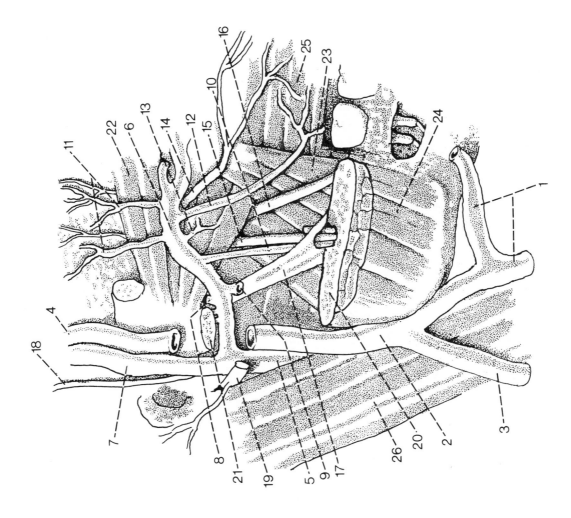

Color and label

1   Facial vein
2   Retromandibular vein
3   External jugular vein
4   Superficial temporal vein
5   External carotid artery
6   Maxillary artery
7   Superficial temporal artery
8   Middle meningeal artery
9   Masseteric artery
10 Inferior alveolar artery
11 Deep temporal arteries
12 Buccal artery
13 Pterygoid branch
14 Buccal nerve
15 Inferior alveolar nerve
16 Lingual nerve
17 Sphenomandibular ligament
18 Auriculotemporal nerve
19 Facial neve
20 Ramus of mandible (cut)
21 Neck of mandible (cut)
22 External pterygoid muscle
23 Medial pterygoid muscle
24 Masseter (cut)
25 Buccinator (partially cut)
26 Sternocleidomastoid muscle

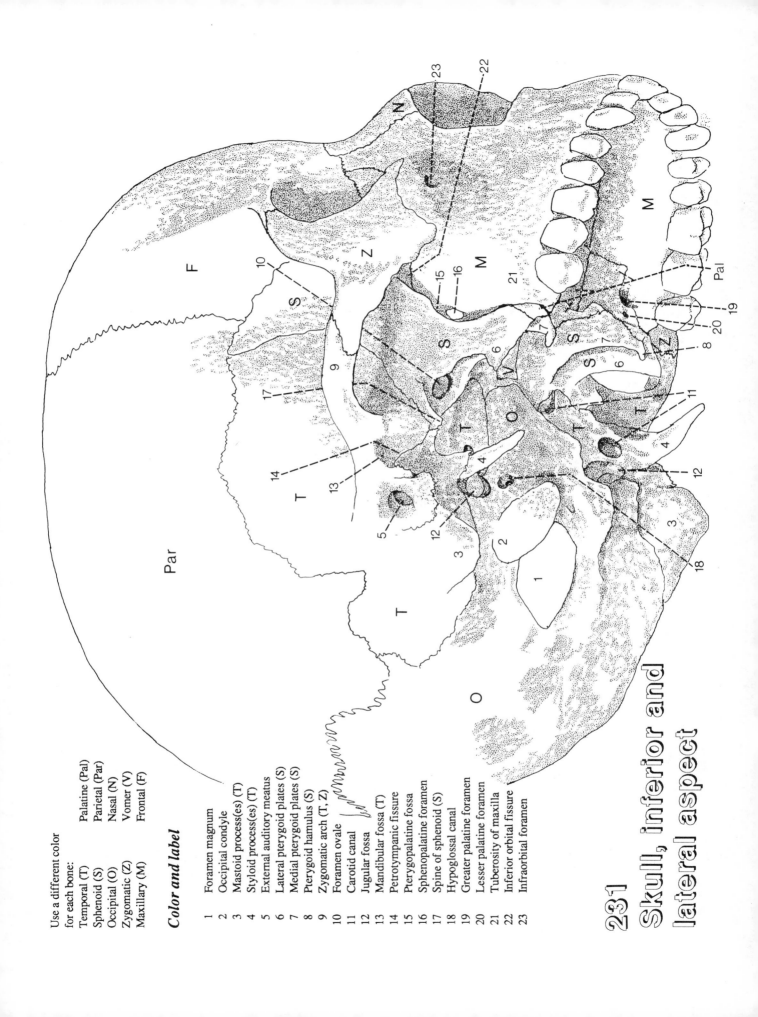

Color and label

1   Foramen magnum
2   Occipital condyle
3   Mastoid process(es) (T)
4   Styloid process(es) (T)
5   External auditory meatus
6   Lateral pterygoid plates (S)
7   Medial pterygoid plates (S)
8   Pterygoid hamulus (S)
9   Zygomatic arch (T, Z)
10 Foramen ovale
11 Carotid canal
12 Jugular fossa
13 Mandibular fossa (T)
14 Petrotympanic fissure
15 Pterygopalatine fossa
16 Sphenopalatine foramen
17 Spine of sphenoid (S)
18 Hypoglossal canal
19 Greater palatine foramen
20 Lesser palatine foramen
21 Tuberosity of maxilla
22 Inferior orbital fissure
23 Infraorbital foramen

231

Skull, inferior and lateral aspect

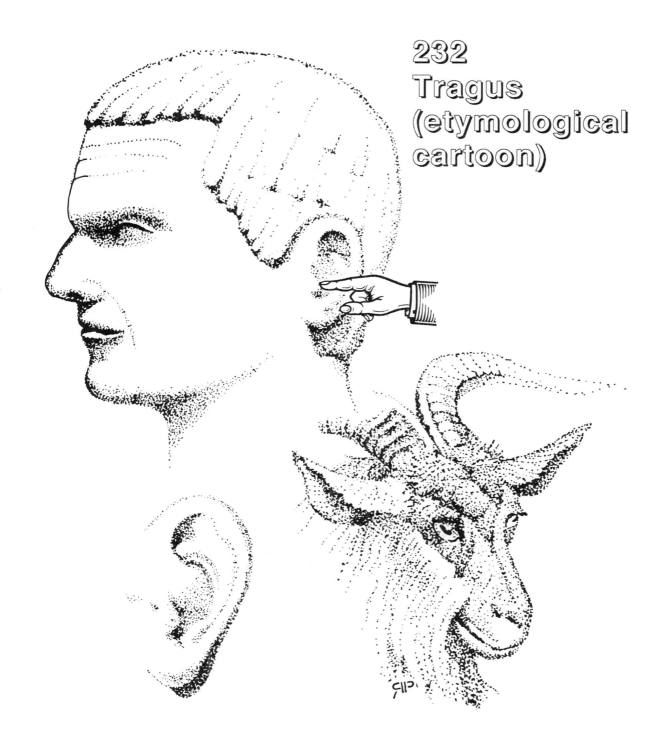

Latin,
billy goat

The tragus of the ear was so named because in some old men it grows a
little tuft of hair that reminded the ancient anatomists of a billy goat's beard.
Tragos is Greek for billy goat and tragus is the Latin. Tragedy originally
meant "goat's song."

233 Mandibular nerve and maxillary artery, I

Color and label

1 Trigeminal ganglion
2 Mandibular nerve
3 Auriculotemporal nerve (notice its two roots surrounding the middle meningeal artery)
4 Middle meningeal artery
5 Buccal nerve (sensory to mucous membrane and skin of cheek)
6 Lingual nerve (supplies general sensation to anterior two-thirds of tongue)
7 Inferior alveolar nerve (cut)
8 Mylohyoid nerve (motor to mylohyoid muscle and anterior belly of digastric muscle)
9 Chorda tympani (branch of facial nerve carrying taste fibers and parasympathetic fibers to lingual nerve; exits skull through petrotympanic fissure)
10 External acoustic meatus nerves
11 Communicating branch with facial nerve
12 Deep temporal nerves (motor to temporalis muscle)
13 Lateral pterygoid nerve
14 Medial pterygoid nerve
15 Masseteric nerve
16 Submandibular ganglion
17 Facial nerve
18 Digastric branch of facial nerve (motor to posterior belly of digastric muscle)
19 Stylohyoid branch of facial nerve
20 Hypoglossal nerve
21 Superior root of ansa cervicalis
22 Internal jugular vein
23 Internal carotid artery
24 External carotid artery
25 Superficial temporal artery
26 Lateral pterygoid muscle (cut)
27 Medial pterygoid muscle (cut)
28 Buccinator muscle (cut and reflected)
29 Anterior belly of digastric muscle
30 Posterior belly of digastric muscle
31 Mylohyoid muscle
32 Submandibular gland (notice its duct crossing the lingual nerve)
33 Sublingual gland
34 Maxillary artery (most of its branches are not shown)
35 Sphenopalatine artery entering nasal cavity through sphenopalatine foramen
36 Infraorbital artery
37 Posterior superior alveolar artery

Mandibular nerve and maxillary artery, II

(See opposite page)

Color and label

1 External carotid artery
2 Maxillary artery
3 Superficial temporal artery
4 Middle meningeal artery
5 Posterior superior alveolar arteries
6 Infraorbital artery
7 Sphenopalatine artery
8 Pterygopalatine fossa
9 Sphenopalatine foramen
10 Mandibular nerve *(exiting foramen ovale)*
11 Deep temporal nerves *(to temporal muscle)*
12 Buccal nerve *(sensory to cheek mucous membrane)*
13 Lingual nerve *(sensory to anterior two-thirds of tongue)*
14 Inferior alveolar nerve *(cut; sensory to teeth in lower jaw)*
15 Mylohyoid nerve *(also to anterior belly of digastric muscle)*
16 Chorda tympani *(nerve; branch of facial nerve carrying taste fibers to tongue and parasympathetic fibers to sublingual and submandibular glands)*
17 Auriculotemporal nerve *(sensory to skin in front of ear and side of head)*
18 Facial nerve
19 Posterior superior alveolar nerve *(from maxillary nerve; sensory to upper posterior teeth)*
20 Carotid canal
21 Jugular foramen
22 Styloid process
23 Occipital condyle
24 Hamulus of medial pterygoid plate
25 Foramen magnum
26 Petrotympanic fissure

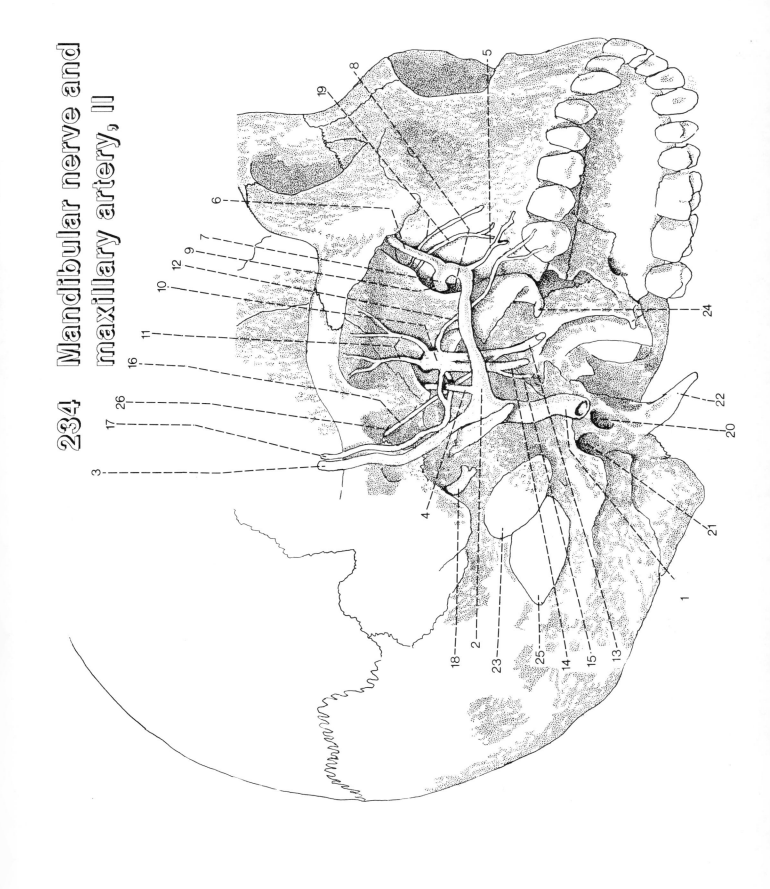

235 Skull, inferior aspect

Color each bone a different color

Temporal (T)   Maxillary (M)
Sphenoid (S)   Palatine (Pal)
Occipital (O)   Vomer (V)
Zygomatic (Z)

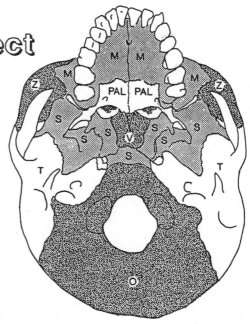

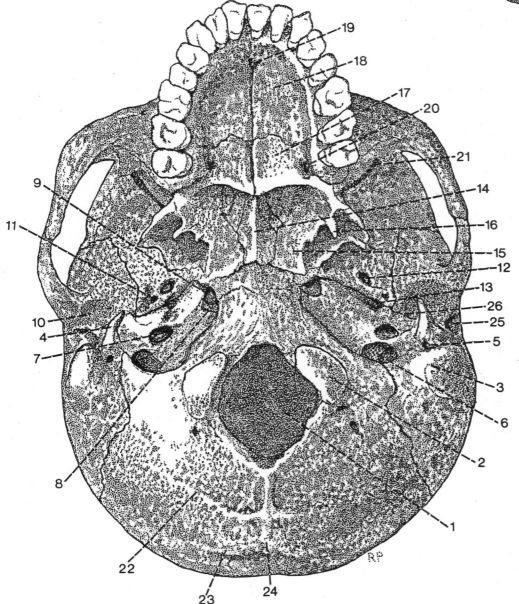

. . . *and label*

1   Foramen magnum
2   Occipital condyle
3   Mastoid process
4   Styloid process
5   Stylomastoid foramen
6   Jugular fossa
7   Carotid canal external aperture
8   Carotid canal internal aperture
9   Foramen lacerum *(plugged up with cartilage in life)*
10 Mandibular fossa
11 Foramen spinosum
12 Foramen ovale
13 Auditory tube sulcus
14 Vomer
15 Medial and lateral pterygoid plates
16 Pterygoid hamulus
17 Horizontal plate of palatine bone
18 Palatine process of maxillary bone
19 Incisive foramen
20 Major palatine foramen
21 Inferior orbital fissure
22 Inferior nuchal line
23 Superior nuchal line
24 External occipital protuberance (inion)
25 External auditory meatus
26 Petrotympanic fissure

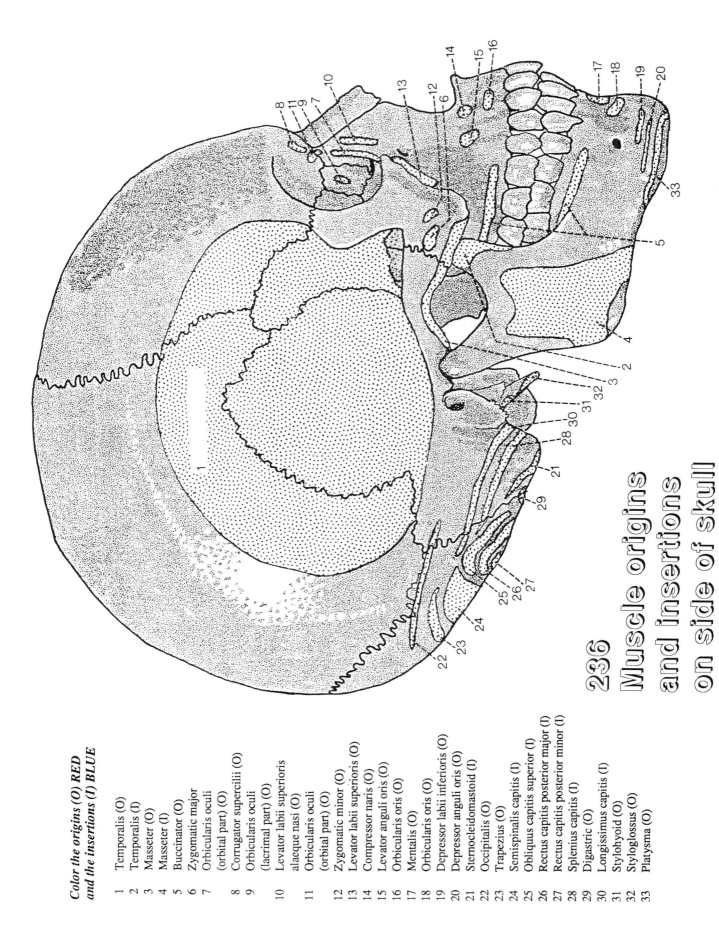

Color the origins (O) RED
and the insertions (I) BLUE

1 Temporalis (O)
2 Temporalis (I)
3 Masseter (O)
4 Masseter (I)
5 Buccinator (O)
6 Zygomatic major
7 Orbicularis oculi
   (orbital part) (O)
8 Corrugator supercilii (O)
9 Orbicularis oculi
   (lacrimal part) (O)
10 Levator labii superioris
   alaeque nasi (O)
11 Orbicularis oculi
   (orbital part) (O)
12 Zygomatic minor (O)
13 Levator labii superioris (O)
14 Compressor naris (O)
15 Levator anguli oris (O)
16 Orbicularis oris (O)
17 Mentalis (O)
18 Orbicularis oris (O)
19 Depressor labii inferioris (O)
20 Depressor anguli oris (O)
21 Sternocleidomastoid (I)
22 Occipitalis (O)
23 Trapezius (O)
24 Semispinalis capitis (I)
25 Obliquus capitis superior (I)
26 Rectus capitis posterior major (I)
27 Rectus capitis posterior minor (I)
28 Splenius capitis (I)
29 Digastric (O)
30 Longissimus capitis (I)
31 Stylohyoid (O)
32 Styloglossus (O)
33 Platysma (O)

236
Muscle origins
and insertions
on side of skull

(See opposite page)

Color and label

1   External carotid artery
2   Maxillary artery
3   Superficial temporal artery
4   Masseteric artery *(to masseter muscle)*
5   Inferior alveolar artery *(with inferior alveolar vein and nerve, supplies teeth in lower jaw)*
6   Pterygoid branches *(supply pterygoid muscles)*
7   Buccal artery *(supplies buccinator and cheek)*
8   Anterior deep temporal artery *(supplies temporalis muscle)*
9   Posterior deep temporal artery *(supplies temporalis muscle)*
10 Posterior superior alveolar artery *(supplies upper back teeth)*
11 Infraorbital artery *(entering orbit)*
12 Sphenopalatine artery *(entering nose through sphenopalatine foramen)*
13 Descending palatine artery
14 Deep auricular artery
15 Anterior tympanic artery
16 Mental artery
17 Lateral pterygoid muscle (superior superficial head)
18 Lateral pterygoid muscle (inferior deep head)
19 Medial pterygoid muscle (superficial head)
20 Medial pterygoid muscle (deep head)
21 Buccinator muscle
22 Masseter muscle *(cut)*
23 Zygomatic arch *(cut)*
24 External auditory meatus
25 Temporomandibular joint capsule
26 Ramus of mandible *(cut, with coronoid process removed)*
27 Middle meningeal artery
28 Sternocleidomastoid muscle

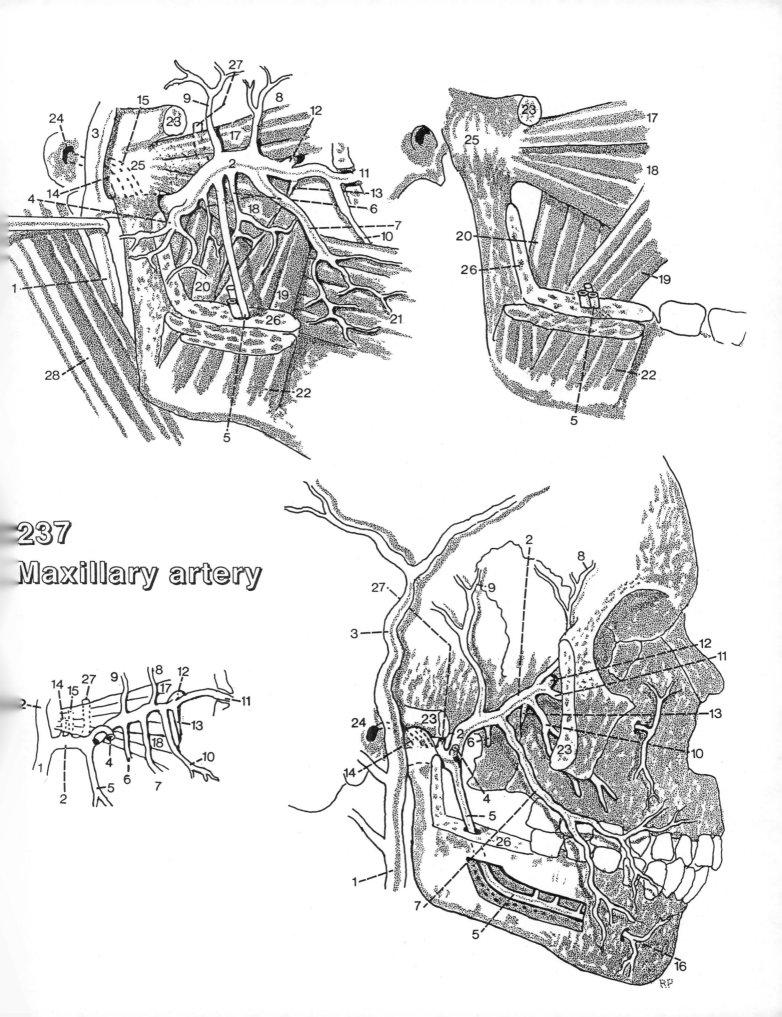

237

Maxillary artery

Head and neck, midsagittal aspect *(See opposite page)*

Color and label

1 Scalp
2 Calvaria of skull
3 Diploë *(spongy marrow of cranial bones)*
4 Superior sagittal sinus *(cut open to show opening of superior cerebral vein)*
5 Falx cerebri
6 Inferior sagittal sinus
7 Crista galli
8 Straight sinus
9 Great cerebral vein
10 Confluence of sinuses
11 Aperture of right transverse sinus
12 Occipital sinus
13 Falx cerebelli
14 Frontal sinus
15 Corpus callosum
16 Anterior cerebral artery
17 Septum pellucidum
18 Fornix
19 Thalamus and interthalamic adhesion
20 Optic chiasm
21 Pituitary gland (hypophysis)
22 Sphenoidal sinus
23 Mamillary body
24 Midbrain (mesencephalon)
25 Mesencephalic tectum
26 Pineal gland
27 Cerebral aqueduct

28 Cerebellum
29 Fourth ventricle
30 Cisterna magna (cerebellomedullary cistern)
31 Basilar artery
32 Left vertebral artery
33 Pons
34 Medulla oblongata
35 Spinal cord
36 Anterior arch of atlas
37 Body and dens of atlas
38 Pharyngeal tonsil
39 Ostium of auditory tube (eustachian tube)
40 Nasal pharynx
41 Middle nasal concha
42 Inferior nasal concha
43 Hard palate
44 Soft palate and uvula
45 Mandible
46 Hyoid bone
47 Genioglossus muscle
48 Geniohyoid muscle
49 Mylohyoid muscle
50 Epiglottis
51 Thyroid cartilage
52 Cricoid cartilage (arch and lamina)
53 Trachea
54 Oral pharynx
55 Laryngeal pharynx
56 Esophagus

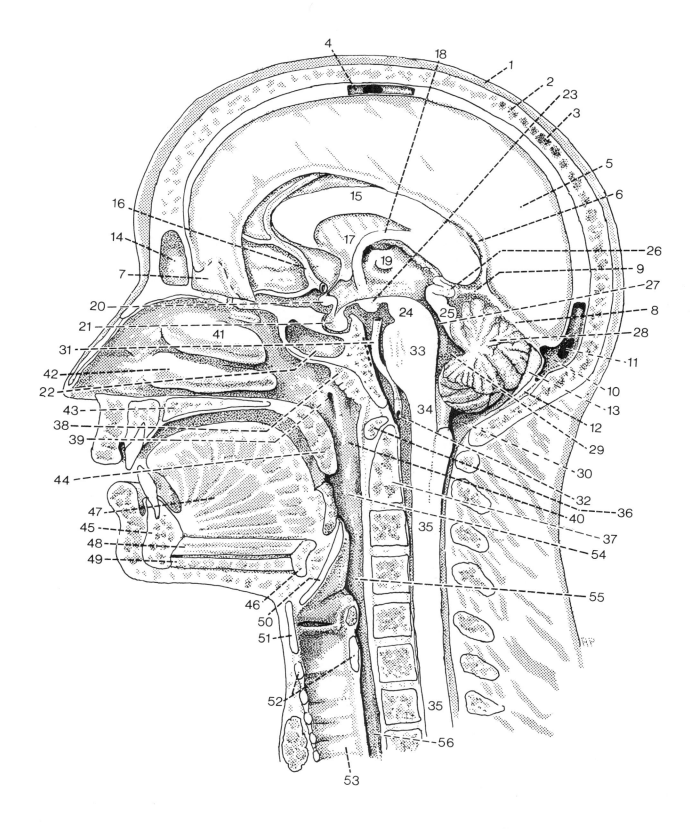

238 Head and neck, midsagittal aspect

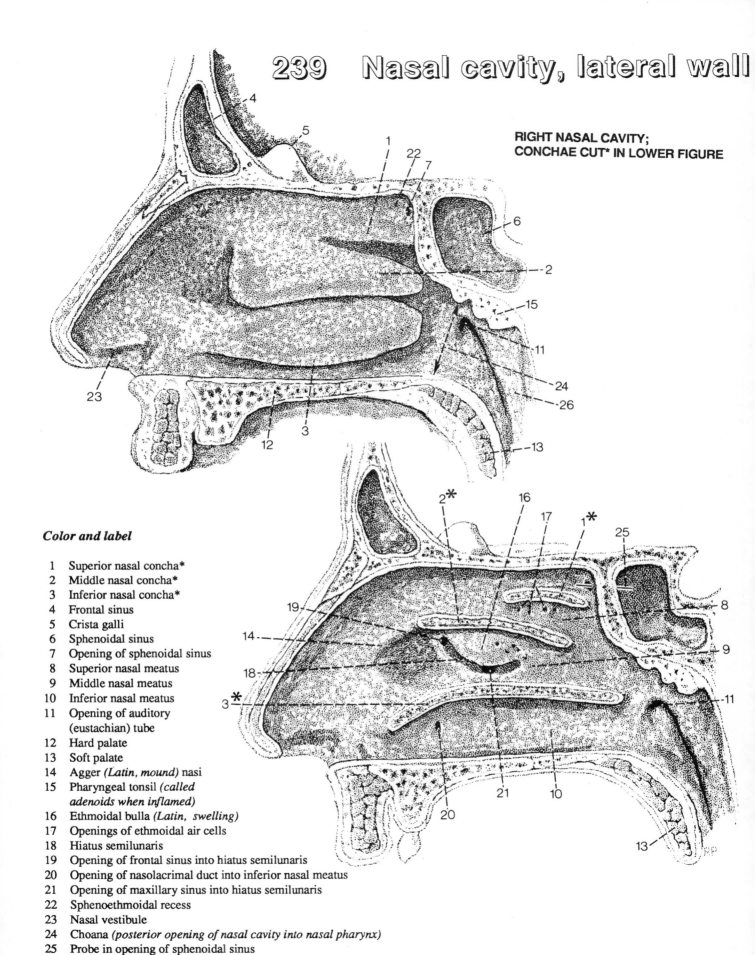

**RIGHT NASAL CAVITY;
CONCHAE CUT* IN LOWER FIGURE**

Color and label

1   Superior nasal concha*
2   Middle nasal concha*
3   Inferior nasal concha*
4   Frontal sinus
5   Crista galli
6   Sphenoidal sinus
7   Opening of sphenoidal sinus
8   Superior nasal meatus
9   Middle nasal meatus
10 Inferior nasal meatus
11 Opening of auditory
    (eustachian) tube
12 Hard palate
13 Soft palate
14 Agger *(Latin, mound)* nasi
15 Pharyngeal tonsil *(called
    adenoids when inflamed)*
16 Ethmoidal bulla *(Latin, swelling)*
17 Openings of ethmoidal air cells
18 Hiatus semilunaris
19 Opening of frontal sinus into hiatus semilunaris
20 Opening of nasolacrimal duct into inferior nasal meatus
21 Opening of maxillary sinus into hiatus semilunaris
22 Sphenoethmoidal recess
23 Nasal vestibule
24 Choana *(posterior opening of nasal cavity into nasal pharynx)*
25 Probe in opening of sphenoidal sinus
26 Nasal pharynx (nasopharynx)

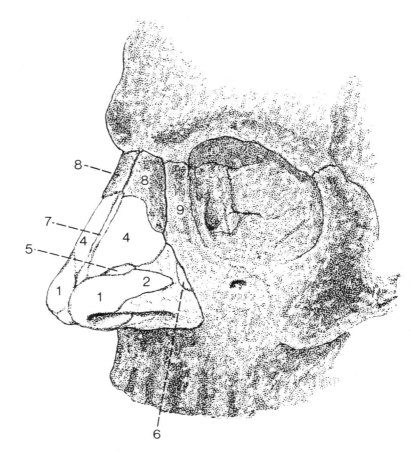

240   Cartilages of the nose

Color and label

1   Greater alar cartilage
    (transparent in lower figure)
2   Lateral crus of greater alar
    cartilage
3   Medial crus of greater alar
    cartilage
4   Lateral nasal cartilage
5   Accessory nasal cartilage
6   Minor alar cartilage
7   Nasal septal cartilage
8   Nasal bone
9   Maxillary bone

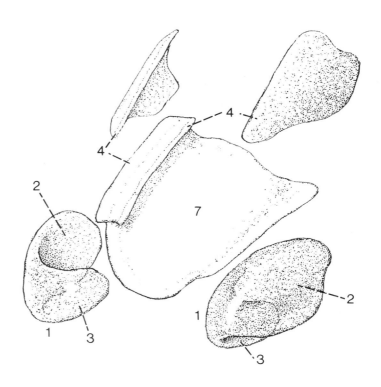

After Spalteholz and Spanner.

Based on and modified from a Somso model.

Color and label

1 Perpendicular plate of ethmoid bone
2 Vomer *(Latin, plowshare)*
3 Nasal spine (of maxilla)
4 Nasal spine (of palatine bone)
5 Palatine process of maxilla
6 Horizontal plate of palatine bone
7 Nasal septal cartilage
8 Greater alar cartilage medial crus *(cut with left lateral crus removed)*
9 Sphenoidal sinus and opening
10 Frontal sinus
11 Soft palate
12 Upper lip
13 Vomeronasal cartilage

RIGHT SIDE OF NASAL CAVITY

Color and label

1 Frontal sinus
2 Frontal bone
3 Nasal bone
4 Lateral nasal cartilage
5 Greater alar cartilage (medial crus)
6 Greater alar cartilage (lateral crus)
7 Maxillary bone
8 Inferior nasal concha *(a separate bone)*
9 Middle nasal concha *(ethmoid)*
10 Superior nasal concha *(ethmoid)*
11 Palatine bone (vertical part)
12 Crista galli *(ethmoid)*
13 Palatine bone (horizontal part)
14 Sphenopalatine foramen
15 Uncinate process *(ethmoid)*
16 Sphenoidal sinus
17 Hypophyseal fossa
18 Medial pterygoid plate and hamulus *(Latin, little hook)*
19 Lateral pterygoid plate
20 Optic nerve and ophthalmic artery
21 Alveolar process of maxillary bone

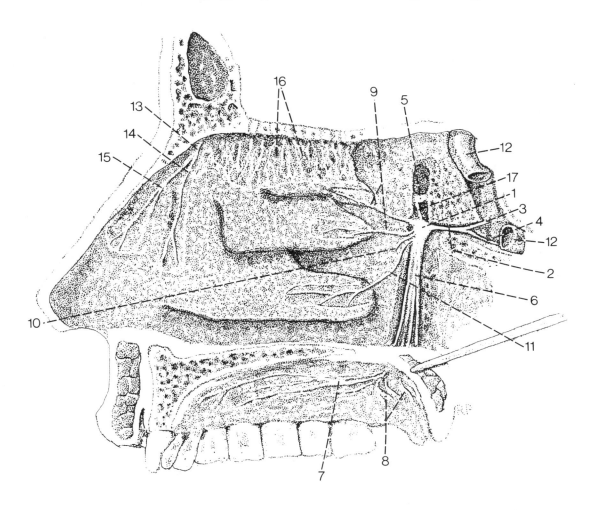

**AND RELATED STRUCTURES VIEWED
FROM INSIDE THE NASAL CAVITY**

Color and label

1 Pterygopalatine ganglion*
2 Nerve of the pterygoid canal
3 Greater petrosal nerve *(para-sympathetic and taste fibers)*
4 Deep petrosal nerve (sympathetic fibers)
5 Maxillary nerve (V_2) in pterygo-palatine fossa*
6 Palatine nerves*
7 Greater palatine nerves
8 Lesser palatine nerves
9 Lateral superior posterior nasal branches of V_2 and pterygo-palatine ganglion

10 Medial superior posterior nasal branches to nasal septum from V_2 and pterygopalatine ganglion
11 Lateral inferior posterior nasal branches of V_2 and pterygo-palatine ganglion
12 Internal carotid artery *(cut)*
13 Internal nasal branches of anterior ethmoidal nerve (V_1)
14 Lateral nasal branches
15 External nasal branches
16 Olfactory nerves
17 Pterygopalatine nerves

*Palatine canal and pterygopalatine
fossa opened from medial aspect.*

After Spalteholz and Spanner.

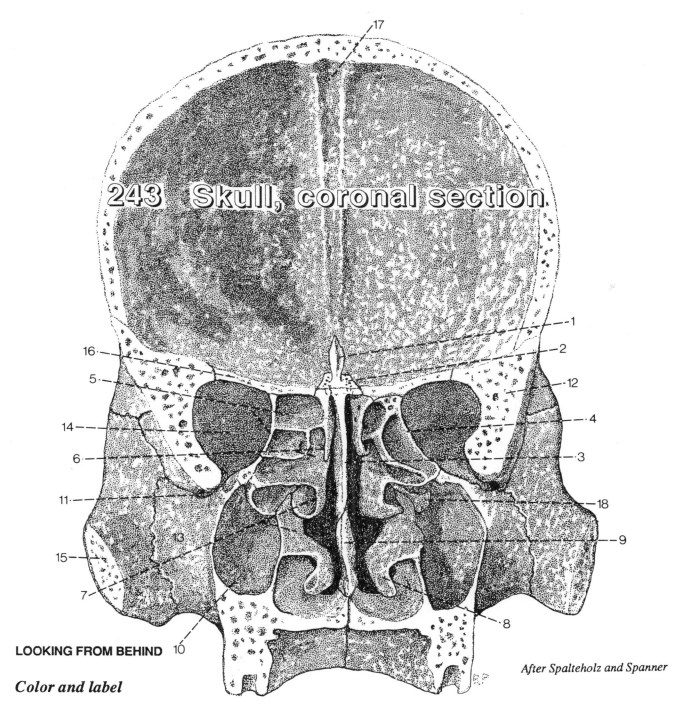

243   Skull, coronal section.

16
5
14
6
11
13
15
7

17

1
2
12
4
3
18
9
8

LOOKING FROM BEHIND   10

After Spalteholz and Spanner

Color and label

1   Crista galli (*Latin, chicken's crest; part of ethmoid*)
2   Cribriform (*Latin, sieve-like*) plate of ethmoid (*contains foramina for olfactory nerves*)
3   Perpendicular plate of ethmoid
4   Orbital plate of ethmoid (*formerly called lamina papyraceus because it was as thin as papyrus*)
5   Ethmoidal air cells (*these number 3–18 on each side*)
6   Superior nasal concha (*Latin, seashell; part of ethmoid*) and superior nasal meatus

7   Middle nasal concha (*part of ethmoid*) and middle nasal meatus
8   Inferior nasal concha (*a separate bone*) and inferior nasal meatus
9   Vomer (*Latin, plowshare*)
10   Maxillary sinus
11   Inferior orbital fissure
12   Greater wing of sphenoid bone
13   Maxillary bone (maxilla)
14   Orbit
15   Zygomatic bone (*zygomatic arch cut*)
16   Orbital part of frontal bone
17   Groove for superior sagittal sinus
18   Uncinate process of ethmoid

**CHEEKS HAVE BEEN CUT
AT CORNERS OF MOUTH**

Color and label

1 Uvula *(Latin, little grape)*
2 Palatine tonsil
3 Palatoglossal arch*
4 Palatopharyngeal arch*
5 Gingiva *(Latin, gum)*
6 Buccinator muscle *(cut)*
7 Frenulum *(Latin, bridle)* of upper lip
8 Frenulum of lower lip
9 Labium superius (upper lip)
10 Labium inferius (lower lip)
11 Dorsum of tongue (dorsum linguae)
12 Hard palate
13 Soft palate
14 Bucca (Latin, cheek) (cut)
15 Isthmus faucius (faucial isthmus)
   *(the posterior opening of the mouth
   into the pharynx)*

*Pillars of the fauces (Latin, throat).

THE PALATE AND RELATED STRUCTURES

Color and label

1 Hard palate (maxilla and palatine bone)
2 Soft palate
3 Hamulus of medial pterygoid plate
4 Palatoglossal muscle (innervated by
   pharyngeal plexus: nerves X, IX)
5 Palatopharyngeus muscle (innervated
   by pharyngeal plexus)
6 Musculus uvulae
7 Palatine tonsil
8 Pterygomandibular raphe
9 Buccinator *(Latin, trumpeter)* muscle
10 Superior pharyngeal constrictor muscle
11 Dorsum of tongue
12 Palatine glands
13 Greater palatine vessels and nerve
14 Lesser palatine vessels and nerve

After Spalteholtz and Spanner.

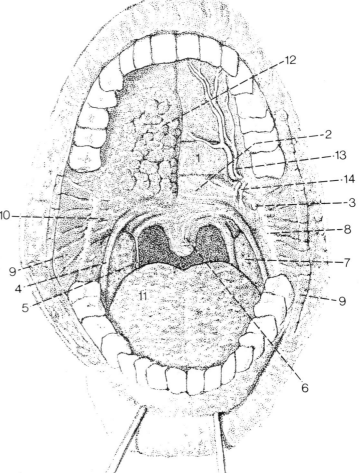

245 Tongue

INFERIOR SURFACE OF THE TONGUE AND RELATED STRUCTURES

Color and label

1 Frenulum of tongue
2 Plica fimbriata
3 Sublingual fold (plica sublingualis)
(contains the openings of the sublingual gland ducts)
4 Sublingual caruncle *(opening of the submandibular duct and main sublingual duct)*

After Spalteholz and Spanner.

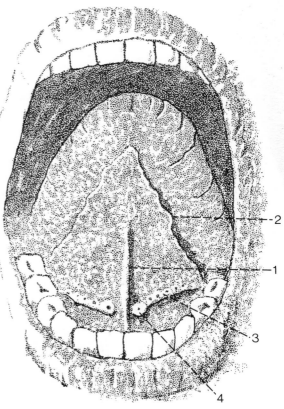

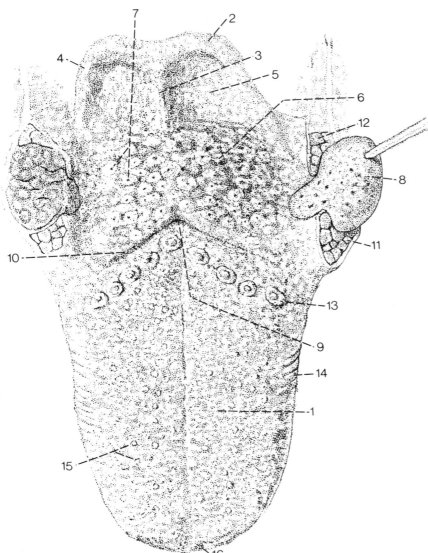

SUPERIOR ASPECT OF THE TONGUE AND RELATED STRUCTURES

Color and label

1 Dorsum of tongue
2 Epiglottis
3 Median glossoepiglottic fold
4 Lateral glossoepiglottic fold
5 Vallecula *(Latin, little valley)* epiglottica
6 Lingual tonsil *(lymph nodules)*
7 Openings of tonsillar crypts
8 Palatine tonsil *(the "tonsils" of childhood)*
9 Foramen cecum *(Latin, blind hole)* linguae
10 Sulcus terminalis
11 Palatoglossal arch and muscle *(cut)*
12 Palatopharyngeal arch and muscle (cut)
13 Vallate papilla *(formerly circumvallate)*
14 Foliate papilla *(Latin, folium, leaf)*
15 Fungiform papilla *(Latin, fungus, mushroom)*
16 Apex of tongue

UPPER FIGURE

Color and label

1 Body of mandible
2 Ramus of mandible
3 Angle of mandible
4 Coronoid process
5 Mandibular notch
6 Condylar process
7 Neck of mandible
8 Pterygoid fovea
9 Head of mandible

10 Mental protuberance
11 Mental tubercle
12 Mental foramen
13 Oblique line
14 Mandibular foramen
15 Lingula of mandible
16 Mylohyoid groove
17 Mylohyoid line

LOWER FIGURE: MANDIBULAR NERVE AND RELATED STRUCTURES

Color and label

1 Mandibular nerve *(V₃ : third branch of trigeminal nerve, nerve V)*
2 Buccal nerve *(sensory to inside of cheek)*
3 Lingual nerve *(pain, touch, temperature to anterior two-thirds of tongue)*
4 Chorda tympani nerve *(cut; taste and preganglionic parasympathetic fibers from nerve VII to lingual nerve)*
5 Submandibular ganglion *(supplies postganglionic parasympathetic fibers to submandibular gland and sublingual gland)*
6 Inferior alveolar nerve *(sensory to teeth and gingiva)*
7 Mylohyoid nerve *(motor to mylohyoid and anterior belly of digastric muscle)*
8 Auriculotemporal nerve *(notice its origin by two roots from the mandibular nerve)*
9 Otic ganglion *(supplies postganglionic parasympathetic fibers to parotid gland)*
10 Origin of genioglossus muscle
11 Geniohyoid muscle *(Greek, genion, chin)*
12 Mylohyoid muscle
13 Hyoid bone *(Greek, yoeides, U-shaped)*
14 Submandibular gland
15 Submandibular duct *(notice its crossing over the lingual nerve)*
16 Sublingual gland *(notice its several ducts, which open at the sublingual fold)*
17 Digastric muscle posterior belly *(cut)* and sling

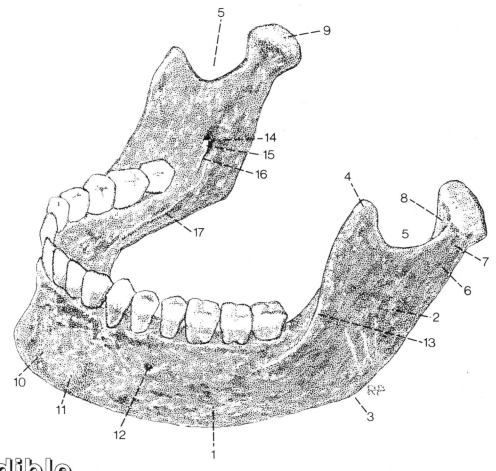

246 Mandible

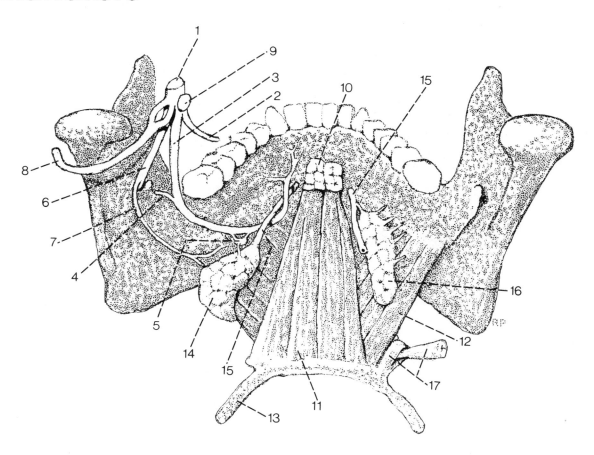

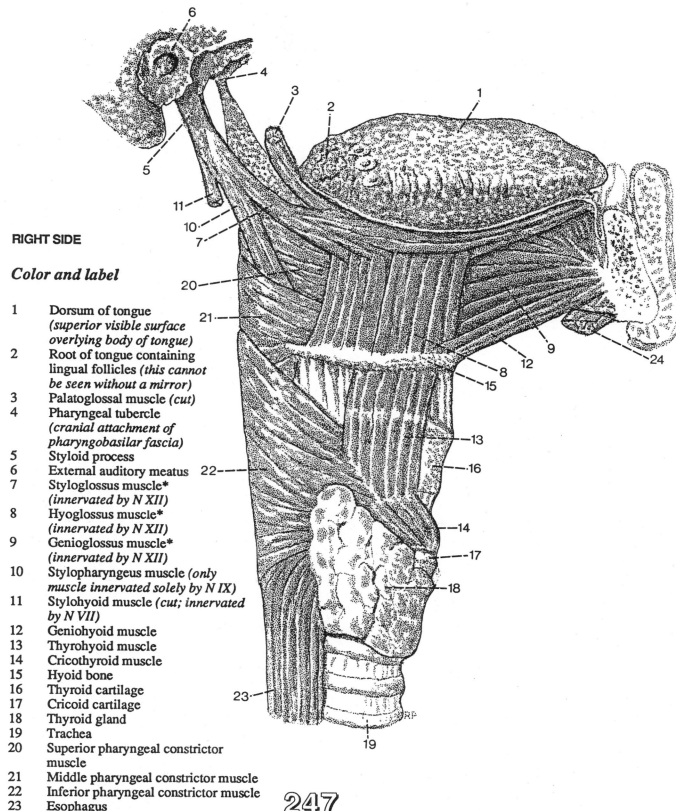

RIGHT SIDE

Color and label

1   Dorsum of tongue
     (*superior visible surface
     overlying body of tongue*)
2   Root of tongue containing
     lingual follicles (*this cannot
     be seen without a mirror*)
3   Palatoglossal muscle (*cut*)
4   Pharyngeal tubercle
     (*cranial attachment of
     pharyngobasilar fascia*)
5   Styloid process
6   External auditory meatus
7   Styloglossus muscle*
     (*innervated by N XII*)
8   Hyoglossus muscle*
     (*innervated by N XII*)
9   Genioglossus muscle*
     (*innervated by N XII*)
10   Stylopharyngeus muscle (*only
     muscle innervated solely by N IX*)
11   Stylohyoid muscle (*cut; innervated
     by N VII*)
12   Geniohyoid muscle
13   Thyrohyoid muscle
14   Cricothyroid muscle
15   Hyoid bone
16   Thyroid cartilage
17   Cricoid cartilage
18   Thyroid gland
19   Trachea
20   Superior pharyngeal constrictor
     muscle
21   Middle pharyngeal constrictor muscle
22   Inferior pharyngeal constrictor muscle
23   Esophagus
24   Anterior belly of digastric muscle (*cut*)

*Extrinsic tongue muscles.

After Wolf-Heidegger.

247
Muscles of the tongue, pharynx and larynx

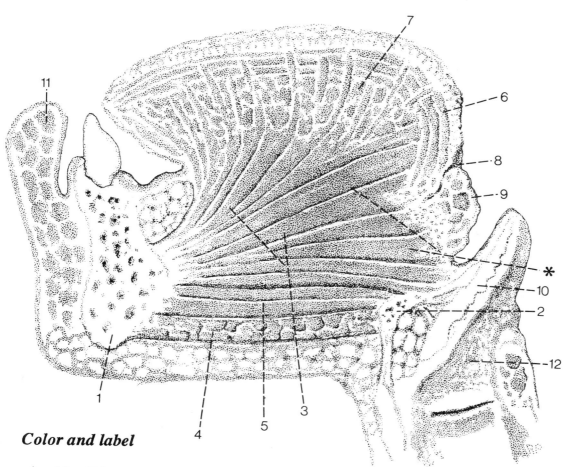

Color and label

1   Mandible
2   Hyoid bone
3   Genioglossus muscle* *(these fibers protrude the tongue)*
4   Mylohyoid muscle *(innervated by N V)*
5   Geniohyoid muscle
6   Superior longitudinal muscle**
7   Transverse lingual muscle**
8   Lingual foramen cecum
9   Lingual tonsil *(follicles)*
10   Epiglottis
11   Lower lip
12   Vestibule of larynx

Extrinsic tongue muscles.
**Intrinsic tongue muscles.*

Color and label

1. Superior longitudinal muscle*
2. Transverse lingual muscle*
3. Vertical lingual muscle*
4. Inferior longitudinal muscle*`
5. Lingual septum
6. Genioglossus muscle**
7. Hyoglossus muscle**
8. Styloglossus muscle**
9. Geniohyoid muscle
10. Mylohyoid *(Greek, myle, mill millstone)* muscle
11. Digastric *(two-bellied)* muscle, anterior belly
12. Platysma muscle
13. Mandible
14. Inferior alveolar nerve, artery, artery, and vein in mandibular canal

15. Buccinator muscle and buccal mucosa
16. Sublingual gland and duct opening at sublingual fold
17. Submandibular gland *(notice that it lies both above and below the myohyoid muscle)*
18. Facial artery
19. Submandibular duct (above) and lingual nerve (below)
20. Hypoglossal nerve and vein
21. Mylohyoid nerve, artery, and vein
22. Deep lingual artery and veins

Intrinsic tongue muscles; arise within tongue and end within tongue.
**Extrinsic tongue muscles; arise outside tongue and end within tongue*

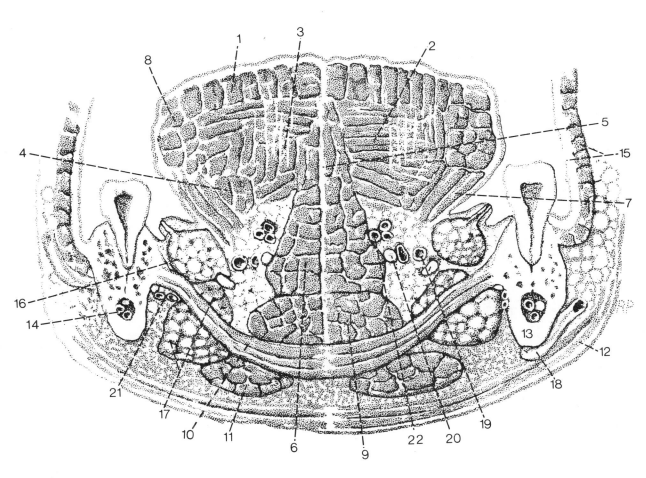

All tongue muscles are innervated by the homolateral (same-side) hypoglossal nerve (N XII)

249   Tongue and related structures, coronal section

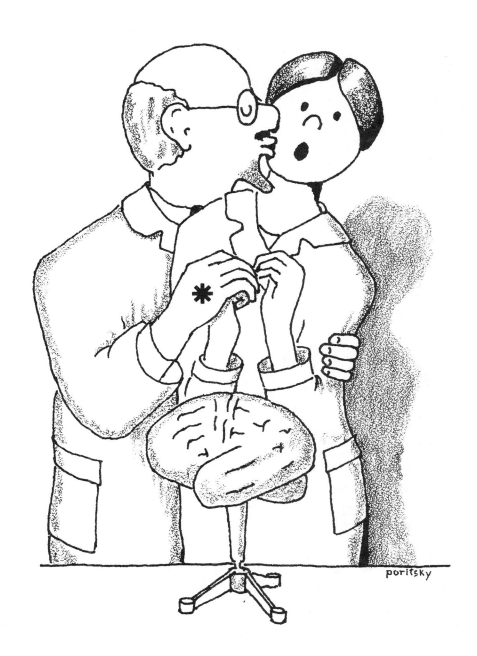

Greek, a joining together

Synapse, the functional connection between nerve cells, was coined by
Sir Charles Sherrington from the Greek synapto, "I join together."

*Brachia conjunctiva, Latin, the arms that come together

251 Oral cavity from inside

**TONGUE AND PHARYNGEAL
MUCOSA AND WALL REMOVED**

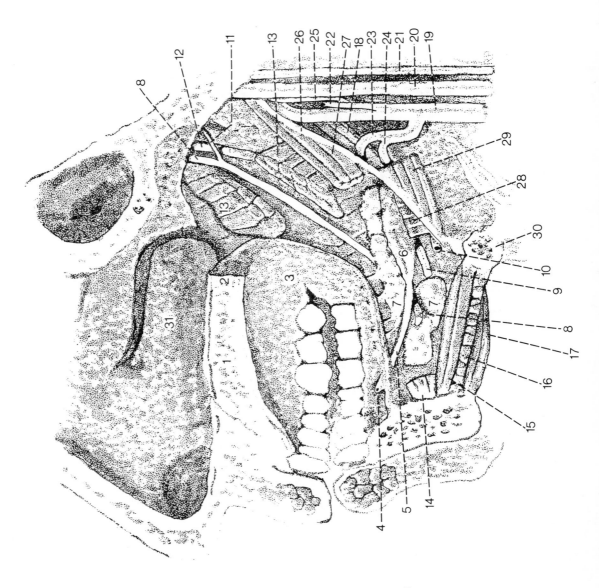

Adapted and modified from Rohan and Yokochi.

Color and label

1. Hard palate
2. Soft palate (*cut and removed*)
3. Oral mucosa
4. Sublingual papilla
5. Submandibular duct
6. Submandibular gland
7. Sublingual gland and ducts
8. Lingual nerve
9. Hypoglossal nerve (*cut*)
10. Deep lingual artery (*cut*)
11. Chorda tympani nerve
12. Inferior alveolar nerve
13. Medial pterygoid muscle (*cut*)
14. Genioglossus muscle origin on mandible
15. Geniohyoid muscle
16. Mylohyoid muscle
17. Anterior belly of digastric muscle
18. Posterior belly of digastric muscle
19. External carotid artery
20. Internal carotid artery
21. Vagus nerve
22. Ascending pharyngeal artery
23. Facial artery
24. Lingual artery
25. Glossopharyngeal nerve (N IX)
26. Stylohyoid ligament
27. Styloglossus muscle (*cut*)
28. Hyoglossus muscle (*cut*)
29. Middle pharyngeal constrictor muscle (*cut*)
30. Hyoid bone
31. Inferior nasal concha

Color and label

1   Levator veli palatini muscle
2   Vagus nerve (N X)
3   Lesion in right vagus nerve
4   Palatoglossal arch
5   Palatopharyngeal arch

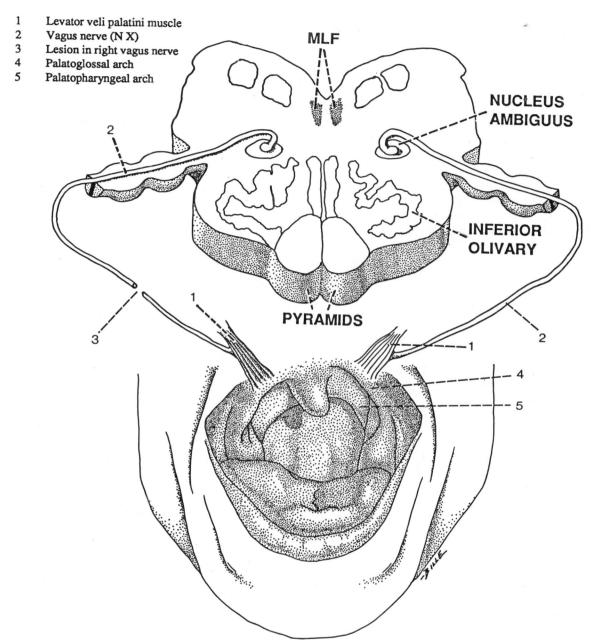

MLF

NUCLEUS
AMBIGUUS

INFERIOR
OLIVARY

PYRAMIDS

252   Levator palatini muscle and soft palate

"Open your mouth and say Ah"

The soft palate is pulled up and back by the levator veli palatini muscle. This happens in speech and in swallowing. The nerve fibers to the levator veli palatini originate from cell bodies in the rostral part of the nucleus ambiguus, which lies in the medulla oblongata. Normally the two levator muscles pull equally on the soft palate, the uvula remains vertical, and the palatoglossal and palatopharyngeal arches on the two sides are symmetrical. If one vagus nerve is damaged, the normal levator veli palatini muscle will pull its half and arches higher than the paralyzed side and the uvula will point to the normal side.

(See opposite page)

Color and label

1   Nasal septum
2   Nasal concha
3   Pharyngeal tonsil
4   Pharyngeal wall *(cut open along posterior raphe)*
5   Nasal pharynx (nasopharynx)
6   Oral pharynx (oropharynx)
7   Laryngeal pharynx (laryngopharynx)
8   Soft palate and uvula
9   Dorsum sellae and clivus *(Latin, slope)* of occipital bone
10   Petrous portion of temporal bone
11   Stylomastoid foramen
12   Styloid process
13   Mastoid process and mastoid air cells
14   Opening of auditory tube
15   Torus tubularis *(Latin, mound of the tube)*
16   Torus of levator veli palatini muscle
17   Pharyngeal recess
18   Palatopharyngeal fold
19   Palatine tonsil
20   Root of tongue (posterior third) with lingual follicles *(tonsil)*
21   Epiglottis
22   Piriform recess
23   Superior laryngeal nerve and vessel under mucous membrane
24   Hyoid bone *(greater horn)*
25   Thyroid cartilage *(superior horn)*
26   Interarytenoid notch
27   Corniculate tubercle *(cartilage)*
28   Cuneiform tubercle *(cartilage)*
29   Aryepiglottic fold
30   Esophagus
31   Thyroid gland and vessels
32   Parathyroid glands
33   Mucous membrane overlying posterior cricoarytenoid muscle and lamina of cricoid cartilage
34   Aditus *(Latin, entrance)* to larynx
35   Vallate papillae
36   Posterior belly of digastric muscle
37   Parotid gland
38   Submandibular gland

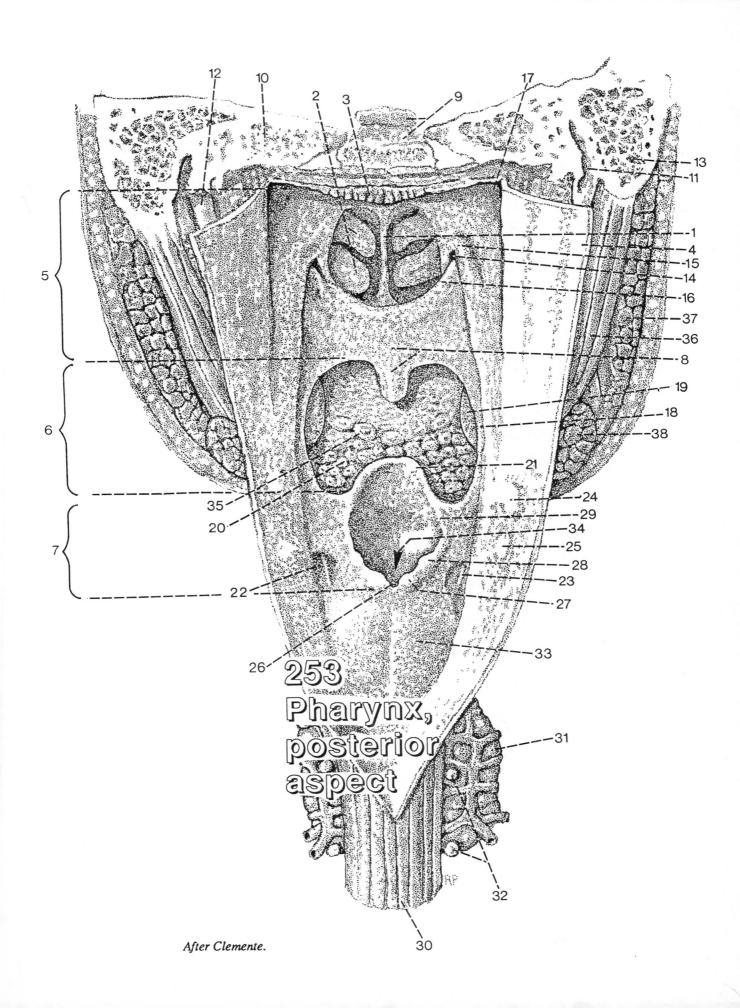

253
Pharynx,
posterior
aspect

After Clemente.

Muscles of the pharynx
(See opposite page)

Color and label

1 Auditory tube *(cartilaginous part)*
2 Tensor veli palatini muscle
3 Levator veli palatini muscle
4 Tendon of tensor veli palatini and palatine aponeurosis
5 Hamulus of medial pterygoid plate
6 Pterygomandibular raphe
7 Buccinator muscle
8 Superior pharyngeal constrictor muscle
9 Palatopharyngeus muscle
10 Salpingopharyngeus muscle
11 Glossopharyngeus *(part of superior constrictor)*
12 Middle pharyngeal constrictor muscle
13 Styloglossus muscle
14 Hyoglossus muscle
15 Stylohyoid ligament
16 Inferior constrictor
17 Mylohyoid muscle
18 Geniohyoid muscle
19 Thyrohyoid membrane
20 Stylopharyngeus muscle
21 Fibers to pharyngoepiglottic fold
22 Longitudinal muscle of pharynx
23 Internal branch of superior laryngeal nerve
24 Thyroid cartilage
25 Cricoid cartilage
26 Trachea
27 Arytenoid cartilage
28 Corniculate cartilage
29 Pharyngeal aponeurosis
30 Cricopharyngeus muscle *(part of inferior constrictor)*
31 Esophageal circular muscle
32 Esophageal longitudinal muscle
33 Pharyngobasilar fascia
34 Hyoid bone

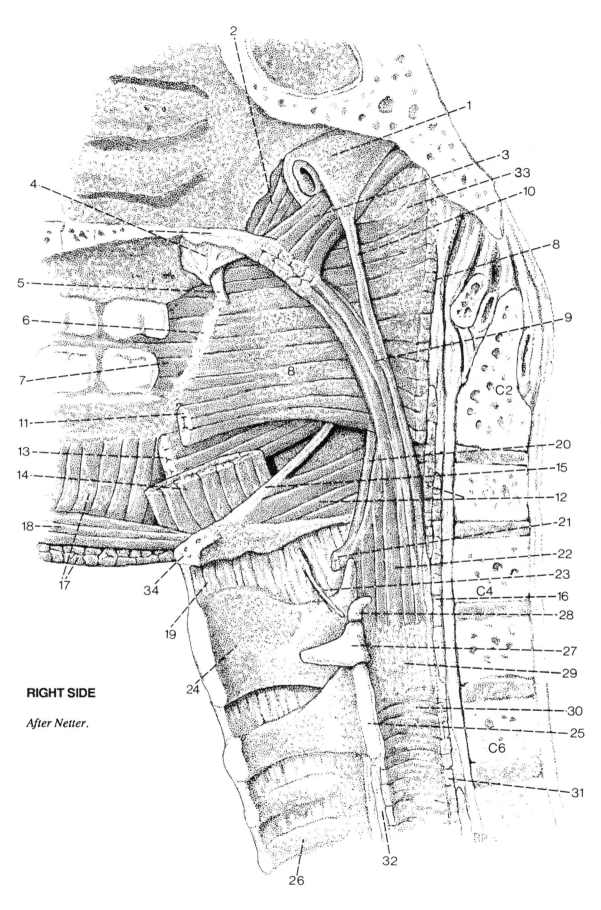

RIGHT SIDE

After Netter.

254   Muscles of the pharynx

Color and label

1   Ciliary ganglion*
2   Pterygopalatine ganglion*
3   Otic ganglion*
4   Submandibular ganglion*
5   Trigeminal nerve sensory root
6   Trigeminal nerve motor root
7   Trigeminal ganglion
8   Nasociliary branch of ophthalmic nerve (V_1)
9   Long ciliary nerve *(sensory to eye)*
10 Short ciliary nerves *(autonomics)*
11 Oculomotor nerve (N III)
12 Oculomotor root to ciliary ganglion *(parasympathetic)*
13 Sympathetic root to ciliary ganglion
14 Internal carotid artery and plexus
15 Maxillary nerve (N V_2)
16 Pterygopalatine nerves
17 Palatine nerves
18 Posterior lateral nasal nerves
19 Nerve of the pterygoid canal (Vidian nerve)
20 Facial nerve (N VII)
21 Greater petrosal nerve *(branch of N VII)*
22 Deep petrosal nerve *(sympathetics)*
23 Lesser petrosal nerve *(branch of N IX)*
24 Lingual nerve *(branch of N V_3)*
25 Chorda tympani nerve *(branch of N VII)*
26 Inferior alveolar nerve *(branch of N V_3)*
27 Glossopharyngeal nerve (N IX)
28 Vagus nerve (N X)
29 Superior larnygeal branch of vagus
30 Superior cardiac branch of vagus
31 Superior cervical sympathetic ganglion
32 Carotid nerve
33 Middle meningeal artery and plexus
34 Maxillary artery and plexus
35 External carotid artery and plexus
36 Carotid sinus nerve *(branch of N IX)*
37 Carotid sinus
38 Common carotid artery
39 Pharyngeal plexus (N IX, N X)
40 Superior cervical sympathetic cardiac nerve
41 Auriculotemporal nerve

These four parasympathetic ganglia contain postganglionic parasympathetic nerve cell bodies upon which preganglionic parasympathetic fibers synapse.

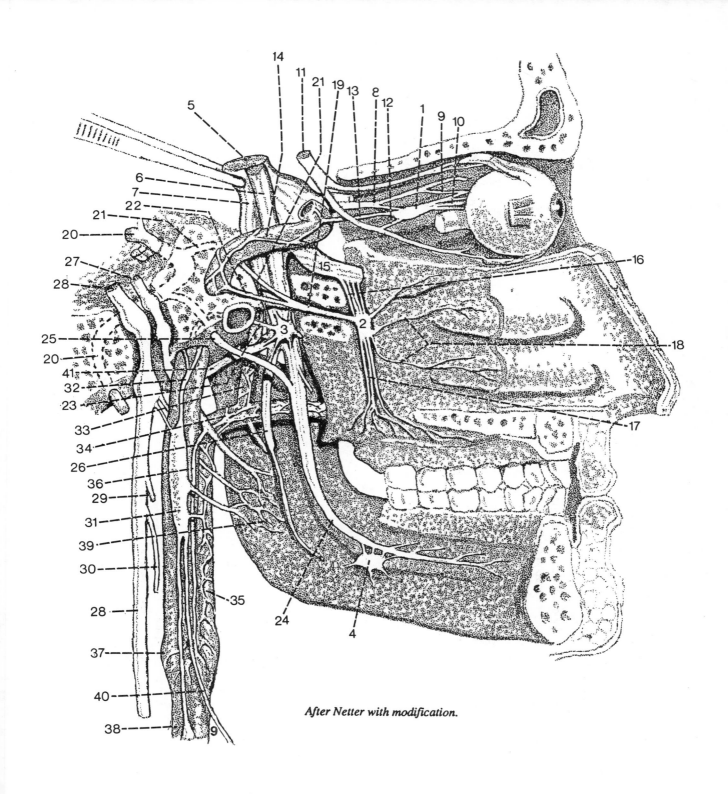

After Netter with modification.

255   Autonomic outflow in the head, I

Color and label

1 Accessory oculomotor nucleus (*old name: Edinger-Westphal nucleus*) with preganglionic parasympathetic neurons and fibers

2 Superior (rostral) salivatory nucleus with preganglionic parasympathetic neurons and fibers

3 Inferior (caudal) salivatory nucleus with preganglionic parasympathetic neurons and fibers

4 Dorsal nucleus of vagus nerve (dorsal vagal nucleus) *formerly dorsal motor nucleus of vagus nerve or nerve X*) with parasympathetic neurons and fibers

5 Ciliary ganglion with postganglionic parasympathetic neurons and fibers

6 Pterygopalatine (*formerly sphenopalatine*) ganglion with parasympathetic neurons and fibers

7 Otic ganglion with postganglionic parasympathetic neurons and fibers

8 Submandibular ganglion with postganglionic parasympathetic neurons and fibers

9 Preganglionic sympathetic cell body in intemediolateral column of thoracic spinal cord

10 Postganglionic sympathetic cell bodies of superior cervical ganglion

11 Oculomotor nerve (N III)

12 Inferior ramus of N III and oculomotor root to ciliary ganglion

13 Short ciliary nerve(s)

14 Trigeminal nerve and ganglion

15 Lacrimal nerve (branch of V_1)

16 Zygomatic facial branch of V_2

17 Facial nerve

18 Greater petrosal nerve

19 Chorda tympani nerve ("*nerve*" *is not used to denote the chorda tympani because when named it was not known to be a nerve; the use of "nerve" here is the author's decision*)

20 Glossopharyngeal nerve (N IX)

21 Tympanic nerve and tympanic plexus

22 Lesser petrosal nerve (*derived from tympanic plexus*)

23 Auriculotemporal nerve (*branch of V_3*)

24 Vagus nerve

25 Superior cardiac branch of vagus nerve

26 Postganglionic parasympathetic fiber to eye

27 Postganglionic parasympathetic fiber to lacrimal gland

28 Postganglionic parasympathetic fibers to nasal glands

29 Postganglionic parasympathetic fibers to palatine glands

30 Postganglionic parasympathetic fibers to submandibular and sublingual glands

31 Postganglionic parasympathetic fiber to paroted gland via auriculotemporal nerve

32 Preganglionic parasympathetic fiber to heart

33 Postganglionic sympathetic fiber to nose via carotid plexus and deep petrosal nerve (*sympathetic fibers pass around parasympathetic ganglia with no interruption*)

34 Midbrain

35 Pons

36 Medulla

Autonomic outflow in the head, II (*See opposite page*)

256

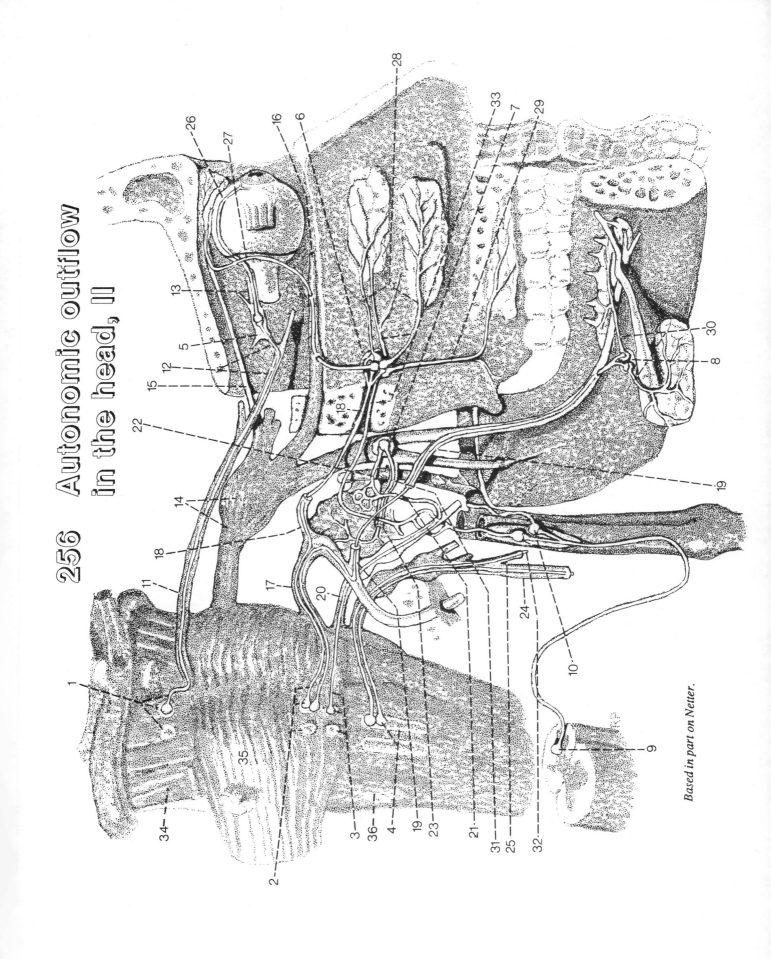

256 Autonomic outflow in the head, II

Based in part on Netter.

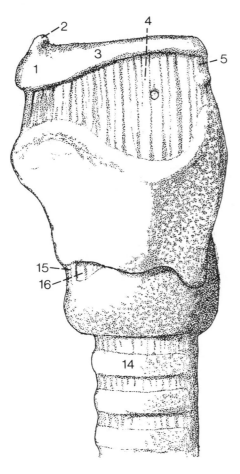

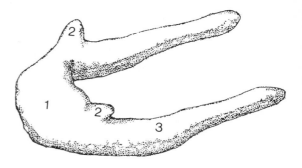

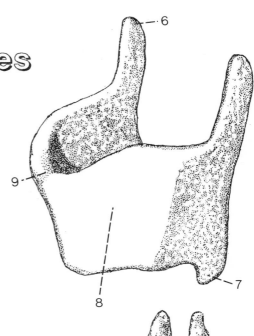

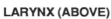

257
Larynx, cartilages

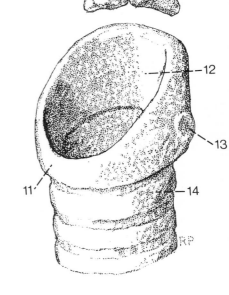

LARYNX (ABOVE)

HYOID BONE AND CARTILAGES OF THE LARYNX (RIGHT)

Color and label

1. Body of hyoid bone
2. Lesser horn (cornu) of hyoid bone
3. Greater horn (cornu) of hyoid bone
4. Thyrohyoid membrane
5. Lateral thyrohyoid ligament
6. Superior horn of thyroid cartilage
7. Inferior horn of thyroid cartilage
8. Lamina of thyroid cartilage
9. Superior thyroid notch
10. Arytenoid *(Greek, arytaina, pitcher, ladle)* cartilage
11. Arch of cricoid cartilage
12. Lamina of cricoid cartilage
13. Facet for inferior horn of thyroid cartilage
14. Tracheal rings
15. Cricothyroid ligament
16. Conus elasticus

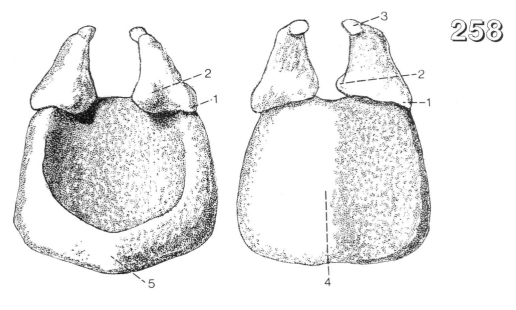

**LEFT, ANTERIOR VIEW;
RIGHT, POSTERIOR VIEW**

Color and label

1 Muscular process of
  arytenoid cartilage
2 Vocal process of
  arytenoid cartilage
3 Corniculate cartilage
4 Lamina of cricoid cartilage
5 Arch of cricoid cartilage

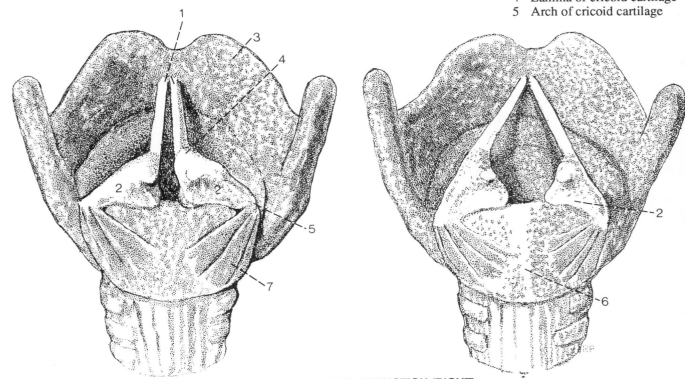

VOCAL LIGAMENTS IN ADDUCTION (LEFT) AND ABDUCTION (RIGHT)

Color and label

1 Vocal ligaments
2 Arytenoid cartilage
3 Thyroid cartilage
4 Vocal process of arytenoid cartilage
5 Muscular process of arytenoid cartilage
6 Lamina of cricoid cartilage
7 Posterior cricoarytenoid muscle *(by pulling the muscular processes
  of arytenoid cartilages posterior the two vocal vocal processes are
  moved away from each other [abducted], thus opening the space between the two vocal ligaments [rima glottidis] into a diamond shape)*

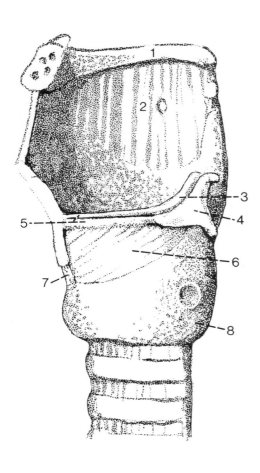

LARYNX PARTIALLY BISECTED

LEFT HALF OF HYOID BONE AND THYROID CARTILAGE REMOVED

Color and label

1 Right half of hyoid bone
2 Right thyrohyoid membrane
3 Right arytenoid cartilage
4 Left arytenoid cartilage
5 Vocal ligaments
6 Conus elasticus
7 Cricothyroid ligament
8 Cricoid cartilage

259
Vocal ligaments
and muscles

MUSCLES OF RIGHT SIDE OF LARYNX

RIGHT HALF OF THYROID CARTILAGE REMOVED

Color and label

1 Aryepiglotticus
2 Thyroarytenoid
3 Arytenoid
4 Lateral cricoarytenoid
5 Cricothyroid (cut)
6 Posterior cricothyroid
7 Thyroepiglotticus

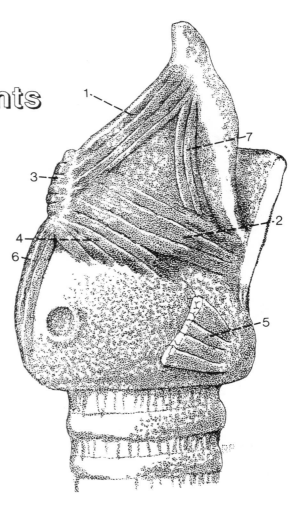

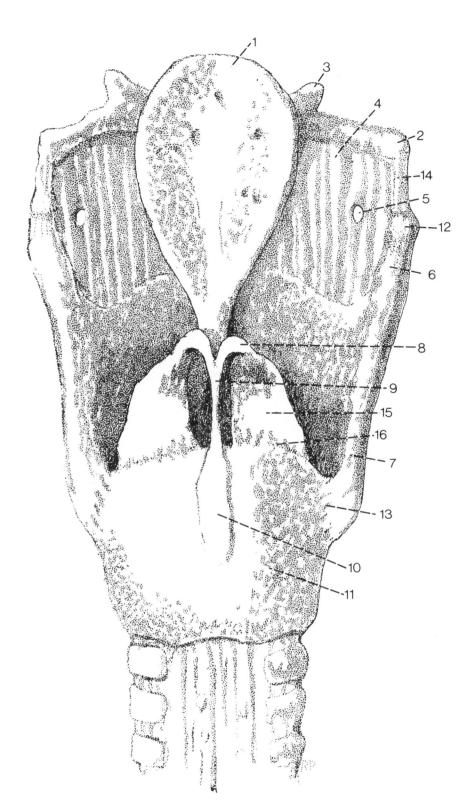

260
Larynx, cartilages, posterior aspect

Color and label

1 Epiglottis
2 Hyoid bone greater horn
3 Hyoid bone lesser horn
4 Thyrohyoid membrane
5 Foramen for internal branch
   of superior laryngeal nerve
   and superior laryngeal artery
6 Superior horn of thyroid cartilage
7 Inferior horn of thyroid cartilage
8 Corniculate cartilage
9 Corniculopharyngeal ligament
10 Cricopharyngeal ligament
11 Lamina of cricoid cartilage
12 Triticeal cartilage
13 Cricothyroid joint and ligament
14 Lateral thyrohyoid ligament
15 Arytenoid cartilage
16 Cricoarytenoid joint and ligament

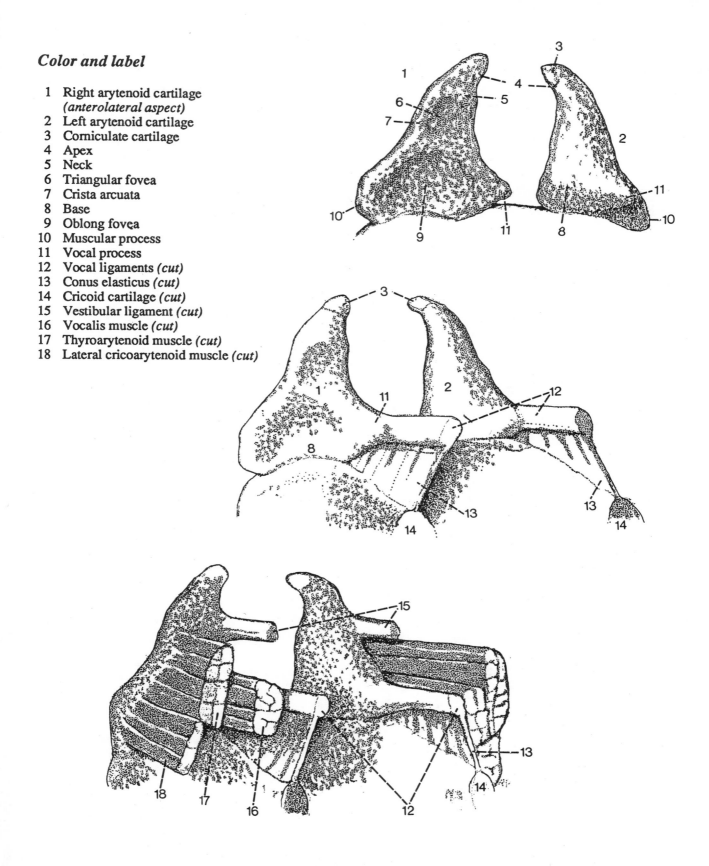

Color and label

1 Right arytenoid cartilage
  (*anterolateral aspect*)
2 Left arytenoid cartilage
3 Corniculate cartilage
4 Apex
5 Neck
6 Triangular fovea
7 Crista arcuata
8 Base
9 Oblong fovea
10 Muscular process
11 Vocal process
12 Vocal ligaments (*cut*)
13 Conus elasticus (*cut*)
14 Cricoid cartilage (*cut*)
15 Vestibular ligament (*cut*)
16 Vocalis muscle (*cut*)
17 Thyroarytenoid muscle (*cut*)
18 Lateral cricoarytenoid muscle (*cut*)

261   Arytenoid cartilages

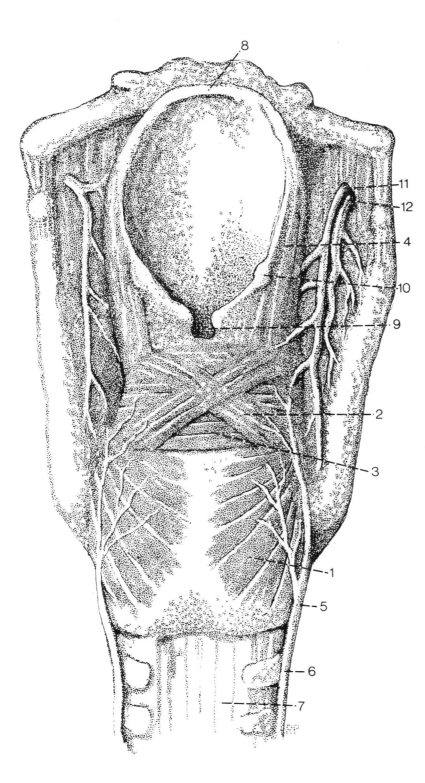

POSTERIOR VIEW

Color and label

1 Posterior cricoarytenoid muscle
2 Oblique arytenoid muscle
3 Transverse arytenoid muscle
4 Aryepiglottic muscle
5 Inferior laryngeal nerve
6 Recurrent laryngeal nerve
7 Membranous tracheal wall and glands
8 Epiglottis
9 Interarytenoid notch
10 Cuneiform tubercle *(over cartilage)*
11 Internal branch of superior laryngeal nerve
12 Superior laryngeal artery

262   Larynx, nerves and muscles

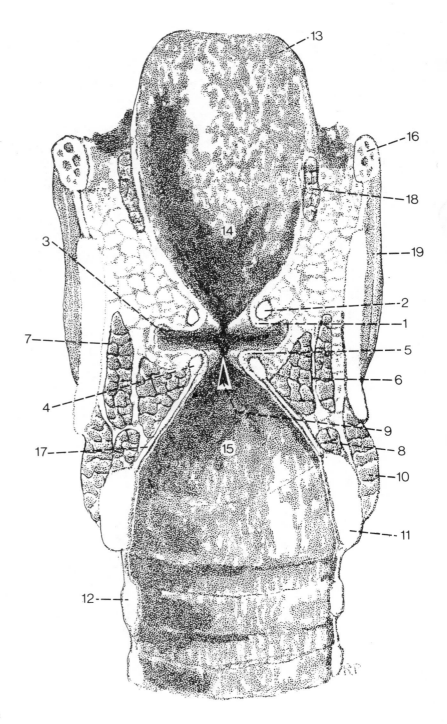

LOOKING FORWARD

Color and label

1 Vestibular fold (*false vocal cord*
2 Vestibular ligament
3 Ventricle of larynx
4 Vocal ligament
5 Vocal fold (*true vocal cord*)
6 Vocalis muscle
7 Thyroarytenoid muscle
8 Lateral cricoarytenoid
9 Rima glottidis (*gap between vocal folds*)
10 Cricothyroid muscle
11 Arch of cricoid cartilage
12 Tracheal rings
13 Epiglottis
14 Vestibule of larynx (*laryngeal cavity above vestibular folds*)
15 Infraglottic space
16 Hyoid bone
17 Conus elasticus
18 Aryepiglottic muscle
19 Thyrohyoid muscle

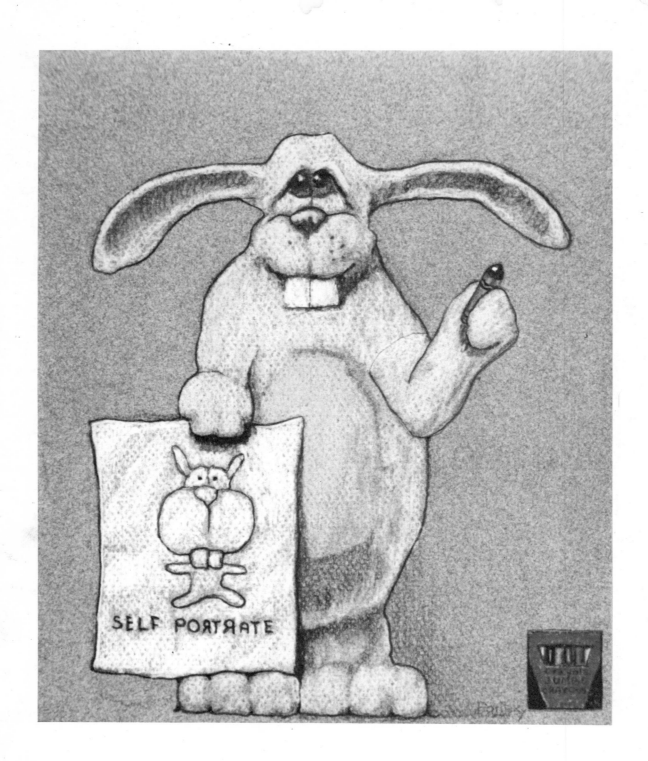